AF616372

Molecular Haematology

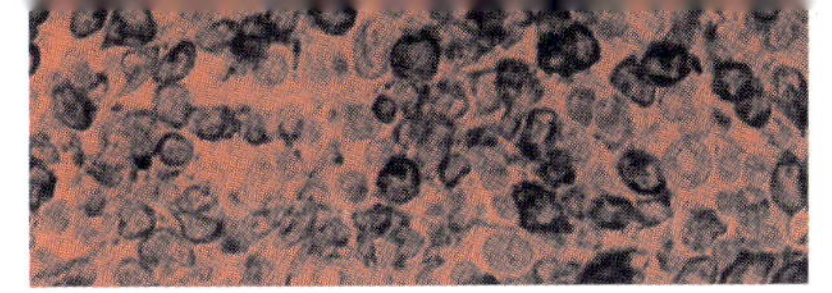

Molecular Haematology

EDITED BY

DREW PROVAN MD MRCP MRCPath
Department of Haematology
Southampton General Hospital
Southampton SO16 6YD, UK

AND

JOHN GRIBBEN MD PhD FRCP FRCPath
Harvard Medical School
Division of Adult Oncology
Dana-Farber Cancer Institute
Boston MA 02115, USA

FOREWORD BY

M.F. PERUTZ

Blackwell
Science

Editorial Offices:
Osney Mead, Oxford OX2 0EL
25 John Street, London WC1N 2BL
23 Ainslie Place, Edinburgh EH3 6AJ
350 Main Street, Malden
MA 02148 5018, USA
54 University Street, Carlton
Victoria 3053, Australia
10, rue Casimir Delavigne
75006 Paris, France

Other Editorial Offices:
Blackwell Wissenschafts-Verlag GmbH
Kurfürstendamm 57
10707 Berlin, Germany

Blackwell Science KK
MG Kodenmacho Building
7–10 Kodenmacho Nihombashi
Chuo-ku, Tokyo 104, Japan

First published 2000

Set by Drew Provan & Excel Typesetters
Co., Hong Kong
Printed and bound in Great Britain.
Printed at the Alden Press, Oxford
and Northampton, and bound
by MPG Books Ltd, Bodmin, Cornwall

A catalogue record for this title
is available from the British Library

ISBN 0-632-05037-3

Library of Congress
Cataloging-in-publication Data

Molecular haematology / edited by
Drew Provan and John Gribben;
foreword by M.F. Perutz.
p. cm.
Includes bibliographical references
and index.
ISBN 0-632-05037-3
1. Blood—Diseases—Molecular
aspects. I. Provan, Andrew.
II. Gribben, John. III. Title: Molecular
hematology.
RC636.M576 2000
616.1′5—dc21 99-16528
CIP

DISTRIBUTORS

Marston Book Services Ltd
PO Box 269
Abingdon, Oxon OX14 4YN
(*Orders*: Tel: 01235 465500
Fax: 01235 465555)

USA
Blackwell Science, Inc.
Commerce Place
350 Main Street
Malden, MA 02148 5018
(*Orders*: Tel: 800 759 6102
781 388 8250
Fax: 781 388 8255)

Canada
Login Brothers Book Company
324 Saulteaux Crescent
Winnipeg, Manitoba R3J 3T2
(*Orders*: Tel: 204 837-2987)

Australia
Blackwell Science Pty Ltd
54 University Street
Carlton, Victoria 3053
(*Orders*: Tel: 3 9347 0300
Fax: 3 9347 5001)

For further information on
Blackwell Science, visit our website:
www.blackwell-science.com

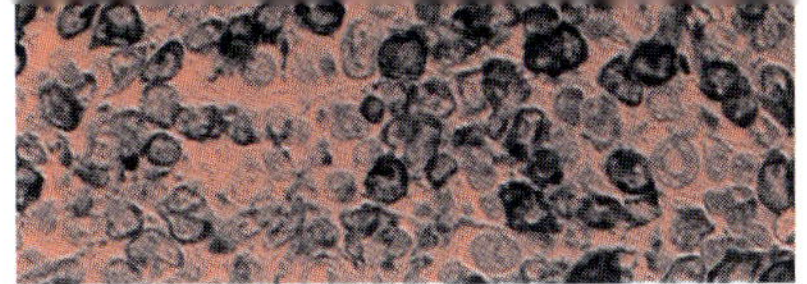

Contents

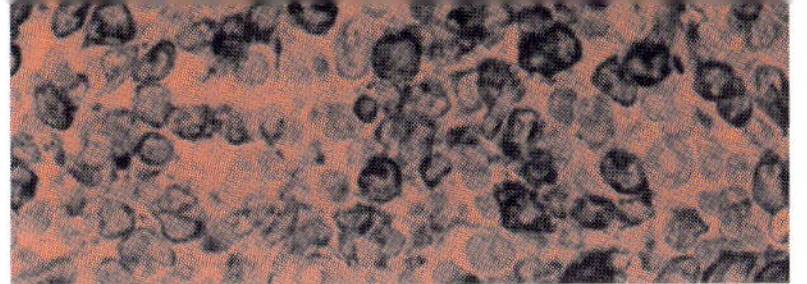

List of contributors

Anthony J Bench MA PhD
Research Associate, Department of Haematology, University of Cambridge, MRC Centre, Hills Road, Cambridge CB2 2QH, UK

James R Berenson MD
Professor of Medicine, UCLA School of Medicine, Chief, Cancer Research, West Los Angeles VA Medical Center, 11301 Wilshire Boulevard, Los Angeles CA 90073, USA

Kim M Champion
Research Assistant, Department of Haematology, University of Cambridge, MRC Centre, Hills Road, Cambridge CB2 2QH, UK

Björn Dahlbäck MD PhD
Professor of Blood Coagulation Research, Department of Clinical Chemistry, University of Lund, University Hospital, Malmo S-20502, Malmo, Sweden

Ian M Franklin PhD FRCP FRCPath
Professor of Transfusion Medicine, Department of Medicine, University of Glasgow, Royal Infirmary, Glasgow G31 2ER, UK

Paul L F Giangrande BSc MD FRCP FRCPath FRCPCH
Consultant Haematologist and Director, Oxford Haemophilia Centre, Churchill Hospital, Oxford OX3 7LJ, UK

Anthony R Green PhD FRCP FRCPath
Wellcome Senior Fellow and Honorary Consultant Haematologist, Department of Haematology, University of Cambridge, MRC Centre, Hills Road, Cambridge CB2 2QH, UK

John G Gribben MD PhD FRCP FRCPath
Associate Professor, Harvard Medical School, Division of Adult Oncology, Dana-Farber Cancer Institute, 44 Binney Street, Boston MA 02115, USA

Andreas Hillarp PhD
Associate Professor and Hospital Chemist, Department of Clinical Chemistry, University of Lund, University Hospital, Malmo S-20502, Malmo, Sweden

A Victor Hoffbrand DM FRCP FRCPath FRCP(Edin) DSc
Emeritus Professor of Haematology and Consultant Haematologist, Royal Free and University College Medical School, Rowland Hill Street, London NW3 2PF, UK

Brian J P Huntly MB ChB MRCP DipRCPath
Clinical Research Fellow, Department of Haematology, University of Cambridge, MRC Centre, Hills Road, Cambridge CB2 2QH, UK

Anastasios Karadimitris MRCP DipRCPath
Research Fellow, Department of Human Genetics, Memorial Sloan-Kettering Cancer Center, 1275 York Avenue, New York NY 10021, USA

Debra M Lillington BSc
Head of Cytogenetics, ICRF Medical Oncology Laboratory, The Medical College of St Bartholomew's Hospital, Charterhouse Square, London EC1M 6BQ, UK

Lucio Luzzatto MD
Courtney Steel Professor and Chairman, Department of Human Genetics, Memorial Sloan-Kettering Cancer Center, 1275 York Avenue, New York NY 10021, USA

Rosemary Mazanet MD PhD
Oracle Partners, L.P. 712 Fifth Avenue, 45th Floor, NYC 10019 and Amgen Inc., Mailstop 99-1-A, One Amgen Center Drive, Thousand Oaks CA 91320, USA

Ken Mills PhD
Senior Lecturer in Haemato-Oncology, University of Wales College of Medicine, Heath Park, Cardiff CF4 4XN, UK

Graham Molineux PhD
Amgen Inc., Mailstop 15-2-A, One Amgen Center Drive, Thousand Oaks CA 91320, USA

Elisabeth P Nacheva MD PhD
Head of Molecular Cytogenetics Laboratory, Department of Haematology, Addenbrookes Hospital, Hills Road, Cambridge CB2 2QQ, UK

Ronald L Nagel MD
Irving D. Karpas Professor of Medicine, Head, Division of Hematology, Albert Einstein College of Medicine, The Bronx, New York 10461, USA

Cristina V Navarrete PhD
Head of Histocompatibility and Immunogenetics, National Blood Service, London and South East, and Honorary Senior Lecturer in Immunology, Royal Free and University College Medical School, University of London, London, UK

David G Oscier MA FRCP FRCPath
Consultant Haematologist, Department of Haematology, The Royal Bournemouth Hospital, Castle Lane East, Bournemouth BH7 7DW, UK

Willem H Ouwehand MD PhD
Lecturer/Honorary Consultant, Division of Transfusion Medicine, Department of Haematology, University of Cambridge, National Blood Service, London and South East, Cambridge, and National Institute for Biological Standards and Control, Potters Bar, UK

Max F Perutz FRS
Director, MRC Laboratory of Molecular Biology, Hills Road, Cambridge CB2 2QH, UK

Drew Provan MD MRCP MRCPath
Senior Lecturer, Department of Haematology, Southampton General Hospital, Tremona Road, Southampton SO16 6YD, UK

Thomas J Schuetz MD PhD
Instructor in Medicine, Dana-Farber Cancer Institute, 44 Binney Street, Boston MA 02115, USA

A Keith Stewart MD FRCP(C)
Associate Professor, Department of Medical Oncology/Hematology, Princess Margaret Hospital, 610 University Avenue, Toronto, Ontario M5G 2M9

Richard M Stone MD
Associate Professor of Medicine and Clinical Director, Leukemia Program, Dana-Farber Cancer Institute, 44 Binney Street, Boston MA 02115, USA

Robert A Vescio MD
Assistant Professor of Medicine, UCLA School of Medicine, West Los Angeles VA Medical Center, 11301 Wilshire Boulevard, Los Angeles CA 90073, USA

David Weatherall FRS
Regius Professor of Medicine, University of Oxford, Institute of Molecular Medicine, John Radcliffe Hospital, Headington, Oxford OX3 9DS, UK

R Gitendra Wickremasinghe PhD
Senior Lecturer in Haematology, Royal Free and University College Medical School, Rowland Hill Street, London NW3 2PF, UK

Dennis Wright MD FRCPath
Emeritus Professor of Pathology, Department of Pathology, Southampton General Hospital, Tremona Road, Southampton SO16 6YD, UK

Bryan D Young BSc PhD
Head, Professor of ICRF Medical Oncology Laboratory, The Medical College of St Bartholomew's Hospital, Charterhouse Square, London EC1M 6BQ, UK

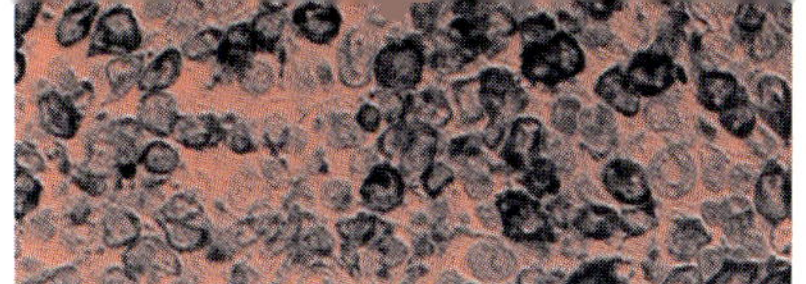

Foreword

In 1968, after a quest lasting 30 years, X-ray analysis of crystalline horse haemoglobin at last reached the stage when I could build a model of its atomic structure. The amino acid sequences of human globin are largely homologous to those of horse globin, which made me confident that their structures are the same. By then, the amino acid substitutions responsible for many abnormal human haemoglobins had been determined. The world authority on them was the late Hermann Lehmann, Professor of Clinical Biochemistry at the University of Cambridge, who worked in the hospital just across the road from our Laboratory of Molecular Biology. I asked him to come over to see if there was any correlation between the symptoms caused by the different amino acids substituted in the abnormal haemoglobin and their positions in the atomic model. The day we spent going through them proved one of the most exciting in our scientific lives. We found haemoglobin to be insensitive to replacements of most amino acid residues on its surface, with the notable exception of sickle cell haemoglobin. On the other hand, we found the molecule to be extremely sensitive to even quite small alterations of internal non-polar contacts, especially those near the haems. Replacements at the contact between the α and β subunits affected respiratory function.

In sickle cell haemoglobin an external glutamate was replaced by a valine. We wrote: '*A non-polar instead at a polar residue at a surface position would suffice to make each molecule adhere to a complementary site at a neighbouring one, that site being created by the conformational change from oxy to deoxy haemoglobin*'. This was soon proved to be correct. We published our findings under the title: 'The Molecular Pathology of Human Haemoglobin'. Our paper marked a turning point because it was the first time that the symptoms of diseases could be interpreted in terms of changes in the atomic structure of the affected protein. In the years that followed, the structure of the contact between the valine of one molecule of sickle cell haemoglobin and that of the complementary site of its neighbour became known in some detail. At a meeting at Arden House near Washington in 1980, several colleagues and I decided to use this knowledge for the design of anti-sickling drugs, but after an effort lasting 10 years, we realised that we were running up against a brick wall. Luckily, the work was not entirely wasted, because we found a series of compounds that lower the oxygen affinity of haemoglobin and we realised that this might be clinically useful. One of those compounds, designed by DJ Abraham at the University of Virginia in Richmond, is now entering phase 3 clinical trials. On the other hand, our failure to find a drug against sickle cell anaemia, even when its cause was known in atomic detail, made me realise the extreme difficulty of finding drugs to correct a malfunction of a protein that is caused by a single amino acid substitution. Most thalassaemias are due not to amino acid substitutions, but to either complete or partial failure to synthesise α- or β-globin chains. Weatherall's chapter shows that, at the genetic level, there may be literally hundreds of different genetic lesions responsible for that failure. Correction of such lesions is now the subject of intensive work in many laboratories.

Early in the next century, the human genome will be complete. It will reveal the amino acid sequences of all the 100 000 or so different proteins of which we are made. Many of these proteins are still unknown. To discover their functions, the next project now under discussion is a billion dollar effort to determine the structures of all the thousands of unknown proteins within 10 years. By then we shall know the identity of the proteins responsible for most of the several thousand different genetic diseases. Will this lead to effective treatment or will medical geneticists be in the same position as doctors were early in this century when the famous physician Sir William Osler confined their task to the establishment of diagnoses? Shall we know the cause of every genetic disease without a cure?

Our only hope lies in somatic gene therapy. AK Stewart's chapter on Molecular Therapeutics describes the many ingenious methods now under development. So far, none of these has produced lasting effects, apparently because the transferred genes are not integrated into the mammalian genome, but a large literature already grown up bears testimony to the great efforts now underway to overcome this problem. My much-loved teacher William Lawrence Bragg used to say '*If you go on hammering away at a problem, eventually it seems to get tired, lies down and lets you catch it.*' Let us hope that somatic gene therapy will soon get tired.

M.F. Perutz
Cambridge

Perutz MF, Lehmann H. (1968) Molecular pathology of human haemoglobin. *Nature*, **219**, 902–909.
Perutz MF, Muirhead H, Cox JM, Goaman LCG. (1968) Three-dimensional Fourier synthesis of horse oxyhaemoglobin at 2.8 Å resolution: the atomic model. *Nature*, **219**, 131–139.

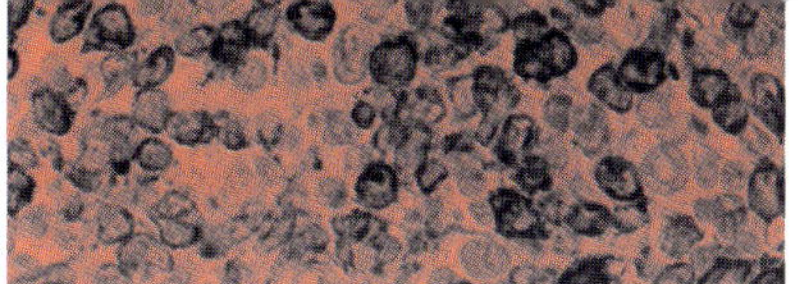

Preface

Molecular biological techniques have revolutionised the diagnosis and management of a wide variety of medical disorders, and have had a major impact on all medical specialties—in many cases the molecular advances are far ahead of any therapeutic developments. Haematology was probably the first branch of medicine to embrace molecular biology through work on haemoglobin, chromosomal rearrangements in malignant and premalignant disorders, and more recently growth factors, oncogenes and molecular therapeutics. Through molecular analysis of abnormal cells we have been able to elucidate the molecular mechanisms underlying many diseases encountered in haematological practice.

However, although there are one or two major texts dealing with molecular aspects of haematological disease (see *Suggested General Reading*), our feeling was that many of our colleagues find such large encyclopaedic tomes rather daunting, perhaps bearing little resemblance to their day-to-day practice. This short book aims to summarise the relevance of molecular advances in our specialty, highlighting the impact molecular biology has had on the diagnostic aspects of disease management as well as therapeutic strategies that have been developed as a direct result of basic molecular biological investigation.

Each of the chapters in *Molecular Haematology* is devoted to one aspect of haematology with coverage from anaemias to gene therapy. Our international team of authors kindly agreed to provide a synopsis of the developments they each saw as being of major importance within their area of expertise. They all managed to write within the tight restrictions we imposed and overall we feel confident that our writers have provided a balanced view of the subject areas.

The book comprises 16 chapters written in a fairly didactic style with illustrations and tables throughout. Rather than choke the text with references, each author has provided a *Further Reading* list with 'key' references for the benefit of the reader.

Molecular haematology is a moving target and already there have been further advances which have not featured in this edition of the book. However, we have attempted to get the book into print as quickly as possible to avoid outdating, which is so common in multi-author texts.

We are very pleased with the final product and we trust that all our contributors will feel that their efforts have been worthwhile. Undoubtedly there will be minor errors and omissions, and we welcome readers' comments and may use these in future editions of the book. Our e-mail addresses can be found below.

Drew Provan (*abp@soton.ac.uk*)
John Gribben (*john_gribben@dfci.harvard.edu*)

Acknowledgements

We would like to thank all our colleagues for agreeing to contribute to the book and for producing such high quality chapters.

Our warm thanks go to the staff at Blackwell Science and in particular, Dr Andy Robinson, Editor-in-Chief, for the enthusiastic manner in which he took this project on, and for his continued patience and encouragement at all stages of the work; Mr Edward Wates, Production Manager Pre-Press, for ensuring the final output matched our expectations, and Beverly King, Editorial Assistant, for keeping things moving along and generally hassling tardy authors. We are most grateful to David Gardner for redrawing all the authors' roughs to such a high standard.

We thank Professor Sally Davies, Central Middlesex Hospital, for her helpful ideas and suggestions.

Suggested general reading

Cox TM, Sinclair J. (1997) *Molecular Biology in Medicine*. Oxford: Blackwell Science.

Hoffbrand AV, Lewis SM, Tuddenham EGD. (eds) (1999) *Postgraduate Haematology*, 4th edn. Oxford: Butterworth-Heinemann.

Jameson JL. (ed) (1998) *Principles of Molecular Medicine*. New York: Humana Press.

Mullis KB. (1990) The unusual origin of the polymerase chain reaction. *Scientific American*, **262**, 56–65.

Stamatoyannopoulos G, Nienhuis AW, Majerus PW, Varmus H. (eds) (1999) *The Molecular Basis of Blood Diseases*, 3rd edn. Philadelphia: W.B. Saunders, *in press*.

Watson JD, Gilman M, Witkowski J, Zoller M. (eds) (1992) *Recombinant DNA*, 2nd edn. New York: Scientific American Books.

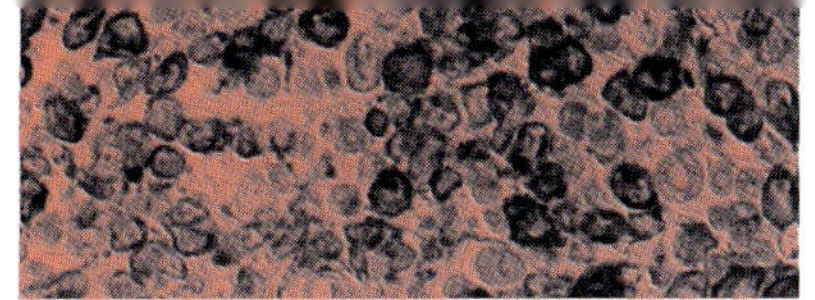

Abbreviations

2,3-DPG	2,3-diphosphoglycerate
Å	Angstrom; 10^{-10} metres
AAV	Adeno-associated virus
ABL	Abelson
ABMT	Autologous bone marrow transplantation
ADA	Adenosine deaminase
AHA	Acute haemolytic anaemia
AIDS	Acquired immunodeficiency syndrome
ALAS2	δ-aminolaevulinate synthase 2
ALG/ATG	Antilymphocyte globulin/antithymocyte globulin
ALL	Acute lymphoblastic leukaemia
AlloBMT	Allogeneic bone marrow transplantation
AML	Acute myeloid leukaemia
APC/R	Activated protein C/resistance
APCs	Antigen-presenting cells
APML	Acute promyelocytic leukaemia, AML M3
APTT	Activated partial thromboplastin time
ASCT	Autologous stem cell transplantation
AT	Antithrombin
ATRA	All-*trans* retinoic acid
BAC	Bacterial artificial chromosome
BCR	Breakpoint cluster region
BFU-E	Burst-forming unit-erythroid
BL	Burkitt's lymphoma
BM	Bone marrow
BMF	Bone marrow failure
BMT	Bone marrow transplant
Cbl	Cobalamin, vitamin B_{12}
CDA	Congenital dyserythropoietic anaemia
CDK	Cyclin-dependent protein kinase
cDNA	Complementary DNA
CDR3	Third complementarity determining region
CFU-E	Erythroid colony-forming unit
CFU-GEMM	Colony-forming units granulocyte-eosinophil-monocyte-macrophage
CFU-GM	Colony-forming units granulocyte-macrophage
CFU-MEG	Megakaryocyte colony-forming unit
CGH	Comparative genomic hybridisation
CLL	Chronic lymphocytic leukaemia
cM	CentiMorgans
CML	Chronic myeloid leukaemia
CMML	Chronic myelomonocytic leukaemia
CMV	Cytomegalovirus
CNS	Central nervous system
CNSHA	Congenital non-spherocytic haemolytic anaemia
CP/CP1	Chronic phase/first chronic phase
CR	Complete remission
CRH	Cytokine receptor homology
CSF	Colony-stimulating factor
CVS	Chorionic villus sampling
der	Derivative
DFS	Disease-free survival
DLBL	Diffuse large B-cell lymphoma
DLI	Donor lymphocyte infusion
DNA	Deoxyribonucleic acid
DOP-PCR	Degenerative oligonucleotide PCR
dTMP	Deoxyribosylthymine monophosphate
dTTP	Deoxyribosylthymine triphosphate
dUMP	Deoxyuridine monophosphate
dUTP	Deoxyuridine triphosphate
eBL	Endemic Burkitt's lymphoma
EBV	Epstein–Barr virus
EGF	Epidermal growth factor
EPO	Erythropoietin
EPOR	Erythropoietin receptor
ET	Essential thrombocythaemia
FA	Fanconi's anaemia
FAB	French–American–British
FISH	Fluorescence *in situ* hybridisation
FITC	Fluorescein isothiocyanate
G6PD	Glucose-6-phosphate dehydrogenase
GAP	GTPase activating protein
G-CSF	Granulocyte colony-stimulating factor
GDP	Guanine diphosphate

Gla	γ-carboxy glutamic acid
GM-CSF	Granulocyte-macrophage colony-stimulating factor
GTP	Guanine triphosphate
GTPase	Enzymatic activity hydrolysing GTP → GDP
GVHD	Graft-versus-host disease
GVL	Graft-versus-leukaemia
HBS	Heparin binding site
HGFs	Haematopoietic growth factors
HHV-8	Human herpesvirus-8
HIV	Human immunodeficiency virus
HLA	Human leucocyte antigen
HLH	Helix–loop–helix
HPA	Human platelet antigen
HPFH	Hereditary persistence of fetal haemoglobin
HSCs	Haematopoietic stem cells
HUMARA	Human androgen receptor assay
IAA	Idiopathic aplastic anaemia
IBMTR	International Bone Marrow Transplant Registry
IF	Intrinsic factor
IFN	Interferon
Ig	Immunoglobulin
IgH	Immunoglobulin heavy chain
IgL	Immunoglobulin light chain
IL	Interleukin
IMF	Idiopathic myelofibrosis
IPSS	International Prognostic Scoring System
IRE	Iron responsive element
ISC	Irreversibly sickled cells
IVS	Intervening sequences
kb	Kilobase pairs (1000 base pairs)
kDa	Kilodalton, unit of molecular mass ≡ 10^3 daltons
KS	Kaposi's sarcoma
KSHV	Kaposi's sarcoma-associated herpesvirus
KSS	Kearns–Sayre syndrome
LCR	Locus control region
LTR	Long terminal repeat
mAbs	Monoclonal antibodies
MALT	Mucosa-associated lymphoid tissue
Mb	Megabase, 1×10^6 bp or nucleotides
M-bcr	Major breakpoint cluster region
MCH	Mean corpuscular haemoglobin
MCHC	Mean corpuscular haemoglobin concentration
MCL	Mantle cell lymphoma
M-CSF	Macrophage colony-stimulating factor
MCV	Mean cell volume
MDR-1	Multidrug resistance gene-1
MDS	Myelodysplastic syndrome
MGUS	Monoclonal gammopathy of undetermined significance
MHC	Major histocompatibility complex
MMLV	Moloney murine leukaemia virus
MPD	Myeloproliferative disease
MRC	Medical Research Council
MRD	Minimal residual disease
mRNA	Messenger RNA
mtDNA	Mitochondrial DNA
MUD	Matched unrelated donor (transplant)
NHL	Non-Hodgkin's lymphoma
NK	Natural killer
NMDP	National Marrow Donor Panel (UK)
NNJ	Neonatal jaundice
NSAIDs	Non-steroidal anti-inflammatory drugs
nt	Nucleotide
ORF	Open reading frame
p50	Partial pressure of O_2 at which Hb is 50% saturated with O_2
PA	Pernicious anaemia
PB	Peripheral blood
PBMCs	Peripheral blood mononuclear cells
PBPC	Peripheral blood progenitor cells
PBSCT	Peripheral blood stem cell transplant
PCR	Polymerase chain reaction
PCV	Packed cell volume
PDGF	Platelet-derived growth factor
PDGFRβ	Platelet-derived growth factor receptor β
Ph	Philadelphia chromosome
PMPS	Pearson's marrow–pancreas syndrome
PNH	Paroxysmal nocturnal haemoglobinuria
PR	Partial remission
PT	Prothrombin time
PV	Polycythaemia (rubra) vera
RA	Refractory anaemia
RAEB	Refractory anaemia with excess blasts
RAEB-T	Refractory anaemia with excess blasts in transformation
RAR	Retinoic acid receptor
RARα	Retinoic acid receptor α
RARS	Refractory anaemia with ringed sideroblasts
RBC	Red blood cells
RNA	Ribonucleic acid
RT-PCR	Reverse transcriptase PCR
RXR	Retinoic X receptor
SA	Sideroblastic anaemia
SAM	S-adenosylmethionine
sBL	Sporadic Burkitt's lymphoma
SCF	Stem cell factor

SCT	Stem cell transplant
SKY	Spectral karyotyping
SRF	Serum response factor
Taq	Heat-stable DNA polymerase from *Thermus aquaticus*
TCII	Transcobalamin II
TCR	T-cell receptor
TdT	Terminal deoxynucleotidyl transferase
TF	Tissue factor
TFPI	Tissue factor pathway inhibitor
TGF-β	Transforming growth factor-β
TIL	Tumour-infiltrating lymphocytes
TNF-α	Tumour necrosis factor-α
TPO	Thrombopoietin
tRNA	Transfer RNA
UV	Ultraviolet
V, D, J, C	Variable, diversity, joining and constant regions
VEGF	Vascular endothelial growth factor
vIRF	Viral interferon regulatory factor
VNTR	Variable number of tandem repeats
YAC	Yeast artificial chromosome

Note: Human gene nomenclature

Throughout the book we have attempted to follow the guidelines for gene nomenclature whereby genotypes are printed in upper case italic and phenotypes are printed in roman case, such that the gene *BCL-2* encodes the protein BCL-2.

The guidelines drawn up as a result of the Nomenclature Meeting held in Toronto on 5 March 1997 may be found on the Internet at:

http://www.gene.ucl.ac.uk/nomenclature/guidelines.html

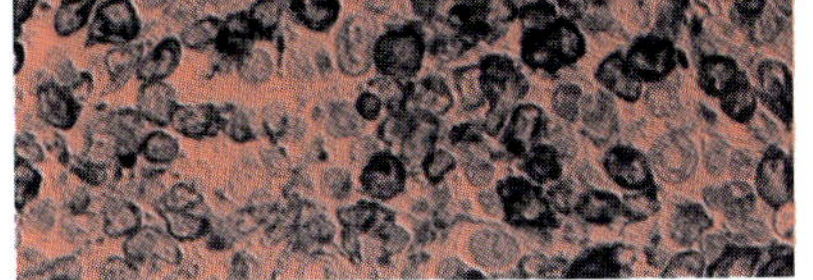

Chapter 1

Beginnings: the molecular pathology of haemoglobin

David Weatherall

Historical background

Linus Pauling first used the term 'molecular disease' in 1949, after the discovery that the structure of sickle cell haemoglobin differed from that of normal haemoglobin. Indeed, it was this seminal observation that led to the concept of *molecular medicine*, that is the description of disease mechanisms at the level of cells and molecules. However, until the development of recombinant DNA technology in the mid-1970s, knowledge of events inside the cell nucleus, notably how genes function, could only be the subject of guesswork based on the structure and function of their protein products. However, as soon as it became possible to isolate human genes and to study their properties, the picture changed dramatically.

Progress over the last 20 years has been driven by technological advances in molecular biology. At first it was possible only to obtain indirect information about the structure and function of genes by DNA/DNA and DNA/RNA hybridisation, that is by probing the quantity or structure of RNA or DNA by annealing reactions with molecular probes. The next major advance was the ability to fractionate DNA into pieces of predictable size with bacterial restriction enzymes. This led to the invention of a technique which played a central role in the early development of human molecular genetics, called Southern blotting after the name of its developer, Edwin Southern. This method allowed the structure and organisation of genes to be studied directly for the first time and led to the definition of a number of different forms of molecular pathology.

Once it was possible to fractionate DNA, it soon became feasible to insert the pieces into vectors that are able to divide within bacteria. The steady improvement in the properties of cloning vectors made it possible to generate libraries of human DNA growing in bacterial cultures. Ingenious approaches were developed to scan the libraries to detect genes of interest; once pinpointed, the appropriate bacterial colonies could be grown to generate larger quantities of DNA carrying a particular gene. Later it became possible to sequence these genes, persuade them to synthesise their products in microorganisms, cultured cells or even other species, and hence to define their key regulatory regions.

The early work in the field of human molecular genetics focused on diseases in which there was some knowledge of the genetic defect at the protein or biochemical level. However, once linkage maps of the human genome became available, following the identification of highly polymorphic regions of DNA, it was possible to search for any gene for a disease, even where the cause was completely unknown. This approach, first called 'reverse genetics' and later rechristened 'positional cloning', led to the discovery of genes for many important diseases.

As even more DNA markers became available, and as methods for sequencing were improved and automated, thoughts turned to the next major goal in this field, that is the Human Genome Project, the complete sequence of the bases that constitute our 100 000 or so genes and all that lies between them. Currently, this is said to be on target for the early part of the new millennium.

During this remarkable period of technical advance, considerable progress has been made towards an understanding of the pathology of disease at the molecular level. It has had a particular impact on haematology, leading to advances in the understanding of gene function and disease mechanisms in almost every aspect of the field.

The inherited disorders of haemoglobin, the thalassaemias and structural haemoglobin variants, the commonest human monogenic diseases, were the first to be studied systematically at the molecular level and a great deal is known about their genotype/phenotype relationships. This field led the way to molecular haematology and, indeed, to the development of molecular medicine. Thus, even though the genetics of haemoglobin is complicated by the fact that different varieties are produced at particular stages of human development, the molecular pathology of the haemoglobinopathies provides an excellent model system for understanding any monogenic disease and the complex interactions between genotype and environment that underlie many multigenic disorders.

In this chapter we will consider the structure, synthesis and genetic control of the human haemoglobins, describe the molecular pathology of the haemoglobin disorders individually, and discuss briefly how the complex interactions of their different genotypes produce a remarkably diverse family of clinical phenotypes. Readers who wish to learn more about the methods of molecular genetics, particularly as applied to the study of haemoglobin disorders, are referred to the reviews cited at the end of this chapter.

The structure, genetic control and synthesis of normal haemoglobin

Structure and function

The varying oxygen requirements during embryonic, fetal and adult life are reflected by the synthesis of different structural haemoglobins at each stage of human development. They all have the same general tetrameric structure, however, consisting of two different pairs of globin chains, each attached to one haem molecule. Adult and fetal haemoglobins have α chains combined with β chains (Hb A, $\alpha_2\beta_2$), δ chains (Hb A_2, $\alpha_2\delta_2$) and γ chains (Hb F, $\alpha_2\gamma_2$). In embryos, α-like chains called ζ chains combine with γ chains to produce Hb Portland ($\zeta_2\gamma_2$), or with ε chains to make Hb Gower 1 ($\zeta_2\varepsilon_2$), while α and ε chains form Hb Gower 2 ($\alpha_2\varepsilon_2$). Fetal haemoglobin is heterogeneous; there are two varieties of γ chains which differ only in their amino acid composition at position 136, which may be occupied by either glycine or alanine; γ chains containing glycine at this position are called $^G\gamma$ chains, those with alanine, $^A\gamma$ chains (Figure 1.1).

The synthesis of haemoglobin tetramers consisting of two unlike pairs of globin chains is absolutely essential for the effective function of haemoglobin as an oxygen carrier. The classical sigmoid shape of the oxygen dissociation curve, which reflects the allosteric properties of the haemoglobin molecule, ensures that at high oxygen tensions in the lungs oxygen is readily taken up, and later released effectively at the lower tensions encountered in the tissues. The shape of the curve is quite different to that of myoglobin, a molecule which consists of a single globin chain with haem attached to it, which, like abnormal haemoglobins that consist of homotetramers of like-chains, has a hyperbolic oxygen dissociation curve.

The transition from a hyperbolic to a sigmoid oxygen dissociation curve, absolutely critical for normal oxygen delivery, reflects co-operativity between the four haem molecules and their globin subunits. When one of them takes on oxygen the affinity of the remaining three increases markedly; this happens because haemoglobin

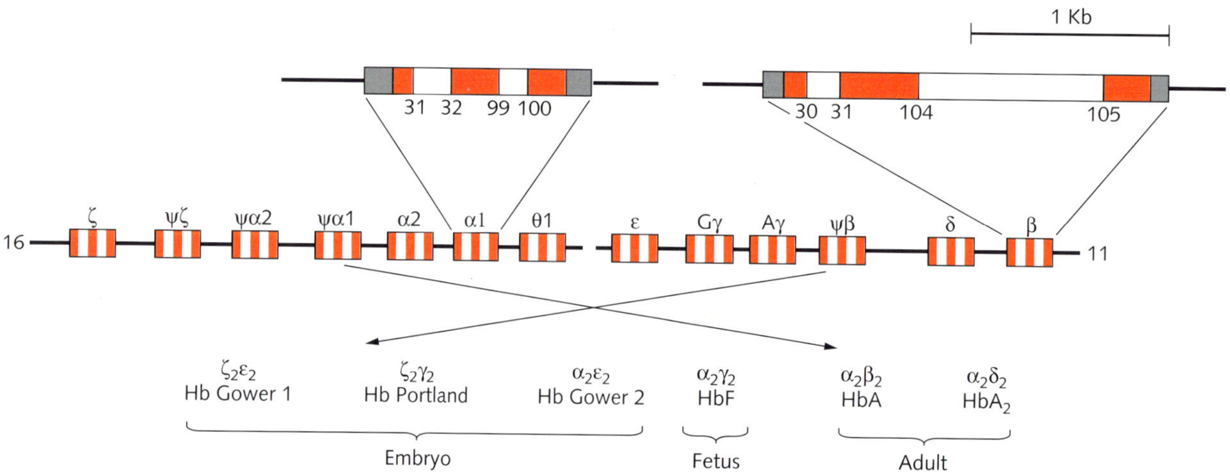

Fig. 1.1 The genetic control of human haemoglobin production in embryonic, fetal and adult life

can exist in two configurations, deoxy (T) and oxy (R), where T and R stand for 'tight' and 'relaxed' states, respectively. The T configuration has a lower affinity than the R for ligands such as oxygen. At some point during the addition of oxygen to the haems, the transition from the T to R configuration occurs and the oxygen affinity of the partially liganded molecule increases dramatically. These allosteric changes result from interactions between the iron of the haem groups and various bonds within the haemoglobin tetramer that lead to subtle spatial changes as oxygen is taken on or given up.

The precise tetrameric structures of the different human haemoglobins, which reflect the primary amino acid sequence of their individual globin chains, are also vital for various adaptive changes which are required to ensure adequate tissue oxygenation. The position of the oxygen dissociation curve can be modified in several ways. For example, oxygen affinity is decreased with increasing CO_2 tensions, the Bohr effect. This facilitates oxygen loading to the tissues, where a drop in pH due to CO_2 influx lowers oxygen affinity; the opposite effect occurs in the lungs. Oxygen affinity is also modified by the level of 2,3-diphosphoglycerate (2,3-DPG) in the red cell. Increasing concentrations shift the oxygen dissociation curve to the right, that is, reduce oxygen affinity, while diminishing concentrations have the opposite effect. 2,3-DPG fits into the gap between the two β chains when it widens during deoxygenation, and interacts with several specific binding sites in the central cavity of the molecule. In the deoxy configuration the gap between the two β chains narrows and the molecule cannot be accommodated. With increasing concentrations of 2,3-DPG, which are found in various hypoxic and anaemic states, more haemoglobin molecules tend to be held in the deoxy configuration and the oxygen dissociation curve is therefore shifted to the right, with more effective release of oxygen.

Fetal red cells have a higher oxygen affinity than adult red cells although, interestingly, purified fetal haemoglobin has a similar oxygen dissociation curve to adult haemoglobin. These differences, which are adapted to the oxygen requirements of fetal life, reflect the relative inability of Hb F to interact with 2,3-DPG compared with Hb A. This is because the γ chains of Hb F lack specific binding sites for 2,3-DPG.

In short, oxygen transport can be modified by a variety of adaptive features in the red cell that include interactions between the different haem molecules, the effects of CO_2 and differential affinities for 2,3-DPG. These changes, together with more general mechanisms involving the cardio-respiratory system, provide the main basis for physiological adaptation to anaemia.

Genetic control of haemoglobin

The α- and β-like globin chains are the products of two different gene families which are found on different chromosomes (Figure 1.1). The β-like globin genes form a linked cluster on chromosome 11, spread over approximately 60 kb (kb = kilobase or 1000 nucleotide bases). The different genes that comprise this cluster are arranged in the order 5′–ε–^{G}γ–^{A}γ–ψβ–δ–β–3′. The α-like genes also form a linked cluster, in this case on chromosome 16, in the order 5′–ζ–ψζ–ψα1–α2–α1–3′. The ψβ, ψζ and ψα genes are pseudogenes, that is they have strong sequence homology with the β, ζ and α genes but contain a number of differences which prevent them from directing the synthesis of any products. They may reflect remnants of genes that were functional at an earlier stage of human evolution.

The structure of the human globin genes is, in essence, similar to that of all mammalian genes. They consist of long strings of nucleotides which are divided into coding regions, or exons, and non-coding inserts called intervening sequences (IVS), or introns. The β-like globin genes contain two introns of 122–130 and 850–900 base pairs between codons 30 and 31, and 104 and 105, respectively (the exon codons are numbered sequentially from the 5′ to the 3′ end of the gene, that is from left to right). Similar, though smaller, introns are found in the α and ζ globin genes. These introns and exons, together with short non-coding sequences at the 5′ and 3′ ends of the genes, represent the major functional regions of the particular genes. However, there are also extremely important regulatory sequences which are essential to subserve these functions, which lie outside the genes themselves.

At the 5′ non-coding (flanking) regions of the globin genes, like all mammalian genes, there are blocks of nucleotide homology. The first, the ATA box, is about 30 bases upstream (to the left) of the initiation codon, that is the start word for the beginning of protein synthesis (*see below*). The second, the CCAAT box, is about 70 base pairs upstream from the 5′ end of the genes. About 80 to 100 bases further upstream there is the sequence GGGGTG, or CACCC, which may be inverted or duplicated. These three highly conserved DNA sequences, called promoter elements, are involved in the initiation of transcription of the individual genes. Finally, at the 3′ non-coding regions of all the globin genes there is the sequence AATAAA which is the signal for cleavage and polyA addition to RNA transcripts (*see below—Gene action and globin synthesis*).

The globin gene clusters also contain several sequences that constitute regulatory elements that interact

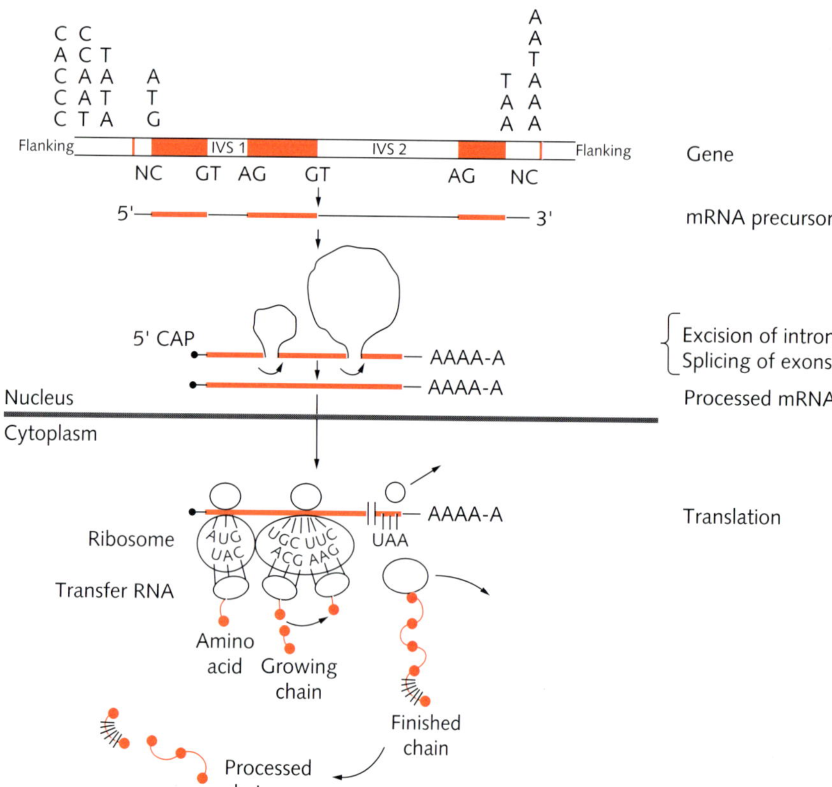

Fig. 1.2 The mechanisms of globin gene transcription and translation

to promote erythroid-specific gene expression and co-ordination of the changes in globin gene activity during development. These include the globin genes themselves and their promoter elements—enhancers—that is, regulatory sequences that increase gene expression despite being located at a considerable distance from the genes, and 'master' regulatory sequences called, in the case of the β globin gene cluster, the locus control region (LCR), and the α genes, HS40 (a nuclease-hypersensitive site in DNA 40 kb from the α globin genes). Each of these sequences has a modular structure made up of an array of short motifs that represent the binding sites for transcriptional activators or repressors.

Gene action and globin synthesis

The flow of information between DNA and protein is summarised in Figure 1.2. When a globin gene is transcribed, messenger RNA (mRNA) is synthesised from one of its strands, a process which begins by the formation of a transcription complex consisting of a variety of regulatory proteins together with an enzyme called RNA polymerase (*see below*). The primary transcript is a large mRNA precursor which contains both intron and exon sequences. While in the nucleus this molecule undergoes a variety of modifications. First, the introns are removed and the exons are spliced together. The intron/exon junctions always have the same sequence, GT at their 5′ end, and AG at their 3′ end. This appears to be essential for accurate splicing; if there is a mutation at these sites this process does not occur. Splicing reflects a complex series of intermediary stages and the interaction of a number of different nuclear proteins. After the exons are joined the mRNAs are modified and stabilised; at their 5′ end a complex CAP structure is formed, while at their 3′ end a string of adenylic acid residues (polyA) is added. The now processed mRNA moves into the cytoplasm where it acts as a template for globin chain production. Because of the rules of base pairing—that is cytosine always pairs with thymine, and guanine with adenine—the structure of the mRNA reflects a faithful copy of the DNA codons from which it is synthesised; the only difference is that, in RNA, uracil (U) replaces thymine (T).

Amino acids are transported to the mRNA template on carriers called transfer RNAs (tRNAs); there are specific tRNAs for each amino acid. Furthermore, because the genetic code is redundant, that is more than one codon can encode for a particular amino acid, there are several different individual tRNAs for different amino acids. Their order in the globin chain is determined by the order of codons in the mRNA. The tRNAs contain three bases, anticodons, which are complementary to mRNA codons for particular amino acids. They carry amino acids to the template where they find the appropriate positioning by codon/anticodon base pairing. When the first tRNA is in position, an initiation complex is formed between several protein initiation factors together with the two subunits which constitute the ribosomes. A second tRNA moves in alongside and the two amino acids which they carry form a peptide bond between them; the globin chain is now two amino acid residues long. This process is continued along the mRNA from left to right, and the growing peptide chain is transferred from one incoming tRNA to the next, that is the mRNA is translated from 5′ to 3′. During this time the tRNAs are held in appropriate steric configuration with the mRNA by the two ribosomal subunits. There are specific initiation (AUG) and termination (UAA, UAG and UGA) codons. When the ribosomes reach the termination codon, translation ceases, the completed globin chains are released, and the ribosomal subunits are recycled. Individual globin chains combine with haem, synthesised through a separate pathway, and then interact with one like and two unlike chains to form a completed haemoglobin tetramer.

Regulation of haemoglobin synthesis

The regulation of globin gene expression is mediated mainly at the transcriptional level, with some fine tuning during translation and post-translational modification of the gene products. DNA that is not involved in transcription is held tightly packaged in a compact, chemically modified form that is inaccessible to transcription factors and polymerases and which is heavily methylated. Activation of a particular gene is reflected by changes in the structure of the surrounding chromatin which can be identified by enhanced sensitivity to nucleases. Erythroid lineage-specific nuclease-hypersensitive sites are found at several locations in the β globin gene cluster. Four are distributed over 20 kb upstream from the ε globin gene in the region of the β globin LCR (Figure 1.3). This vital regulatory region is able to establish a transcriptionally active domain spanning the entire β globin gene cluster. Several enhancer sequences have been identified in this cluster. A variety of regulatory proteins bind to the LCR, and to the promoter regions of the globin genes and to the enhancer sequences. It is thought that the LCR and other enhancer regions become

Fig. 1.3 The position of the major regulatory regions in the β and α globin gene clusters
The arrows indicate the position of the erythroid lineage-specific nuclease-hypersensitive sites. (HS = hypersensitive.)

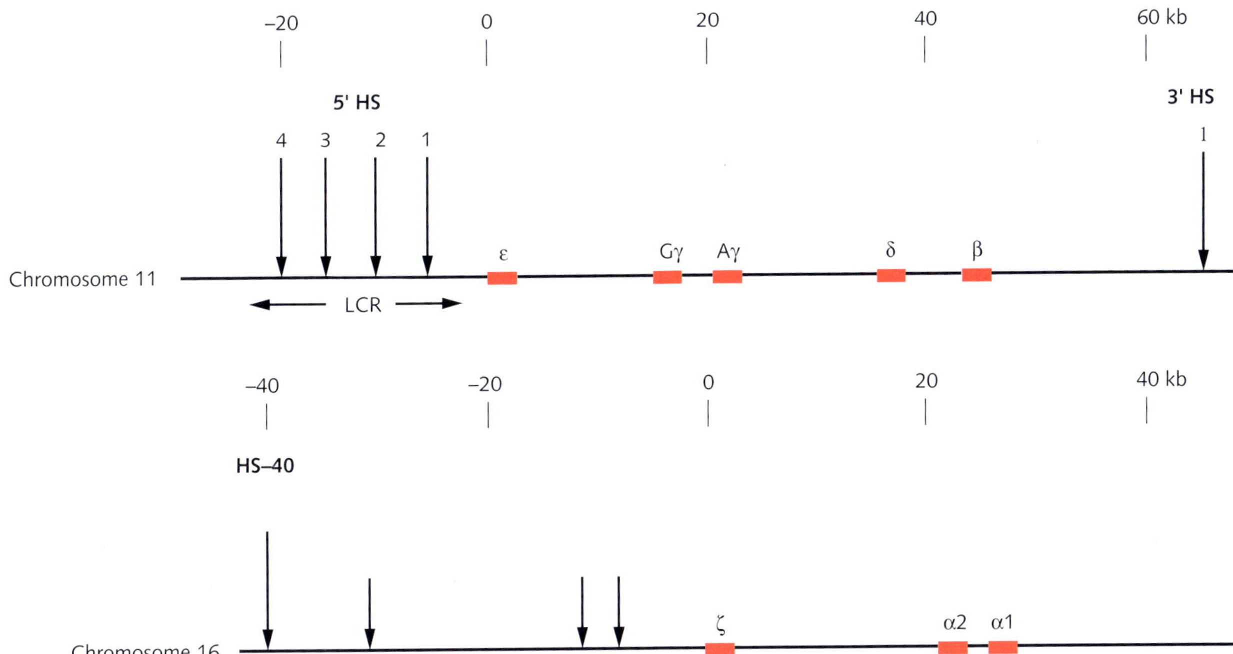

opposed to the promoters to increase the rate of transcription of the genes to which they are related. All these regulatory regions bind a variety of erythroid-specific transcription factors, notably GATA-1 and NFE-E2, as well as other factors which are more ubiquitous in their tissue distribution. It is the interaction between these factors and the enhancers and promoters which sets the level of gene expression.

The binding of haematopoietic-specific factors activates the LCR which renders the entire β globin gene cluster transcriptionally active. These factors also bind to the enhancer and promoter sequences, which work in tandem to regulate the expression of the individual genes in the clusters. It is likely that some of the transcriptional factors are developmental-stage-specific, and hence may be responsible for the differential expression of the embryonic, fetal and adult globin genes. The α globin gene cluster also contains an element, HS40, which has some structural features in common with the β LCR, although it is different in aspects of its structure. A number of enhancer-like sequences have also been identified, although it is becoming clear that there are fundamental differences in the pattern of regulation of the two globin gene clusters.

In addition to the different regulatory sequences outlined above, there are also sequences which may be involved specifically with 'silencing' of genes, notably those for the embryonic haemoglobins, during development.

Some degree of regulation is also mediated by differences in the rates of initiation and translation of the different mRNAs, and at the post-transcriptional level by differential affinity for different protein subunits. However, this kind of post-transcriptional fine tuning probably plays a relatively small role in determining the overall output of the globin gene products.

Regulation of developmental changes in globin gene expression

During development, the site of red cell production moves from the yolk sac to the fetal liver and spleen, and hence to bone marrow in the adult. Embryonic, fetal and adult haemoglobin synthesis are approximately related in time to these changes in the site of erythropoiesis, although it is quite clear that the various switches, between embryonic and fetal, and fetal and adult haemoglobin synthesis, are beautifully synchronised throughout these different sites. Fetal haemoglobin synthesis declines during the later months of gestation and Hb F is replaced by Hbs A and A_2 by the end of the first year of life.

Despite a great deal of research, very little is known about the regulation of these different switches from one globin gene to another during development. Work from a variety of different sources suggests that there may be specific regions in the α and β globin gene clusters that may be responsive to the action of transcription factors, some of which may be developmental-stage-specific. However, proteins of this type have not yet been isolated, and nothing is known about their regulation and how it is mediated during development.

The molecular pathology of haemoglobin

As is the case for most monogenic diseases, the inherited disorders of haemoglobin fall into two major classes. First, there are those that result from a reduced output of one or other globin genes, the *thalassaemias*. Second, there is a wide range of conditions that result from the production of *structurally abnormal globin chains*; the type of disease depends on how the particular alteration in protein structure interferes with its stability or function. Of course, no biological classification is entirely satisfactory; those which attempt to define the haemoglobin disorders are no exception. There are some structural haemoglobin variants which happen to be synthesised at a reduced rate and hence are associated with a clinical picture similar to thalassaemia. And there are other classes of mutations which simply interfere with the normal transition from fetal to adult haemoglobin synthesis, a family of conditions that is given the general title 'hereditary persistence of fetal haemoglobin'. Furthermore, because these diseases are all so common, and occur together in particular populations, it is not uncommon for an individual to inherit a gene for one or other form of thalassaemia and a structural haemoglobin variant. The rather heterogeneous group of conditions that results from all these different mutations and interactions is summarised in Table 1.1.

Over recent years determination of the molecular pathology of the two common forms of thalassaemia, α and β, has provided a remarkable picture of the repertoire of mutations that can underlie human monogenic disease. Similarly, studies of the relationship between structure and function in the structurally abnormal haemoglobins have provided a great deal of information about normal human haemoglobin function.

In the sections that follow we will describe, in outline, the different forms of molecular pathology that underlie these conditions.

Table 1.1 The thalassaemias and related disorders.

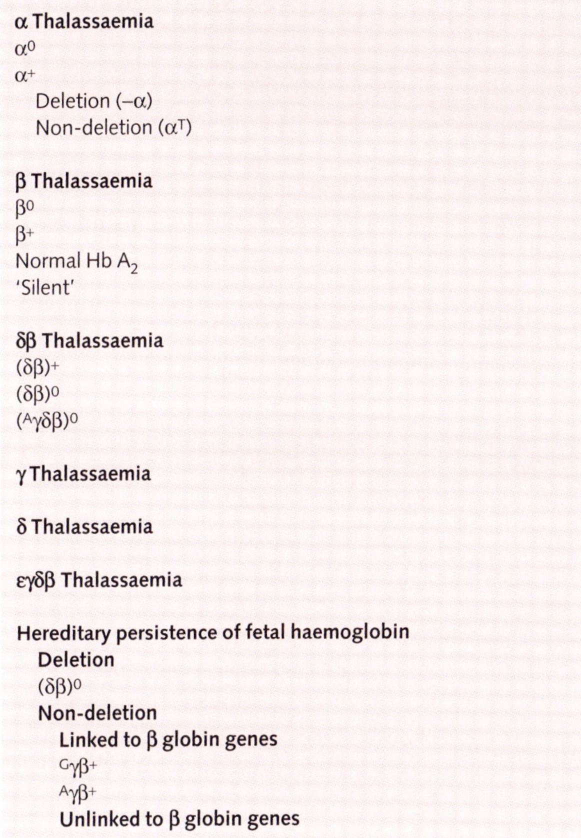

α Thalassaemia
α^0
α^+
Deletion (–α)
Non-deletion (α^T)
β Thalassaemia
β^0
β^+
Normal Hb A_2
'Silent'
δβ Thalassaemia
$(\delta\beta)^+$
$(\delta\beta)^0$
$(^{A}\gamma\delta\beta)^0$
γ Thalassaemia
δ Thalassaemia
εγδβ Thalassaemia
Hereditary persistence of fetal haemoglobin
Deletion
$(\delta\beta)^0$
Non-deletion
Linked to β globin genes
$^{G}\gamma\beta^+$
$^{A}\gamma\beta^+$
Unlinked to β globin genes

The β thalassaemias

There are two main classes of β thalassaemia, β^0 thalassaemia, in which there is an absence of β globin chain production, and β^+ thalassaemia, in which there is a variable reduction in the output of β globin chains. As shown in Figure 1.4, mutations of the β globin genes may cause a reduced output of gene product at the levels of transcription, mRNA processing, translation, or through the stability of the globin gene product.

Defective β globin gene transcription

There are a variety of mechanisms that interfere with the normal transcription of the β globin genes. First, the genes may be either completely or partially deleted. Overall, deletions of the β globin genes are not commonly found in patients with β thalassaemia, with one exception: a 619 bp deletion involving the 3′ end of the gene is found frequently in the Sind populations of India and Pakistan, where it constitutes about 30% of the β thalassaemia alleles. Other deletions are extremely rare.

A much more common group of mutations, that results in a moderate decrease in the rate of transcription of the β globin genes involves single nucleotide substitutions in or near the TATA box at about –30 nucleotides (nt) from the transcription start site, or in the proximal or distal promoter elements at –90 nt and –105 nt. These mutations result in decreased β globin mRNA production, ranging from 10 to 25% of the normal output. Thus, they are usually associated with the mild forms of β^+ thalassaemia. They are particularly common in African populations, an observation which explains the unusual mildness of β thalassaemia in this racial group. One particular mutation, C → T at position –101 nt to the β globin gene, causes an extremely mild deficit of β

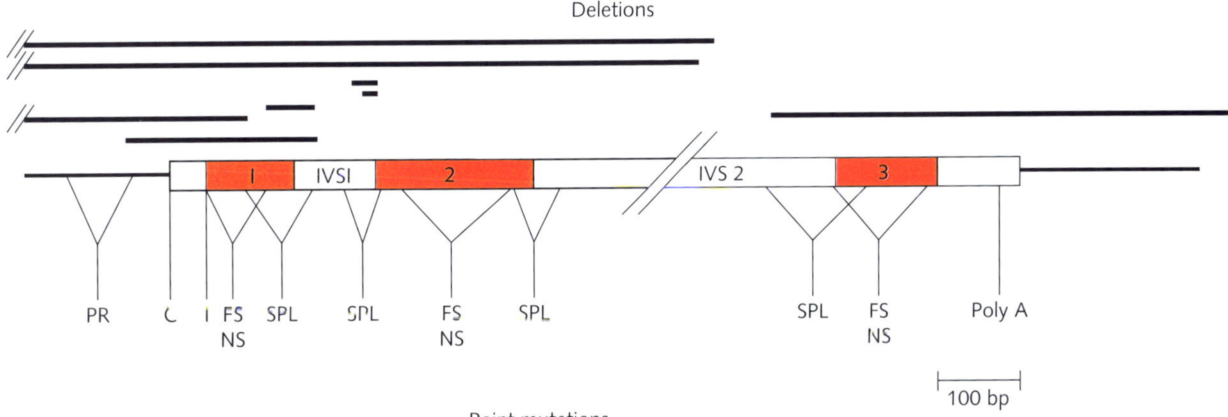

Fig. 1.4 The mutations of the β globin gene that underlie β thalassaemia
The heavy black lines indicate the length of the deletions. The point mutations are designated as follows: PR = promoter; C = CAP site; I = initiation codon; FS, NS = frameshift and nonsense mutations; SPL = splice mutations; PolyA = polyA addition site mutations.

globin mRNA. Indeed, this allele is so mild that it is completely silent in carriers and can only be identified by its interaction with more severe β thalassaemia alleles in compound heterozygotes.

Mutations that cause abnormal processing of mRNA

As mentioned earlier, the boundaries between exons and introns are marked by the invariant dinucleotides GT at the donor (5′) site, and AG at the acceptor (3′) site. Mutations, that is base changes, that affect either of these sites completely abolish normal splicing and produce the phenotype of β^0 thalassaemia. The transcription of genes carrying these mutations appears to be normal, but there is a complete inactivation of splicing at the altered junction.

Another family of mutations involves what are called 'splice site consensus sequences'. Although only the GT dinucleotide is invariant at the donor splice site, there is conservation of adjacent nucleotides and a common, or consensus, sequence of these regions can be identified. Mutations within this sequence can reduce the efficiency of splicing to varying degrees because they lead to alternate splicing at the surrounding cryptic sites. For example, mutations of the nucleotide at position 5 of IVS-1 (the first intervening sequence), G → C or T, result in a marked reduction of β chain production and in the phenotype of severe β^+ thalassaemia. On the other hand, the substitution of C for T at position 6 in IVS-1 leads to only a mild reduction in the output of β chains.

Another mechanism that leads to abnormal splicing involves 'cryptic splice sites', that is regions of DNA which, if mutated, assume the function of a splice site at an inappropriate region of the mRNA precursor. For example, a variety of mutations activate a cryptic site which spans codons 24–27 of exon 1 of the β globin gene. This site contains a GT dinucleotide, and adjacent substitutions that alter it so that it more closely resembles the consensus donor splice site result in its activation, even though the normal splice site is intact. A mutation at codon 24 GGT → GGA, though it does not alter the amino acid which is normally found in this position in the β globin chain (glycine), allows some splicing to occur at this site instead of the exon/intron boundary. This results in the production of both normal and abnormally spliced β globin mRNA and hence in the clinical phenotype of severe β thalassaemia. Interestingly, mutations at codons 19, 26 and 27 result in both a reduced production of normal mRNA due to abnormal splicing, and to an amino acid substitution when the mRNA which is spliced normally is translated into protein. The abnormal haemoglobins produced are haemoglobins Malay, E and Knossos, respectively. All these variants are associated with a mild β^+ thalassaemia-like phenotype. These mutations illustrate how sequence changes in coding rather than intervening sequences influence RNA processing, and underline the importance of competition between potential splice site sequences in generating both normal and abnormal varieties of β globin mRNA.

Cryptic splice sites in introns may also carry mutations that activate them even though the normal splice sites remain intact. A common mutation of this kind in Mediterranean populations involves a base substitution at position 110 in IVS-1. This region contains a sequence similar to a 3′ acceptor site, though it lacks the invariant AG dinucleotide. The change of the G to A at position 110 creates this dinucleotide. The result is that about 90% of the RNA transcript splices to this particular site, and only 10% to the normal site, again producing the phenotype of severe β^+ thalassaemia (Figure 1.5). Several other β thalassaemia mutations have been described which generate new donor sites within IVS-2 of the β globin gene.

Another family of mutations that interferes with β globin gene processing involves the sequence AAUAAA in the 3′ untranslated regions which is the signal for cleavage and polyadenylation of the β globin gene transcript. Somehow, these mutations destabilise the transcript. For example, a T → C substitution in this sequence leads to only one tenth of the normal amount of β globin mRNA transcript and hence to the phenotype of a moderately severe β^+ thalassaemia. Another example of a mutation which probably leads to defective processing of function of β globin mRNA is the single base substitution, A → C, in the CAP site. It is not yet understood how this mutation causes a reduced rate of transcription of the β globin gene.

There is also another small subset of rare mutations which involve the 3′ untranslated region of the β globin gene and are associated with relatively mild forms of β thalassaemia. It is thought that these interfere in some way with transcription but the mechanism is unknown.

Mutations which result in abnormal translation of β globin mRNA

There are three main classes of mutations of this kind. Base substitutions that change an amino acid codon to a chain termination codon prevent the translation of β globin mRNA and result in the phenotype of β^0 thalassaemia. Several mutations of this kind have been described; the commonest, involving codon 17, occurs widely throughout Southeast Asia. Similarly, a codon 39

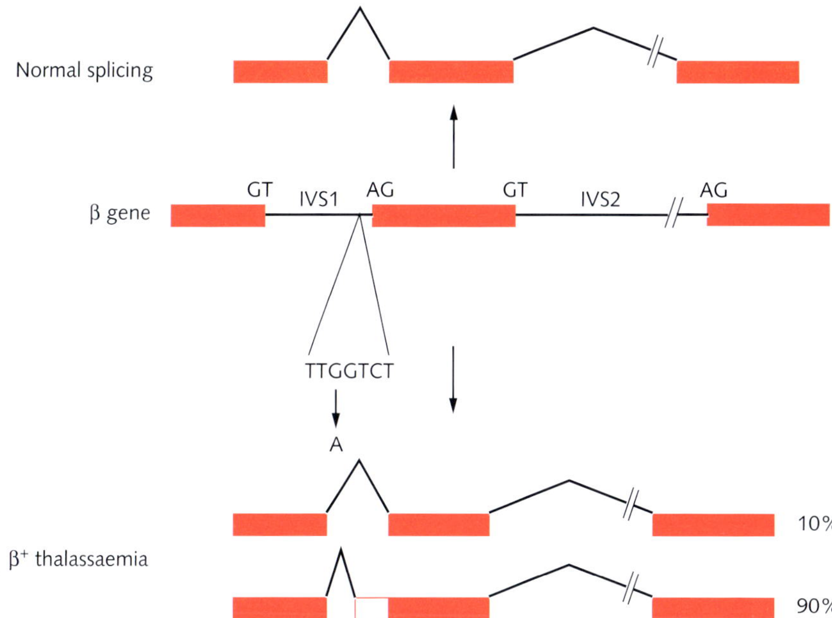

Fig. 1.5 The generation of a new splice site in an intron as the mechanism for a form of β+ thalassaemia
For details see text.

mutation is encountered frequently in the Mediterranean region.

The second class involves the insertion or deletion of one, two or four nucleotides in the coding region of the β globin gene. These disrupt the normal reading frame, cause a frameshift, and hence interfere with the translation of β globin mRNA. The end result is the insertion of anomalous amino acids after the frameshift until a termination codon is reached in the new reading frame. This type of mutation always leads to the phenotype of β^0 thalassaemia.

Finally, there are several mutations which involve the β globin gene initiation codon and which, presumably, reduce the efficiency of translation.

Unstable β globin chain variants

Some forms of β thalassaemia result from the synthesis of highly unstable β globin chains which are incapable of forming haemoglobin tetramers, and which are rapidly degraded, leading to the phenotype of β^0 thalassaemia. Indeed, in many of these conditions no abnormal globin chain product can be demonstrated by protein analysis and the molecular pathology has to be interpreted simply on the basis of a derived sequence of the variant β chain obtained by DNA analysis.

Recent studies have provided some interesting insights into how complex clinical phenotypes may result from the synthesis of unstable β globin products. For example, there is a spectrum of disorders that result from mutations in exon 3 which give rise to a moderately severe form of β thalassaemia in heterozygotes. It is now clear that these conditions result from the synthesis of long, unstable β chains that precipitate in the red cell precursors. We shall return to the pathophysiology of these conditions later. Indeed, it is now clear that the whole family of disorders results from the production of unstable β chains, which may be either truncated, of normal length or elongated, and which give rise to a wide spectrum of conditions ranging from mild hypochromic anaemia to severe, dominantly inherited β thalassaemia.

The molecular pathology of the α thalassaemias

The molecular pathology of the α thalassaemias is more complicated than that of the β thalassaemias, simply because there are two α globin genes per haploid genome. Thus, the normal α globin genotype can be written αα/αα. As in the case of β thalassaemia, there are two major varieties of α thalassaemia, α^+ and α^0 thalassaemia. In α^+ thalassaemia one of the linked α globin genes is lost, either by deletion (–) or mutation (T); the heterozygous genotype can be written –α/αα or $\alpha^T\alpha$/αα. In α^0 thalassaemia the loss of both α globin genes nearly always results from a deletion; the heterozygous genotype is therefore written – –/αα. In populations where specific deletions are particularly common—Southeast Asia (SEA) or the Mediterranean region (MED)—it is useful to add the appropriate superscript as follows: $--^{SEA}$/αα or $--^{MED}$/αα. It follows that when we speak

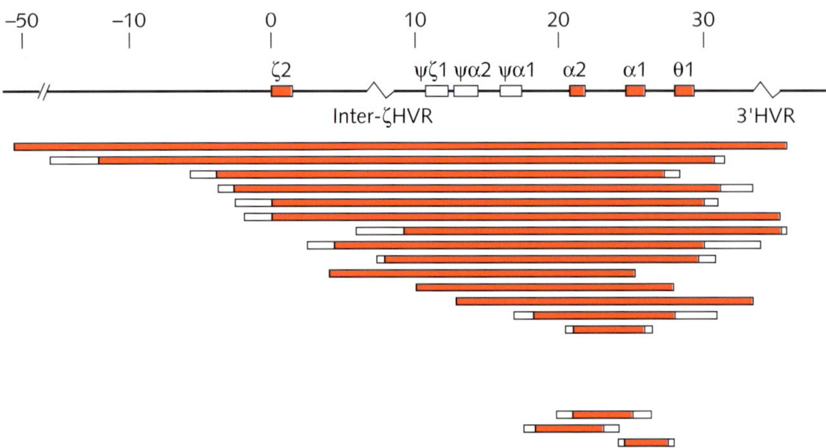

Fig. 1.6 Some of the deletions that underlie α^0 and α^+ thalassaemia
The heavy black lines indicate the length of the deletions. The unshaded regions indicate uncertainty about the precise breakpoints. The three small deletions at the bottom of the figure represent the common α^+ thalassaemia deletions.

of an 'α thalassaemia gene' what we are really referring to is a haplotype, i.e. the state and function of both of the linked α globin genes.

α^0 thalassaemia

Three main molecular pathologies, all involving deletions, have been found to underlie the α^0 thalassaemia phenotype. The majority of cases result from deletions that remove both α globin genes and a varying length of the α globin gene cluster (Figure 1.6). Occasionally, however, the α globin gene cluster is intact but is inactivated by a deletion which involves the major regulatory region HS40, 40 kb upstream from the α globin genes. Finally, the α globin genes may be lost as part of a truncation of the tip of the short arm of chromosome 16.

As well as providing us with an understanding of the molecular basis for α^0 thalassaemia, detailed studies of these deletions have yielded more general information about the mechanisms that underlie this form of molecular pathology. For example, it has been found that the 5′ breakpoints of a number of deletions of the α globin gene cluster are located approximately the same distance apart and in the same order along the chromosome as their respective 3′ breakpoints; similar findings have been observed in deletions of the β globin gene cluster. These deletions seem to have resulted from illegitimate recombination events which have led to the deletion of an integral number of chromatin loops as they pass through their nuclear attachment points during chromosomal replication. Another long deletion has been characterised in which a new piece of DNA bridges the two breakpoints in the α globin gene cluster. The inserted sequence originates upstream from the α globin gene cluster, where it normally is found in an inverted orientation to that found between the breakpoints of the deletion. Thus it appears to have been incorporated into the junction in a way that reflects its close proximity to the deletion breakpoint region during replication. Other deletions seem to be related to the family of Alu-repeats, simple repeat sequences that are widely dispersed throughout the genome; one deletion appears to have resulted from a simple homologous recombination between two repeats of this kind that are usually 62 kb apart.

A number of forms of α^0 thalassaemia result from terminal truncations of the short arm of chromosome 16 to a site about 50 kb distal to the α globin genes. The telomeric consensus sequence TTAGGGn has been added directly to the site of the break. Since these mutations are stably inherited, it appears that telomeric DNA alone is sufficient to stabilise the ends of broken chromosomes.

The molecular pathology of α^+ thalassaemia

As mentioned earlier, the α^+ thalassaemias result from the inactivation of one of the duplicated α globin genes, either by deletion or point mutation.

α^+ thalassaemia due to gene deletions

There are two common forms of α^+ thalassaemia due to loss of one or other of the duplicated α globin genes, $-\alpha^{3.7}$ and $-\alpha^{4.2}$, where the 3.7 and 4.2 indicate the size of the deletions. The way in which these deletions have been generated reflects the underlying structure of the α globin gene complex (Figure 1.7). Each α gene lies within a boundary of homology, approximately 4 kb long, probably generated by an ancient duplication event. The homologous regions, which are divided by small inserts,

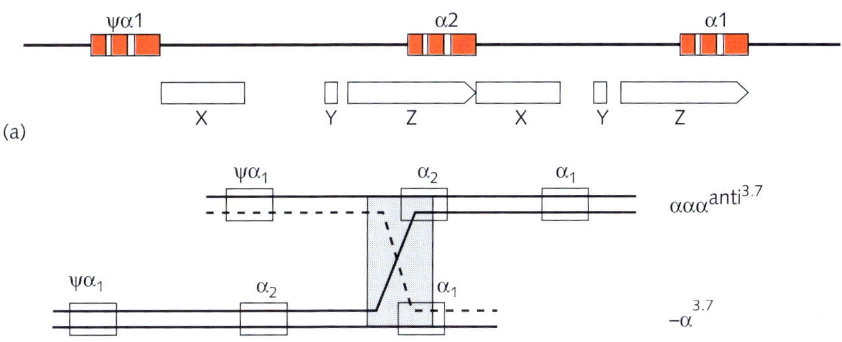

(b) Rightward crossover

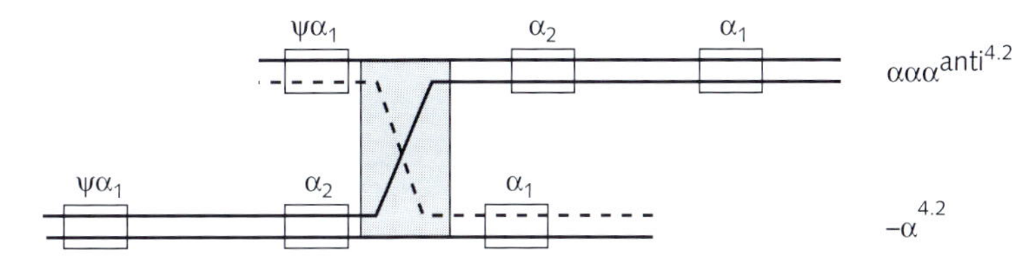

(c) Leftward crossover

Fig. 1.7 Mechanisms of the generation of the common deletion forms of α^+ thalassaemia
(a) The normal arrangement of the α globin genes, with the regions of homology X, Y and Z.
(b) The crossover which generates the $-\alpha^{3.7}$ deletion.
(c) The crossover which generates the $-\alpha^{4.2}$ deletion.

are designated X, Y and Z. The duplicated Z boxes are 3.7 kb apart and the X boxes are 4.2 kb apart. As the result of misalignment and reciprocal crossover between these segments at meiosis, a chromosome is produced with either a single (−α) or triplicated (ααα) α globin gene. As shown in Figure 1.7, if crossover occurs between homologous Z boxes 3.7 kb of DNA are lost, an event which is described as a rightward deletion, $-\alpha^{3.7}$. A similar crossover between the two X boxes deletes 4.2 kb, the leftward deletion, $-\alpha^{4.2}$. The corresponding triplicated α gene arrangements are called $\alpha\alpha\alpha^{\text{anti } 3.7}$ or $\alpha\alpha\alpha^{\text{anti } 4.2}$. A variety of different points of crossing over within the Z boxes give rise to different length deletions, still involving 3.7 kb.

Non-deletion types of α^+ thalassaemia

These disorders result from single or oligonucleotide mutations of the particular α globin gene. Most of them involve the α2 gene but, since the output from this locus is 2–3 times greater than that from the α1 gene, this may simply reflect ascertainment bias due to the greater phenotypic effect and, possibly, a greater selective advantage.

Overall, these mutations interfere with α globin gene function in a similar way to those that affect the β globin genes. They affect either transcription, translation or post-translational stability of the gene product. Since the principles are the same as for β thalassaemia, we do not need to describe them in detail, with one exception, a mutation which has not been observed in the β globin gene cluster. It turns out that there is a family of mutations that involves the α2 globin gene termination codon, TAA. Each specifically changes this codon so that an amino acid is inserted instead of the chain terminating. This is followed by 'read-through' of α globin mRNA which is not normally translated until another in-phase termination codon is reached. The result is an elongated α chain with 31 additional residues at the C terminal end. Five haemoglobin variants of this type have been identified. The commonest, haemoglobin Constant Spring, occurs at a high frequency in many parts of Southeast Asia. It is not absolutely clear why the read-through of normally untranslated mRNAs leads to a reduced output from the α2 gene, although there is considerable evidence that it in some way destabilises the mRNA.

α thalassaemia/mental retardation syndromes

There is a family of mild forms of α thalassaemia which is quite different to that described in the previous section and which is associated with varying degrees of mental retardation. Recent studies indicate that there are two quite different varieties of this condition, one encoded on chromosome 16 (ATR-16), the other on the X chromosome (ATR-X).

The ATR-16 syndrome is characterised by a relatively

mild mental handicap with a variable constellation of facial and skeletal dysmorphisms. These individuals have long deletions involving the α globin gene cluster, but removing at least one to two Mb. This condition can arise in several ways, including unbalanced translocation involving chromosome 16, truncation of the tip of chromosome 16, and the loss of the α globin gene cluster and parts of its flanking regions by other mechanisms.

The ATR-X syndrome results from mutations in a gene on the X chromosome for a transcription factor, *XH2*, which is one of a family of highly conserved DNA helicases, proteins with a variety of functions involved with transcription and other aspects of gene regulation. It seems likely that the product of this gene is involved in α globin gene transcription but that it is also an important player in early fetal development, particularly of the urogenital system and brain. Many different mutations of this gene, involving either its helicase or zinc-finger motifs, underlie this important disorder.

Rarer forms of thalassaemia and related disorders

There are a variety of other conditions that involve the β globin gene cluster which, although less common than the β thalassaemias, provide some important information about mechanisms of molecular pathology and therefore should be mentioned briefly.

The δβ thalassaemias

Like the β thalassaemias, the δβ thalassaemias, which result from defective δ and β chain synthesis, are subdivided into the $(\delta\beta)^+$ and $(\delta\beta)^0$ forms.

The $(\delta\beta)^+$ thalassaemias result from the unequal crossing over between the δ and β globin gene loci at meiosis with the production of δβ fusion genes. The resulting δβ fusion chain products combine with α chains to form a family of haemoglobin variants called the haemoglobin Lepores, after the family name of the first patient of this kind to be discovered. Because the synthesis of these variants is directed by genes with the 5′ sequences of the δ globin genes, which have defective promoters, they are synthesised at a reduced rate and result in the phenotype of a moderately severe form of δβ thalassaemia.

The $(\delta\beta)^0$ thalassaemias nearly all result from long deletions involving the β globin gene complex. Sometimes they involve the $^A\gamma$ globin chains and hence the only active locus remaining is the $^G\gamma$ locus. In other cases the $^G\gamma$ and $^A\gamma$ loci are left intact and the deletion simply removes the δ and β globin genes; in these cases both $^G\gamma$ and $^A\gamma$ globin genes remain functional. For some reason, these long deletions allow persistent synthesis of the γ globin genes at a relatively high level during adult life which helps to compensate for the absence of β and δ globin chain production. They are classified according to the kind of fetal haemoglobin that is produced, and hence into two varieties, $^G\gamma(^A\gamma\delta\beta)^0$ and $^G\gamma^A\gamma(\delta\beta)^0$ thalassaemia; in line with other forms of thalassaemia, they are best described by what is not produced, i.e. $(^A\gamma\delta\beta)^0$ and $(\delta\beta)^0$ thalassaemia, respectively. Homozygotes produce only fetal haemoglobin, while heterozygotes have a thalassaemic blood picture together with about 5–15% haemoglobin F.

Hereditary persistence of fetal haemoglobin (HPFH)

Genetically determined persistent fetal haemoglobin synthesis in adult life is of no clinical importance except that its genetic determinants can interact with the β thalassaemias or structural haemoglobin variants; the resulting high level of haemoglobin F production often ameliorates these conditions. The different forms of HPFH result from either long deletions involving the δβ globin gene cluster, similar to those that cause $(\delta\beta)^0$ thalassaemia, or from point mutations that involve the promoters of the $^G\gamma$ or $^A\gamma$ globin genes. In the former case there is no β globin chain synthesis and therefore these conditions are classified as $(\delta\beta)^0$ HPFH. In cases in which there are promoter mutations involving the γ globin genes, there is increased γ globin chain production in adult life associated with some β and δ chain synthesis *in cis*, i.e. directed by the same chromosome, to the HPFH mutations. Thus depending on whether the point mutations involve the promoter of the $^G\gamma$ or $^A\gamma$ globin genes, these conditions are called $^G\gamma\beta^+$ HPFH and $^A\gamma\beta^+$ HPFH, respectively.

There is another family of HPFH-like disorders in which the genetic determinant is not encoded in the β chain cluster. In one case the determinant encodes on chromosome 6, although its nature is as yet to be determined.

It should be pointed out that all these conditions are very heterogeneous and that many different deletions or point mutations have been discovered that produce the rather similar phenotypes of $(\delta\beta)^0$ or $^G\gamma$ or $^A\gamma\beta^+$ HPFH.

Structural haemoglobin variants

Over 700 structural haemoglobin variants have been described, most of which are of no clinical significance. Only if the underlying mutation interferes with the stability or function of the haemoglobin molecule is there any important clinical accompaniment.

The majority of these variants result from missense

mutations, that is base substitutions which produce a codon change which encodes for a different amino acid in the affected globin chain. Rarely, structural variants result from more subtle alterations in the structure of the α or β globin genes. Shortened chains may result from internal deletions of their particular genes, while elongated chains result either from duplications within genes or frameshift mutations which allow the chain termination codon to be read through and additional amino acids to be added to the C terminal end.

Genotype/phenotype relationships for the inherited disorders of haemoglobin

It is now necessary briefly to relate the remarkably diverse molecular pathology described in the previous sections to the phenotypes observed in patients with these diseases. It will not be possible to describe all these complex issues here. Rather we shall focus on those aspects that illustrate the more general principles of how abnormal gene action is reflected in a particular clinical picture. Perhaps the most important question that we will address is why patients with apparently identical genetic lesions have widely differing disorders, a problem that still bedevils the whole field of medical genetics, even in the molecular era.

The β thalassaemias

As we have seen, the basic defect that results from the 170 or more different mutations that underlie these conditions is reduced β globin chain production. α globin chain synthesis proceeds normally and hence there is imbalanced globin chain output with an excess of α chains (Figure 1.8). Unpaired α chains precipitate in both red cell precursors and their progeny with the production of inclusion bodies. These interfere with normal red cell maturation and survival in a variety of complex ways. Their attachment to red cell membrane causes alterations in its structure, and their degradation products, notably haem, haemin (oxidised haem) and iron, result in oxidative damage to the red cell contents and membrane. These interactions result in intramedullary destruction of red cell precursors and in a shortened survival of such cells as they reach the peripheral blood. The end result is an anaemia of varying severity. This, in turn, causes tissue hypoxia and the production of relatively large amounts of erythropoietin which lead to a massive expansion of the ineffective bone marrow, resulting in bone deformity, a hypermetabolic state with wasting and malaise, and bone fragility.

A large proportion of haemoglobin in the blood of β thalassaemics is the fetal variety. Normal individuals produce about 1% of Hb F, unevenly distributed among their red cells. In the bone marrow of β thalassaemics, any red cell precursors that synthesise γ chains come under strong selection because they combine with α chains to produce fetal haemoglobin and therefore the degree of globin chain imbalance is reduced. Furthermore, the likelihood of γ chain production seems to be increased in a highly stimulated erythroid bone marrow. It seems likely that these two factors combine to increase the relative output of haemoglobin F in this disorder. However, it has a higher oxygen affinity than haemoglobin A and hence patients with β thalassaemia are not able to adapt to low haemoglobin levels as well as those who have adult haemoglobin.

The greatly expanded, ineffective erythron leads to an increased rate of iron absorption and this, combined with iron received by blood transfusion, leads to progressive iron loading of the tissues, with subsequent liver, cardiac and endocrine damage.

The constant bombardment of the spleen with abnormal red cells leads to its hypertrophy. Hence there is progressive splenomegaly with an increased plasma volume and trapping of part of the circulating red cell mass in the spleen. This leads to worsening of the anaemia. All these pathophysiological mechanisms except for iron loading can be reversed by regular blood transfusion which, in effect, shuts off the ineffective bone marrow and its consequences.

Thus it is possible to relate nearly all the important features of the severe forms of β thalassaemia to the primary defect in globin gene action. But can we also explain their remarkable clinical diversity? Part of it reflects the different mutations of the β globin genes. For example, some of the promoter or splice mutations cause an extremely mild form of β^+ thalassaemia. Many β thalassaemics are compound heterozygotes for either two severe β thalassaemia alleles, a severe and mild allele, or different mild alleles, and this also accounts for a considerable amount of clinical diversity of the disease.

What of patients who have the same mutations at their β loci yet have completely different clinical phenotypes? The co-inheritance of α thalassaemia, which reduces the magnitude of the excess of α globin chains in β thalassaemia, may ameliorate the clinical course. This remarkable experiment of nature provides unequivocal confirmation that the major pathophysiological mechanism that underlies β thalassaemia is imbalanced globin chain synthesis. In other patients, particularly those who are homozygous for β^0 thalassaemia yet run a particularly mild course, it is apparent that an unusually efficient production of fetal haemoglobin is the major

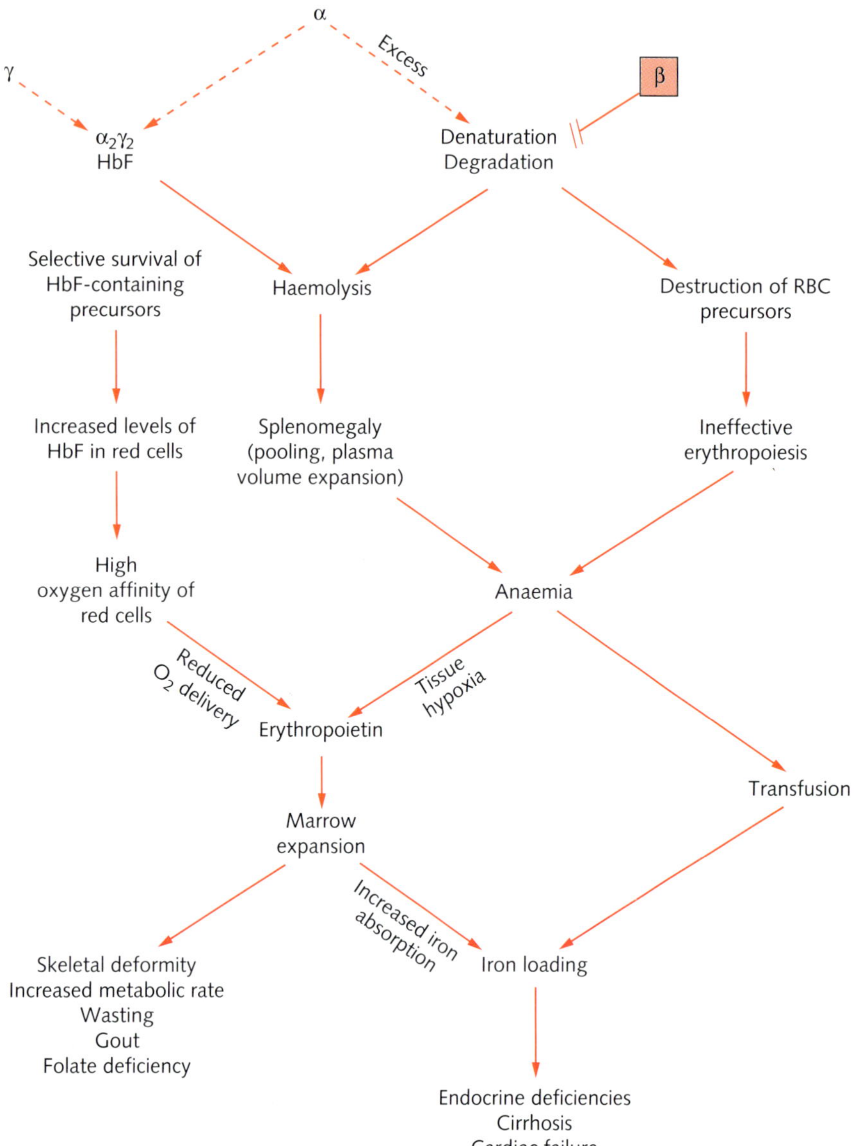

Fig. 1.8 The pathophysiology of β thalassaemia

ameliorating factor. Although in some cases it is possible to demonstrate the co-segregation of a gene for HPFH, in many patients this is not possible and currently we do not understand the remarkable variability of haemoglobin F response associated with this disease. Another possible mechanism that might be involved in modifying the phenotype is a genetic polymorphism involving the rate of proteolysis of excess α globin chains; it has not yet been possible to obtain any firm data which would point to the existence of this type of genetic variability.

In short, while we have a reasonable idea of how the β thalassaemia phenotype is modified, many questions remain and a considerable amount of the clinical variability of the disease remains unexplained.

The α thalassaemias

The pathophysiology of the α thalassaemias differs from that of the β thalassaemias mainly because of the properties of the excess globin chains that are produced as a result of defective α chain synthesis. While the excess α chains produced in β thalassaemia are unstable and precipitate, this is not the case in the α thalassaemias, in which excess γ chains or β chains are able to form the soluble homotetramers, $γ_4$ (Hb Bart's) and $β_4$ (Hb H)

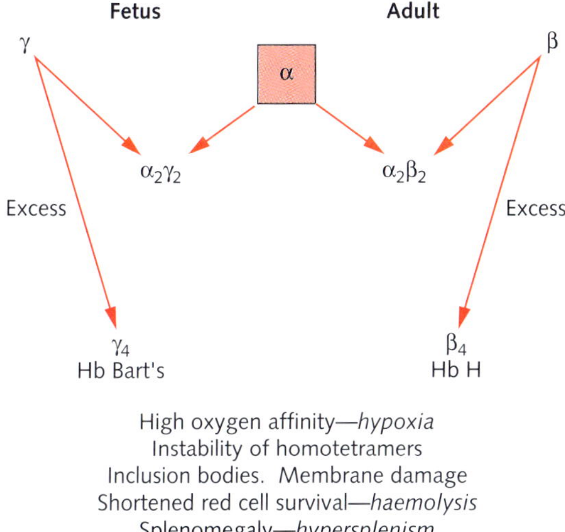

Fig. 1.9 The pathophysiology of α thalassaemia

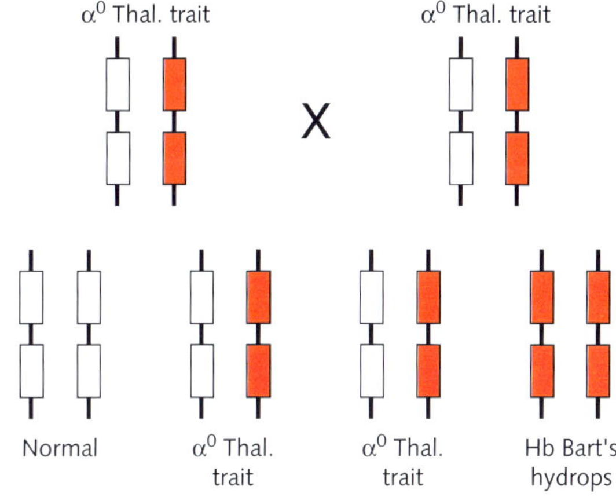

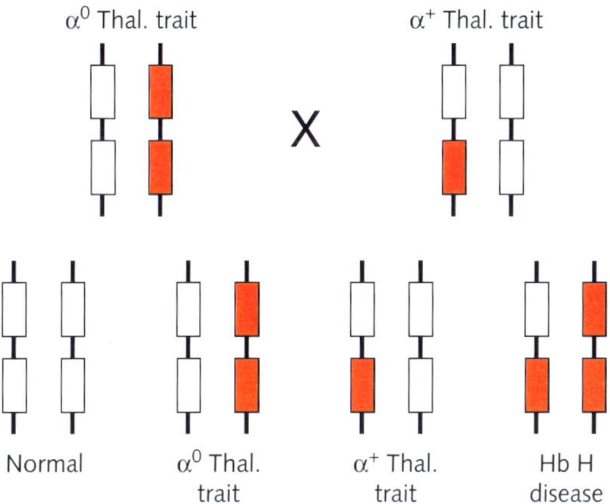

Fig. 1.10 The genetics of the common forms of α thalassaemia The light boxes represent normal α genes and the shaded boxes deleted α genes. The mating shown at the top shows how two $α^0$ thalassaemia heterozygotes can produce a baby with the haemoglobin Bart's hydrops syndrome. The mating at the bottom is between an $α^0$ and an $α^+$ thalassaemia trait; one in four of their offspring will have haemoglobin H disease.

(Figure 1.9). Although these variants, particularly Hb H, are unstable and precipitate in older red cell populations, they remain soluble sufficiently long for the red cells to mature and develop relatively normally. Hence there is far less ineffective erythropoiesis in the α thalassaemias and the main cause of the anaemia is haemolysis associated with the precipitation of Hb H in older red cells. In addition, of course, there is a reduction in normal haemoglobin synthesis which results in hypochromic, microcytic erythrocytes. Another important factor in the pathophysiology of the α thalassaemias is the fact that Hbs Bart's and H are useless oxygen carriers, having an oxygen dissociation curve similar to that of myoglobin. Hence the circulating haemoglobin level may give a false impression of the oxygen-delivering capacity of the blood and patients may be symptomatic at relatively high haemoglobin levels.

The different clinical phenotypes of the α thalassaemias are an elegant example of the effects of gene dosage (Figure 1.10). The heterozygous state for $α^+$ thalassaemia is associated with minimal haematological changes. That for $α^0$ thalassaemia, that is the loss of two α globin genes, is characterised by moderate hypochromia and microcytosis, similar to that of the β thalassaemia trait. It does not matter whether the α genes are lost on the same chromosome or on opposite pairs of homologous chromosomes. Hence the homozygous state for $α^+$ thalassaemia, −α/−α, has a similar phenotype to the heterozygous state for $α^0$ thalassaemia (− −/αα).

The loss of three α globin genes, which usually results from the compound heterozygous states for $α^0$ and $α^+$ thalassaemia, is associated with a moderately severe anaemia with the production of varying levels of haemoglobin H. This condition, haemoglobin H disease, is characterised by varying anaemia and splenomegaly with a marked shortening of the red cell survival.

Finally, the homozygous state for $α^0$ thalassaemia (− −/− −) is characterised by death *in utero* or just after birth, with the clinical picture of hydrops fetalis. These babies produce no α chains and their haemoglobin consists mainly of Bart's with a variable persistence of embryonic haemoglobin. This is reflected by gross intrauterine hypoxia; although these babies may have haemoglobin values as high as 8–9 g/dl, most of it is unable to release its oxygen. This is reflected by the hydropic changes, a massive outpouring of nucleated red cells, and hepatosplenomegaly with persistent haematopoiesis in the liver and spleen.

Structural haemoglobin variants

While the majority of the structural haemoglobin variants produce no clinical disability, a few, notably the sickling, and the rare variants are associated with instability or abnormal oxygen transport (*discussed in detail in Chapter 10*).

The sickling disorders

The sickling disorders are comprised of the homozygous state for the sickle cell gene, sickle cell anaemia, and the compound heterozygous state for the sickle cell gene and various structural haemoglobin variants, or β thalassaemia. The chronic haemolysis and episodes of vascular occlusion and red cell sequestration that characterise sickle cell anaemia can all be related to the replacement of the normal $\beta 6$ glutamic acid by valine in haemoglobin S. This causes a hydrophobic interaction with another haemoglobin molecule, triggering an aggregation into large polymers. It is this change that causes the sickling distortion of the red blood cell and hence a marked decrease in its deformability. The resulting rigidity of the red cells is responsible for the vaso-occlusive changes that lead to many of the most serious aspects of all the sickling disorders.

The different conformations of sickle cells, that is banana shaped or resembling a holly leaf, reflect different orientations of bundles of fibres along the long axis of the cell, the three-dimensional structure of which is constituted by a rope-like polymer composed of 14 strands. The rate and extent of polymer formation depends on the degree of oxygenation, the cellular haemoglobin concentration, and the presence or absence of haemoglobin F. The latter inhibits polymerisation and hence tends to ameliorate sickling. Polymerisation of haemoglobin S causes damage to the red cell membrane, the result of which is an irreversibly sickled cell. Probably the most important mechanism is cellular dehydration consequent on abnormalities of potassium/chloride co-transport and Ca^{2+}-activated potassium efflux. This is sufficient to trigger the Ca^{2+}-dependent (Gardos) potassium channel, providing a mechanism for the loss of potassium and water leading to cellular dehydration.

The vascular pathology of the sickling disorders is not entirely related to the rigidity of sickled red cells, however. There is now a wealth of evidence that abnormal interactions between sickled cells and the vascular endothelium play a major role in the pathophysiology of the sickling disorders.

Unstable haemoglobin variants

There are a variety of different mechanisms underlying haemoglobin stability resulting from amino acid substitutions in different parts of the molecule. The first is typified by amino acid substitutions in the vicinity of the haem pocket, all of which lead to a decrease in the stability of the binding of haem to globin. A second group of unstable variants results from amino acids that simply disrupt the secondary structure of the globin chains. About 75% of globin is in the form of α helix, in which proline cannot participate except as part of one of the initial three residues. At least 11 unstable haemoglobin variants have been described that result from the substitution of proline for leucine, five that are caused by an alanine to proline change, and three in which proline is substituted for histidine. Another group of variants that causes disruption of the normal configuration of the haemoglobin molecule involves internal substitutions that somehow interfere with its stabilisation by hydrophobic interactions. Finally, there are two groups of unstable haemoglobins that result from gross structural abnormalities of the globin subunits; many are due to deletions involving regions at or near interhelical corners. A few of the elongated globin chain variants are also unstable.

Abnormal oxygen transport

There is a family of haemoglobin variants that is associated with a high oxygen affinity and hereditary polycythaemia. Most result from amino acid substitutions that affect the equilibrium between the R and T states (*see earlier section—Structure and function*). Thus many of them result from amino acid substitutions at the α_1/β_2 interface, the C terminal end of the β chain, and at the 2,3-DPG binding sites.

Congenital cyanosis due to haemoglobin variants

There is a family of structural haemoglobin variants that is designated haemoglobin M, to indicate congenital methaemoglobinaemia, and further defined by their place of discovery. The iron atom of haem is normally linked to the imidazole group of the proximal histidine residue of the α and β chains. There is another histidine residue on the opposite side, near the sixth co-ordination position of the haem iron; this, the so-called distal histidine residue, is the normal site of binding of oxygen.

Several M haemoglobins result from the substitution of a tyrosine for either the proximal or distal histidine residues in the α or β chains.

Postscript

In this short account of the molecular pathology of haemoglobin we have considered how mutations at or close to the α or β globin genes result in a diverse family of clinical disorders due to the defective synthesis of haemoglobin or its abnormal structure. Work in this field over the last 20 years has given us a fairly good idea of the repertoire of different mutations that underlie single gene disorders and how these are expressed as discrete clinical phenotypes. Perhaps more importantly, however, the globin field has taught us how the interaction of a limited number of genes can produce a remarkably diverse series of clinical pictures, and something of the basis for how monogenic diseases due to the same mutation may vary widely in their clinical expression.

Further reading

Bunn HF, Forget BG. (1986) *Hemoglobin: Molecular, Genetic and Clinical Aspects*. Philadelphia: W.B. Saunders.

Fritsch EF, Wozney JM. (1987) Methods of molecular genetics. In: Stamatoyannopoulos G, Nienhuis AW, Majerus PW, Varmus H, eds. *The Molecular Basis of Blood Diseases*, 2nd edn. Philadelphia: W.B. Saunders, pp. 3–32.

Grosveld F, Dillon N, Higgs D. (1993) The regulation of human globin gene expression. *Clinical Haematology*, **6**, 31–55.

Higgs DR. (1993) α-Thalassaemia. *Clinical Haematology*, **6**, 117–150.

Huisman THJ. (1993) The structure and function of normal and abnormal haemoglobins. *Clinical Haematology*, **6**, 1–30.

Huisman THJ, Carver MFH, Erol Baysal E. (1997) *A Syllabus of Thalassemia Mutations*. Augusta, GA: The Sickle Cell Anemia Foundation.

Jankowski JAZ, Polak JM. (1996) *Clinical Gene Analysis and Manipulation*. Cambridge: Cambridge University Press.

Stamatoyannopoulos G, Nienhuis AW. (1999) Hemoglobin switching. In: Stamatoyannopoulos G, Nienhuis AW, Majerus PW, Varmus H, eds. *The Molecular Basis of Blood Diseases*, 3rd edn. Philadelphia: W.B. Saunders, *in press*.

Strachan T. (1992) *The Human Genome*. Oxford: BIOS Scientific Publishers Ltd.

Thein SL. (1993) β-thalassaemia. *Clinical Haematology*, **6**, 151–176.

Weatherall DJ. (1999) Thalassemia. In: Stamatoyannopoulos G, Nienhuis AW, Majerus PW, Varmus H, eds. *The Molecular Basis of Blood Diseases*, 3rd edn. Philadelphia: W.B. Saunders, *in press*.

Weatherall DJ, Clegg JB, Higgs DR, Wood WG. (1999) The hemoglobinopathies. In: Scriver CR, Beaudet AL, Sly WS, Valle D, eds. *The Metabolic Basis of Inherited Disease*, 8th edn. New York: McGraw-Hill, *in press*.

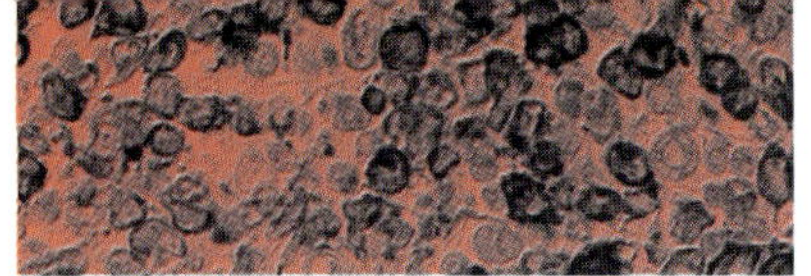

Chapter 2 Molecular cytogenetics

Debra M Lillington & Bryan D Young

Introduction

Conventional cytogenetics has played a major role in uncovering many of the genetic changes associated with haematological malignancies. Indeed, the study of these diseases has been important to our understanding of malignancy as a whole. Although leukaemias and lymphomas constitute a small part of all human malignancy, the number of genes identified through chromosomal translocations in these diseases greatly exceeds those identified in other cancers, and the advent of molecular and biological techniques with the introduction of fluorescently labelled DNA molecules is transforming this field. While conventional cytogenetics will continue to play a major role in the front line investigation of leukaemias, increasingly fluorescence techniques are yielding great benefits. DNA probes can be labelled with a variety of fluorochromes and the fate of any individual fragment of DNA can be assessed by *in situ* hybridisation to both metaphase and interphase cells.

These new techniques will be particularly applicable to the investigation of complex karyotypes. While conventional G-banded analysis can readily determine the presence of the well-known chromosomal translocations, it can be difficult to fully characterise the abnormalities on G-banding alone when complex rearrangements have occurred. As more DNA probes are generated through the human genome project, molecular cytogenetics will have greater application to the analysis of leukaemia and lymphomas. It is well established that certain cytogenetic subgroups have a major impact on prognosis and therefore such molecular approaches will continue to have a role to play in the clinical management of patients.

Numerical abnormality detection

Gains and losses of whole chromosomes are frequent events in the leukaemic karyotype. Normally these can be readily assessed by conventional cytogenetic analysis. However, where there is a low mitotic index, it will be more appropriate to apply fluorescence *in situ* hybridisation techniques. The simplest way to assess the number of any individual chromosome present in a cell is to use a probe corresponding to the alphoid repeat sequences (also termed α-satellite DNA) present at the centromere of each human chromosome. Such probes have the advantage that they give strong signals with little background and normally little cross reaction with other chromosomes. Thus it is possible to use such a probe to assess the number of chromosomes present in an interphase leukaemic cell. Plate 2.1 (facing page 128) illustrates the detection of an extra copy of the X chromosome in a patient with acute lymphoblastic leukaemia with a hyperdiploid karyotype. Where part of a chromosome has been deleted this will not be detected by this approach and an alternative strategy will be required. This approach will also not detect the occurrence of chromosome translocations. Combinations of probes can be used to assess a series of chromosomes simultaneously. Such probes are commercially available for most human chromosome centromeres. Although this approach is suitable for detecting the presence of abnormal cells when they are present in large numbers, it is less appropriate for the detection of residual leukaemic cells against a normal cell background; this is because there is a proportion of false positive results due to spurious signals over a nucleus. By using multiple probes simultaneously it has been possible to achieve a much greater level of sensitivity. For example, in one study three simultaneously labelled probes were used and it was possible to detect a leukaemic clone down to dilutions of 10^{-4}. Thus by combining probes it is possible to apply this approach to the detection of minimal residual disease (*see Chapter 4*).

Detection of translocations by fluorescence *in situ* hybridisation (FISH)

The molecular cloning of many of the chromosomal translocation breakpoints occurring in haematological malignancy has not only led to the identification of the genes involved, but has provided new reagents with considerable diagnostic potential. A variety of molecular biological techniques can be deployed to exploit the unique clonal nature of these events in the diagnosis and monitoring of the presence of the malignant cell. The polymerase chain reaction (PCR) can yield highly efficient detection of the gene fusions when the breakpoints are within certain defined regions. This can be performed on DNA when the breaks are clustered at the genomic DNA level. For example, the t(14;18) typical of follicular lymphoma can be readily detected by this means. More commonly it is necessary to use mRNA, after conversion to cDNA, as a template in order to overcome the problem of breakpoints occurring within large introns (this is termed reverse transcriptase PCR, *RT-PCR*). Such PCR-based approaches to translocation detection have the advantage that a very high level of sensitivity can be achieved. However, there is a concomitant risk of contamination when high levels of sensitivity are sought, and this is especially difficult to eliminate when RT-PCR is used since sequence analysis cannot distinguish the contaminant molecule from the one under investigation.

A variety of strategies can be used to detect translocations by FISH. The simplest approach is to use a probe which spans the expected breakpoint. This may be a *yeast artificial chromosome* (YAC), a *bacterial artificial chromosome* (BAC) or *cosmid* probe, depending on the gene target. The presence of a translocation will be indicated by the splitting of the hybridisation signal on the affected chromosome. Part of the signal will be retained on the centromeric side of the breakpoint and part of the signal will be transferred on the telomeric side of the breakpoint. A third hybridisation signal will be visible on the unaffected chromosome. This approach is particularly useful where multiple different chromosome partners can be involved, as with the *MLL* gene for which over 20 possible translocations have been described. Thus a suspected 11q23 abnormality can be investigated using a *MLL* gene probe and information about the translocation obtained without any knowledge of the partner chromosome. An example is illustrated in Plate 2.2 in which a t(11;22) translocation is shown to involve the region containing the MLL gene.

When the two partners in a translocation are well characterised, it is possible to use combinations of fluorochromes to detect the gene fusion. In this approach the probe for one gene is detected with one fluorochrome (red) and the probe for the other is simultaneously detected with a second fluorochrome (green). When a translocation is present the red and green signals are fused to give a single yellow signal. Typically the red and green signals are also present on the two unaffected chromosomes. The probes are usually selected to lie outside the translocation breakpoint so the results are not confused by split signals. The detection of the t(9;22) translocation by this approach is illustrated in Plate 2.3a in which the co-localisation of the signals can be seen in both a metaphase cell and in an interphase cell. The detection of the t(15;17) translocation only in interphase cells is illustrated in Plate 2.3b. Co-localisation in interphase nuclei is particularly appropriate for analysis of translocations in samples with a low mitotic index. A particular example of an event which is suitable for this analysis is the t(11;14) translocation which is found in about 70% of mantle cell lymphoma. Detection of this event by conventional cytogenetic analysis is often difficult due to the lack of metaphase cells. Molecular techniques are also hindered by the fact that breakpoints can be scattered over 1 Mb. By using a probe telomeric to the 11q13 breakpoint region and a probe centromeric to the immunoglobulin heavy chain (IgH) breakpoints at 14q32, a high proportion of t(11;14) translocations may be detected by co-localisation of signals in interphase cells (*see* Monteil *et al.*, 1996).

The co-localisation of signals in interphase nuclei can result in a level of false positive results due to the superposition of signals by chance. A refinement of this approach involves the use of a third differently labelled probe which will reduce the level of false positives. This method has been applied to the t(9;22) translocation and separate identification of the Philadelphia (Ph) chromosome and the derivative 9 chromosome has been shown to result in a low level of false positives allowing the detection of residual disease. Alternatively, commercial probes exist in which one of the probes spans the breakpoint region; hence if a translocation truly exists a fusion and an extra signal will be generated.

The direct visualisation of chromosomal breakpoints has been made possible by *in situ* hybridisation to DNA fibres. DNA molecules or fibres can be released from frozen tissue or intact cells and hybridised with a combination of probes to a breakpoint region. By labelling

Table 2.1 Translocations associated with specific haematological malignancies.

Translocation	Disease	Reference
t(11;14)	Mantle cell lymphoma	Monteil *et al.*, 1996 Vaandrager *et al.*, 1996 Cuneo *et al.*, 1997
t(8;14)	Burkitt's lymphoma	Siebert *et al.*, 1998
t(14;18)	Follicular lymphoma	Takashima *et al.*, 1997
t(3;14)	B-NHL	Ueda *et al.*, 1997
t(2;5)	ALCL	Johnson *et al.*, 1997 Mathew *et al.*, 1997
t(15;17)	APML	Mancini *et al.*, 1995 Fischer *et al.*, 1996
t(8;21)	AML	Hagemeijer *et al.*, 1998 Paskulin *et al.*, 1998
inv(16)	AML	Dierlamm *et al.*, 1998
t(8;16)	AML	Giles *et al.*, 1997
t(11;n)	AML, ALL	Kearney *et al.*, 1992
t(9;22)	CML, ALL	Sinclair *et al.*, 1997

each probe with alternate fluorescent colours, a potential barcode pattern is generated along the chromatin fibre. This approach has been applied to the detection of the t(11;14) chromosome translocation in mantle cell lymphoma. DNA probes covering several hundred kilobase pairs are hybridised to the DNA fibres and chromosome translocations are detected by splitting of the barcode pattern along the fibre. By examining the pattern of breaks it is possible to determine the position of a breakpoint within this region. Thus, the application of *in situ* hybridisation to DNA fibres is a powerful method for the detection of breakpoints which may be scattered over a large region.

FISH can be particularly valuable for revealing the presence of cryptic translocations. In rare instances a leukaemia, which by morphology belongs to a certain subgroup, may lack the hallmark translocation. FISH has been used to reveal the presence of cryptic t(15;17) fusions in a series of acute promyelocytic leukaemias which, by conventional analysis, lacked this translocation (*discussed in* Grimwade *et al.*, 1997).

The applications of FISH to detect the more common translocations in haematological malignancies are listed in Table 2.1.

Chromosome painting

Conventional cytogenetics can often indicate that an abnormality may exist on a chromosome without being able to pinpoint accurately the nature of the aberration. Candidate probes can be used in *in situ* hybridisation experiments on such marker chromosomes in an attempt to define the aberration. However, where the precise details of the aberration are unknown, it is more efficient to use a chromosome probe mixture which hybridises to the complete length of the chromosome. This technique is known as *chromosome painting*.

The availability of physically separated human chromosomes, either in the form of somatic cell hybrids or as flow sorted chromosome populations, has provided DNA pools from which such chromosome paints can be created. In order to provide sufficient quantities of probe, it has been necessary to develop universal PCR amplification methods. It is important that such methods are as representative as possible so that the full length of a chromosome will be evenly highlighted. Two alternative approaches have been adopted. Firstly, oligonucleotide primers based on repeat sequences, such as the Alu-repeat family, have been used to amplify the intervening sequences. This method is particularly appropriate for the amplification of sequences from somatic cell hybrids since the human sequences will be selectively amplified. Secondly, an alternative approach is the use of oligonucleotide primers incorporating a short degenerate sequence (degenerate oligonucleotide PCR or *DOP-PCR*) to amplify sequences non-specifically. This method has been particularly useful where the chromosomes have been physically separated by flow sorting.

Both approaches yield fragments of amplified DNA forming a pool of sequences which is representative of the full length of the chromosome. When labelled and used in *in situ* hybridisation experiments, the signals obtained highlight the length of the chromosome and should not cross react with other chromosomes. Variations in signals along the lines of the chromosome can be introduced when Alu-PCR is used, due to the variation in the frequency of Alu-repeats along the length of human chromosomes.

Chromosome painting is used when a marker chromosome of uncertain origin is observed in a tumour cell. Translocations will be observed as the splitting of the signal and joining on to other chromosomes. Two-colour chromosome painting can be particularly informative where translocations are observed as the fusion between the two fluorochromes. Plate 2.4 illustrates how the analysis of a t(2;15) translocation can be performed against the background of a complex karyotype.

24-colour analysis of the karyotype (M-FISH or SKY)

Conventional chromosome analysis has relied on the skill and training of the cytogeneticist to interpret the G-banded karyotype. This approach has been extremely productive in the study of leukaemias and lymphomas and has led to the identification of key translocation events important in the pathogenesis of these malignancies. However, it is also known that some events are undetected by conventional analysis. For example, the t(12;21) translocation, one of the commonest events in childhood B-cell acute lymphoblastic leukaemia (ALL), was not discovered until 1994. The introduction of whole chromosome painting has helped in the description of subtle chromosome changes. However, the application of a chromosome paint requires some prior knowledge of the affected chromosome.

Recent technical advances have allowed the principle of chromosome painting to be extended to the point where all chromosomes can be simultaneously identified. A key advance has been the use of combinatorial labelling in which each chromosome probe DNA is labelled with a unique combination of a small number of fluorochromes. After combinatorial labelling, from not more than five fluorochromes it is possible to combine the 24 differently labelled chromosome paints into a single hybridisation step. In order to distinguish the resultant signals on the hybridised metaphase cell, two different strategies have been developed. In one approach (known as M-FISH) a series of optical filters is used to collect images from each of the five fluorochrome signals separately, after which these separate images are combined and merged into a composite image in which each chromosome is assigned a distinctive pseudo-colour based on its fluorochrome combination. In a different approach (known as *spectral karyotyping* or SKY) an interferometer is used to determine, after Fourier transformation, the spectral characteristics of each pixel of the image. With both methods the contribution of each chromosome paint to the image can be determined and thus a pseudo-colour assigned to each appropriate point on the image. In this way the contribution of each human chromosome i.e. the 22 autosomes and the X and the Y sex chromosomes, can be displayed using 24 different pseudo-colours. Chromosomal identification can be further aided by the simultaneous acquisition of a DAPI (4′,6-diamidino-2-phenylindole) banded image. The ability to identify every human chromosome in a single step will have wide clinical utility and should complement standard cytogenetics, particularly for the characterisation of complex or subtle abnormalities.

Plate 2.5 illustrates the use of M-FISH to analyse the karyotype of a case of ALL. The t(8;22) translocation can be clearly visualised in addition to a complex three-way translocation involving chromosomes 1, 4 and 9. In a recent study using the spectral karyotyping technique, 15 cases of haematological malignancy with unidentified chromosome aberrations have been analysed. Additional cytogenetic information was derived including the identification of marker chromosomes and the detection of subtle chromosomal translocations, which had been unsuspected by conventional analysis. For example, a marker chromosome previously only identified as add(19) could be characterised as a translocation involving chromosome 19 and chromosomes 2 and 10.

This approach has recently been extended to the analysis of mouse chromosomes. With this approach it has been possible to identify previously hidden chromosome aberrations in t(12;15)-positive plasmacytomas.

Although this approach will undoubtedly have a major impact on the analysis of the karyotype of solid tumours where the alterations tend to be more frequent and more complex, it will still have an important role to play in haematological malignancies. For example, a proportion of leukaemias are reported as having apparently normal karyotypes. SKY or M-FISH could help to uncover previously unknown cryptic alterations. These approaches will also be important in the refining of known constitutional abnormalities of the type encountered in pre- and post-natal diagnostics.

Comparative genomic hybridisation

Comparative genomic hybridisation (CGH) was developed almost 6 years ago, and since then has gained acceptance as a molecular cytogenetic tool which can provide an extensive analysis of the entire genome in a single step. In essence, this method provides information on those regions gained or lost in the DNA of a tumour specimen. Tumour DNA is usually labelled with one fluorochrome (green) and hybridised to normal metaphase chromosomes after being mixed with a reference normal DNA which has been labelled with a different fluorochrome (red). The resultant ratio of the two signals observed on the length of the chromosomes reflects the differences in copy number between the tumour and reference DNA samples. Thus, amplified regions in the tumour DNA are indicated by an increased green/red ratio whereas deletions result in a reduced ratio.

In recent years technical enhancements to CGH have led to its application to a wide variety of tumours. These advances have included the labelling of DNA with nucleotides directly coupled to fluorochromes, the production of the target metaphase cells in a controlled and standardised manner and the introduction of commercial software packages specifically designed for CGH. Furthermore, the introduction of a universal amplification step has meant that CGH can be performed on small microdissected fragments of tissue or on single cells. Thus CGH is of great value when the amount of tissue is limited and where it is not possible to obtain metaphase cells directly from the tumour. However, certain limitations also apply—CGH will not easily detect changes which involve regions of less than ~5–10 Mb of DNA, unless they involve high-level amplifications. Contamination of the tumour sample with normal cells can also lead to degradation of the signal. In practice the sample should consist of at least 50% tumour cells. CGH has been applied to a variety of haematological malignancies. Although reciprocal chromosome translocations, which are frequent events in leukaemias and lymphomas, would remain undetected with this technique, CGH has been of considerable value in identifying the frequency and pattern of chromosomal gains and losses. The minimal size of deletion which can be detected by this method has been investigated using samples from B-cell leukaemias with previously determined 11q deletions. It was found that deletions down to 10–12 Mb could be readily visualised.

Plate 2.6 illustrates the use of CGH to analyse the changes taking place in a case of follicular lymphoma. Green arrows highlight the regions amplified in the tumour DNA and red arrows show the regions lost in the tumour.

Childhood ALL has been investigated by CGH. The pattern found in hyperdiploid ALL generally agreed with that established by conventional karyotyping, although examples of CGH revealing abnormalities in cases with previously normal karyotypes have been reported. A series of cases of refractory acute myeloid leukaemia (AML) has been investigated by CGH and losses at 5q and 7q were found in agreement with previous cytogenetic studies identifying these events as important in this class of leukaemia. However, losses were also found at 12p suggesting that events critical to the development of refractory AML may also take place in this region.

Clonal chromosomal changes have not been well documented in multiple myeloma and plasma cell leukaemias due to the low mitotic index of these cells and CGH may be very informative in helping to define the critical regions suitable for further study. In one study, losses on 13q and 14q and gains on 1q and chromosome 7 occurred in 50–60% of samples examined. In another the gain of chromosome 19 was particularly noted in addition to losses of chromosome 13. It was also found that, whereas chromosome abnormalities could be found in only 43% of cases by G-banded analysis, CGH detected abnormalities in up to 70% of the same cases. CGH can be of particular value in defining a minimal region of deletion if sufficient cases are analysed. Thus 13q and 6q deletions in multiple myeloma have been narrowed to 13q14–21 and 6q21, respectively.

Chronic lymphocytic leukaemia (CLL) has been investigated in a study combining CGH with conventional karyotyping and a high level of concordance was found between the two techniques. The most frequent aberration was found to be loss of 11q14–24 occurring in 25% of cases suggesting that events in this region could be important in the pathogenesis of CLL (*see* Karhu *et al.*, 1997).

The occurrence of reciprocal chromosomal translocations in malignant lymphoma has been well documented. However, the application of CGH is revealing the importance of chromosomal gains and losses in lymphomagenesis. A series of diffuse large B-cell lymphomas (DLBL) was studied by CGH and nine sites of chromosomal amplification were identified, six of these being confirmed by Southern analysis using candidate gene probes. Similarly, a series of mantle cell lymphomas (MCL) has been examined and a gain of 3q was the most common abnormality (50% of cases). A deletion at 11q22 was found in one-third of cases of MCL and it was also noted that the mean number of aberrations was higher in the more aggressive variants of MCL. In the study by Monni *et al.* (1998), the changes were different from those found in other types of non-Hodgkin's lymphoma.

Primary large B-cell lymphomas of the gastrointestinal tract have also been studied by CGH and the most frequent abnormalities were gains of all or part of chromosomes 11, 12, 1q and 3q. Losses of parts of 6q and parts of 17p were also noted. It was concluded that the pattern of gain and loss was distinct from that reported for low grade (mucosa-associated lymphoid tissue, MALT) lymphomas of the stomach and bowel. One case of a high-level amplification involved 2p13–15 and the involvement of the *REL* gene was demonstrated by Southern analysis. Amplifications of *REL* have been described previously in extranodal lymphomas. Follicular lymphoma, which is characterised by the t(14;18) translocation, has also been investigated by CGH. Genomic abnormalities were detected in 80% of cases examined and these included gains of chromosomes 18q, X, 7, 2, 6p and 8q, and losses involving 6q and 17p.

The value of CGH in pinpointing regions of the genome important in haematological malignancy is already clear. Although these data will provide a valuable starting point, other techniques will have to be invoked in order to identify the critical target genes. Future developments may include the application of the CGH principle to arrayed target sequences and the screening by automatic scanning methods. This would potentially avoid the requirement for normal metaphase cells with the variability which that introduces.

Conclusions

G-banded analysis has been pivotal in identifying recurrent abnormalities in malignant disease and has led to the identification of the genes involved in many diseases. The introduction of FISH techniques has been immensely successful in complementing and indeed providing more accurate characterisation of cytogenetic abnormalities. The major limiting factor with routine cytogenetics is the reliance on the ability to achieve dividing metaphase cells. FISH can be applied to all cells and, in CGH, a genome analysis of chromosomal imbalance can be performed directly on the DNA extracted from the tumour of interest. M-FISH is particularly applicable to the analysis of complex karyotypes, and future developments include combining the use of telomere probes with M-FISH which will enable both subtle and complex rearrangements to be detected.

Further reading

Detection of numerical abnormalities

Kasprzyk A, Secker-Walker LM. (1997) Increased sensitivity of minimal residual disease detection by interphase FISH in acute lymphoblastic leukemia with hyperdiploidy. *Leukemia*, **11**, 429–435.

Detection translocations using FISH

Cuneo A, Bigoni R, Negrini M *et al.* (1997) Cytogenetic and interphase cytogenetic characterization of atypical chronic lymphocytic leukemia carrying BCL1 translocation. *Cancer Research*, **57**, 1144–1150.

Dierlamm J, Stul M, Vranckx H *et al.* (1998) FISH identifies inv(16)(p13q22) masked by translocations in three cases of acute myeloid leukemia. *Genes, Chromosomes and Cancer*, **22**, 87–94.

Fischer K, Scholl C, Salat J *et al.* (1996) Design and validation of DNA probe sets for a comprehensive interphase cytogenetic analysis of acute myeloid leukemia. *Blood*, **88**, 3962–3971.

Giles RH, Dauwerse JG, Higgins C *et al.* (1997) Detection of CBP rearrangements in acute myelogenous leukemia with t(8;16). *Leukemia*, **11**, 2087–2096.

Grimwade D, Gorman P, Duprez E *et al.* (1997) Characterization of cryptic rearrangements and variant translocations in acute promyelocytic leukemia. *Blood*, **90**, 4876–4885.

Hagemeijer A, de Klein A, Wijsman J *et al.* (1998) Development of an interphase fluorescent *in situ* hybridization (FISH) test to detect t(8;21) in AML patients. *Leukemia*, **12**, 96–101.

Johnson PW, Leek J, Swinbank K *et al.* (1997) The use of fluorescent *in situ* hybridization for detection of the t(2;5)(p23;q35) translocation in anaplastic large-cell lymphoma. *Annals of Oncology*, **8 Suppl. 2**, 65–69.

Kearney L, Bower M, Gibbons B *et al.* (1992) Chromosome 11q23 translocations in both infant and adult acute leukemias are detected by *in situ* hybridisation with a yeast artificial chromosome. *Blood*, **80**, 1659–1665.

Mancini M, Nanni M, Cedrone M *et al.* (1995) Combined cytogenetic, FISH and molecular analysis in acute promyelocytic leukaemia at diagnosis and in complete remission. *British Journal of Haematology*, **91**, 878–884.

Mathew P, Sanger WG, Weisenburger DD *et al.* (1997) Detection of the t(2;5)(p23;q35) and NPM–ALK fusion in non-Hodgkin's lymphoma by two-color fluorescence *in situ* hybridization. *Blood*, **89**, 1678–1685.

Monteil M, Callanan M, Dascalescu C, Sotto JJ, Leroux D. (1996) Molecular diagnosis of t(11;14) in mantle cell lymphoma using two-colour interphase fluorescence *in situ* hybridization. *British Journal of Haematology*, **93**, 656–660.

Paskulin GA, Philips G, Morgan R *et al.* (1998) Pre-clinical evaluation of probes to detect t(8;21) AML minimal residual disease by fluorescence *in situ* hybridization. *Genes, Chromosomes and Cancer*, **21**, 144–151.

Siebert R, Matthiesen P, Harder S *et al.* (1998) Application of interphase fluorescence *in situ* hybridization for the detection of the Burkitt translocation t(8;14)(q24;q32) in B-cell lymphomas. *Blood*, **91**, 984–990.

Sinclair PB, Green AR, Grace C, Nacheva EP. (1997) Improved sensitivity of BCR-ABL detection: a triple-probe three-color fluorescence *in situ* hybridization system. *Blood*, **90**, 1395–1402.

Takashima T, Itoh M, Ueda Y *et al.* (1997) Detection of 14q32.33 translocation and t(11;14) in interphase nuclei of chronic B-cell leukemia/lymphomas by *in situ* hybridization. *International Journal of Cancer*, **72**, 31–38.

Ueda Y, Nishida K, Miki T *et al.* (1997) Interphase detection of BCL6/IgH fusion gene in non-Hodgkin lymphoma by fluorescence *in situ* hybridization. *Cancer Genetics and Cytogenetics*, **99**, 102–107.

Vaandrager JW, Schuuring E, Zwikstra E *et al.* (1996) Direct visualization of dispersed 11q13 chromosomal translocations in mantle cell lymphoma by multicolor DNA fiber fluorescence *in situ* hybridization. *Blood*, **88**, 1177–1182.

Chromosome painting

Suijkerbuijk RF, Matthopoulos D, Kearney L *et al.* (1992) Fluorescent *in situ* identification of human marker chromosomes using flow sorting and Alu element-mediated PCR. *Genomics*, **13**, 355–362.

Telenius H, Pelmear AH, Tunnacliffe A *et al.* (1992) Cytogenetic analysis by chromosome painting using DOP-PCR amplified flow-sorted chromosomes. *Genes, Chromosomes and Cancer*, **4**, 257–263.

Colour analysis of chromosomes

Coleman AE, Schrock E, Weaver Z *et al.* (1997) Previously hidden chromosome aberrations in t(12;15)-positive BALB/c plasmacytomas uncovered by multicolor spectral karyotyping. *Cancer Research*, **57**, 4585–4592.

Liyanage M, Coleman A, du Manoir S *et al.* (1996) Multicolour spectral karyotyping of mouse chromosomes. *Nature Genetics*, **14**, 312–315.

Schrock E, du Manoir S, Veldman T *et al.* (1996) Multicolor spectral karyotyping of human chromosomes. *Science*, **273**, 494–497.

Schrock E, Veldman T, Padilla-Nash H *et al.* (1997) Spectral karyotyping refines cytogenetic diagnostics of constitutional chromosomal abnormalities. *Human Genetics*, **101**, 255–262.

Speicher MR, Gwyn Ballard S, Ward DC. (1996) Karyotyping human chromosomes by combinatorial multi-fluor FISH. *Nature Genetics*, **12**, 368–375.

Veldman T, Vignon C, Schrock E, Rowley JD, Ried T. (1997) Hidden chromosome abnormalities in haematological malignancies detected by multicolour spectral karyotyping. *Nature Genetics*, **15**, 406–410.

Comparative genomic hybridisation

Avet-Loiseau H, Andree-Ashley LE, Moore D *et al.* (1997) Molecular cytogenetic abnormalities in multiple myeloma and plasma cell leukemia measured using comparative genomic hybridization. *Genes, Chromosomes and Cancer*, **19**, 124–133.

Avet-Loiseau H, Vigier M, Moreau A *et al.* (1997) Comparative genomic hybridization detects genomic abnormalities in 80% of follicular lymphomas. *British Journal of Haematology*, **97**, 119–122.

Barth TFE, Dohner H, Werner CA *et al.* (1998) Characteristic pattern of chromosomal gains and losses in primary large B-cell lymphomas of the gastrointestinal tract. *Blood*, **91**, 4321–4330.

Bentz M, Plesch A, Stilgenbauer S, Dohner H, Lichter P. (1998) Minimal sizes of deletions detected by comparative genomic hybridization. *Genes, Chromosomes and Cancer*, **21**, 172–175.

Cigudosa JC, Rao PH, Calasanz MJ *et al.* (1998) Characterization of nonrandom chromosomal gains and losses in multiple myeloma by comparative genomic hybridization. *Blood*, **91**, 3007–3010.

El-Rifai W, Elonen E, Larramendy M, Ruutu T, Knuutila S. (1997) Chromosomal breakpoints and changes in DNA copy number in refractory acute myeloid leukemia. *Leukemia*, **11**, 958–963.

Forozan F, Karhu R, Kononen J, Kallioniemi A, Kallioniemi OP. (1997) Genome screening by comparative genomic hybridization. *Trends in Genetics*, **13**, 405–409.

Haas O, Henn T, Romanakis K, du Manoir S, Lengauer C. (1998) Comparative genomic hybridization as part of a new diagnostic strategy in childhood hyperdiploid acute lymphoblastic leukemia. *Leukemia*, **12**, 474–481.

Houldsworth J, Mathew S, Rao PH *et al.* (1996) REL proto-oncogene is frequently amplified in extranodal diffuse large cell lymphoma. *Blood*, **87**, 25–29.

Joos S, Otano-Joos MI, Ziegler S *et al.* (1996) Primary mediastinal (thymic) B-cell lymphoma is characterized by gains of chromosomal material including 9p and amplification of the REL gene. *Blood*, **87**, 1571–1578.

Kallioniemi A, Kallioniemi OP, Sudar D *et al.* (1992) Comparative genomic hybridization for molecular cytogenetic analysis of solid tumors. *Science*, **258**, 818–821.

Karhu R, Knuutila S, Kallioniemi OP *et al.* (1997) Frequent loss of the 11q14-24 region in chronic lymphocytic leukemia: a study by comparative genomic hybridization. Tampere CLL Group. *Genes, Chromosomes and Cancer*, **19**, 286–290.

Karhu R, Siitonen S, Tanner M *et al.* (1997) Genetic aberrations in pediatric acute lymphoblastic leukemia by comparative genomic hybridization. *Cancer Genetics and Cytogenetics*, **95**, 123–129.

Monni O, Oinonen R, Elonen E *et al.* (1998) Gain of 3q and deletion of 11q22 are frequent aberrations in mantle cell lymphoma. *Genes, Chromosomes and Cancer*, **21**, 298–307.

Paszek-Vigier M, Talmant P, Mechinaud F *et al.* (1997) Comparative genomic hybridization is a powerful tool, complementary to cytogenetics, to identify chromosomal abnormalities in childhood acute lymphoblastic leukaemia. *British Journal of Haematology*, **99**, 589–596.

Rao PH, Houldsworth J, Dyomina K *et al.* (1998) Chromosomal and gene amplification in diffuse large B-cell lymphoma. *Blood*, **92**, 234–240.

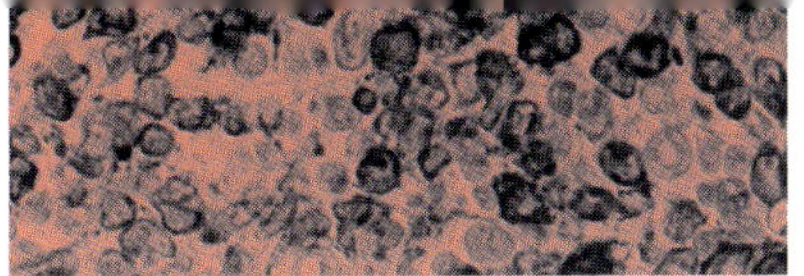

Chapter 3 Molecular basis of leukaemia and lymphoma

R Gitendra Wickremasinghe & A Victor Hoffbrand

Introduction

Haematopoiesis is regulated by a set of cytokines which modulate the survival, proliferation and differentiation of stem and progenitor cells (*Chapter 15*). Binding of these polypeptides to their cognate cell-surface receptors results in the activation of biochemical signal transduction pathways. These pathways culminate in the activation of specific transcription factors and the consequent expression of specific genes whose protein products trigger cell proliferation or promote differentiation towards mature blood cells. Differentiation within the haematopoietic lineage is linked to a concomitant loss of the ability to proliferate. While growth factors and cytokines sometimes promote cell survival via triggering expression of specific anti-apoptotic genes, the modulation of the biochemical activities of pre-existing survival-regulating proteins also plays an important role in this process.

Mutation, translocation or inversion of genes whose products regulate proliferation, differentiation or cell survival results in the generation of abnormal signalling molecules or in the enhanced expression of regulatory proteins. These abnormal genes are referred to as *oncogenes* and their normal counterparts as *proto-oncogenes*. Oncogenes contribute to malignant transformation through promotion of uncontrolled cell proliferation, blockade of normal differentiation or the prevention of apoptosis (programmed cell death).

In contrast to proto-oncogenes, tumour suppressor genes (or anti-oncogenes) encode proteins which negatively regulate proliferation. Functional inactivation of both copies of a tumour suppressor gene by deletion or mutation is usually required to promote malignant transformation. Thus, tumour suppressor genes are genetically recessive in transformation whereas oncogenes are dominant. Members of cancer-prone families may inherit a deletion of one locus of a tumour suppressor gene, thereby increasing the probability that deletion or mutation of the remaining locus will contribute to malignant transformation via generation of a cell which is unable to synthesise a protein important in the negative regulation of cell proliferation.

The mechanisms responsible for the uncontrolled expansion of leukaemia and lymphoma cells are closely related to the regulatory mechanisms of normal haematopoietic cells. These pathways are therefore outlined here.

Mechanisms which regulate cell proliferation in the haematopoietic system

Activation of receptor protein tyrosine kinase consequent to ligand binding

A subset of cytokine receptors are transmembrane proteins whose intracellular domains possess a protein tyrosine kinase (PTK) domain. The amino-terminal ligand-binding domains are presented on the extracellular face of the plasma membrane (Figure 3.1). A transmembrane α-helix bridges the ligand-binding domain to the PTK domain. The C-terminal tail of the receptor possesses several tyrosine residues which are potential substrates for the receptor's own PTK activity. However, steric constraints prevent intramolecular phosphorylation of these tyrosine residues. The receptors for

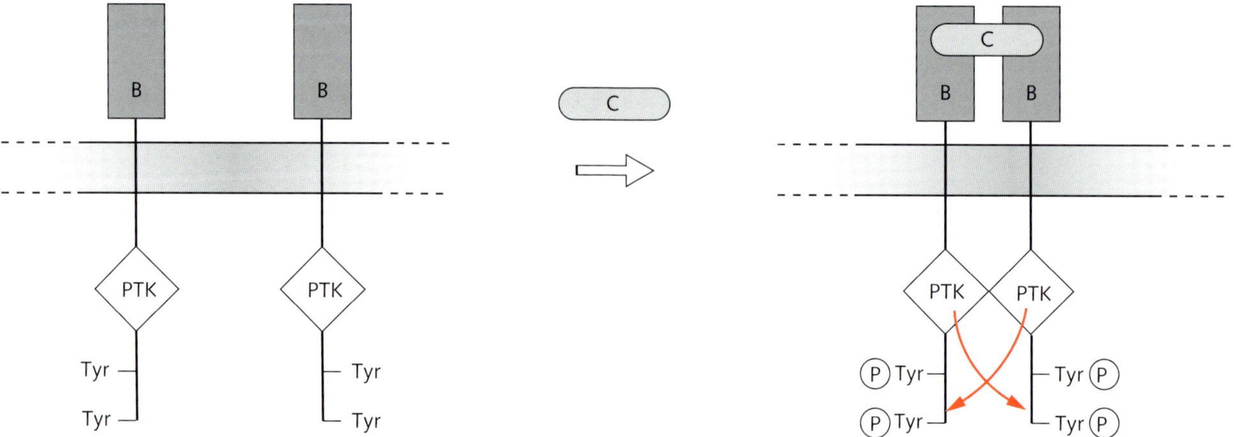

Fig. 3.1 Activation of cytokine receptors with intrinsic protein tyrosine kinase activity
C, cytokine; B, cytokine-binding domain; PTK, protein tyrosine kinase domain; Tyr, tyrosine residue.

macrophage colony-stimulating factor (M-CSF) and stem cell factor (SCF; kit ligand) contain an intrinsic PTK activity.

Binding of a growth factor molecule to the ligand-binding domains of two receptor molecules initiates receptor dimerisation. The resulting juxtaposition of intracellular domains promotes intermolecular phosphorylation of the tyrosine residues of one partner by the PTK activity of the other (Figure 3.1). These tyrosine phosphorylation events constitute the initial biochemical response following growth factor binding and are crucial to the induction of subsequent signal transduction pathways.

Signalling by SH2 domain-containing proteins

The SRC homology 2 (SH2) domain is a modular structure which is found in a large number of proteins involved in signal transduction. These domains share an ability to bind tightly to phosphorylated tyrosine residues and thereby mediate protein–protein interactions. A subset of proteins involved in signalling are enzymes containing intrinsic SH2 domains. Another subset of SH2 proteins lack any intrinsic catalytic activity but act as adaptor proteins by specifically binding signalling enzymes. Different SH2 domains have subtly different structures, allowing them to discriminate between target phosphotyrosine residues in a manner dependent on the surrounding amino acid sequence. Therefore, activated, tyrosine-phosphorylated growth factor receptors can bind several SH2-containing proteins and consequently activate multiple signalling pathways (Figure 3.2). Individual receptors bind different subsets of SH2-containing proteins however, and therefore activate different combinations of intracellular pathways.

Binding of signalling proteins to receptors results in their translocation to the inner face of the plasma membrane, thereby promoting their interactions with membrane-localised substrates. Furthermore, recruitment to receptors also promotes phosphorylation of at least some of these proteins by the receptor's PTK activity, thereby modulating their biochemical activity. Signalling mechanisms initiated by some SH2-containing proteins are described below.

Phospholipase C_γ

Phospholipase C_γ contains an intrinsic SH2 domain and is located in the cytoplasm of unstimulated cells. It is translocated to growth factor receptors following activation of the receptors by ligand binding (Figure 3.2). Translocation greatly enhances the access of the enzyme to its membrane-localised inositol lipid substrate. Consequent cleavage of the lipid results in the generation of two potent second messenger molecules, diacylglycerol and inositol trisphosphate. Diacylglycerol is an allosteric activator of the serine/threonine-specific enzyme, protein kinase C. Inositol trisphosphate binds to receptors located on the endoplasmic reticulum and consequently triggers the release of stored Ca^{2+} ions. The resulting increase in cytoplasmic Ca^{2+} concentration synergises with protein kinase C activation in modulating gene

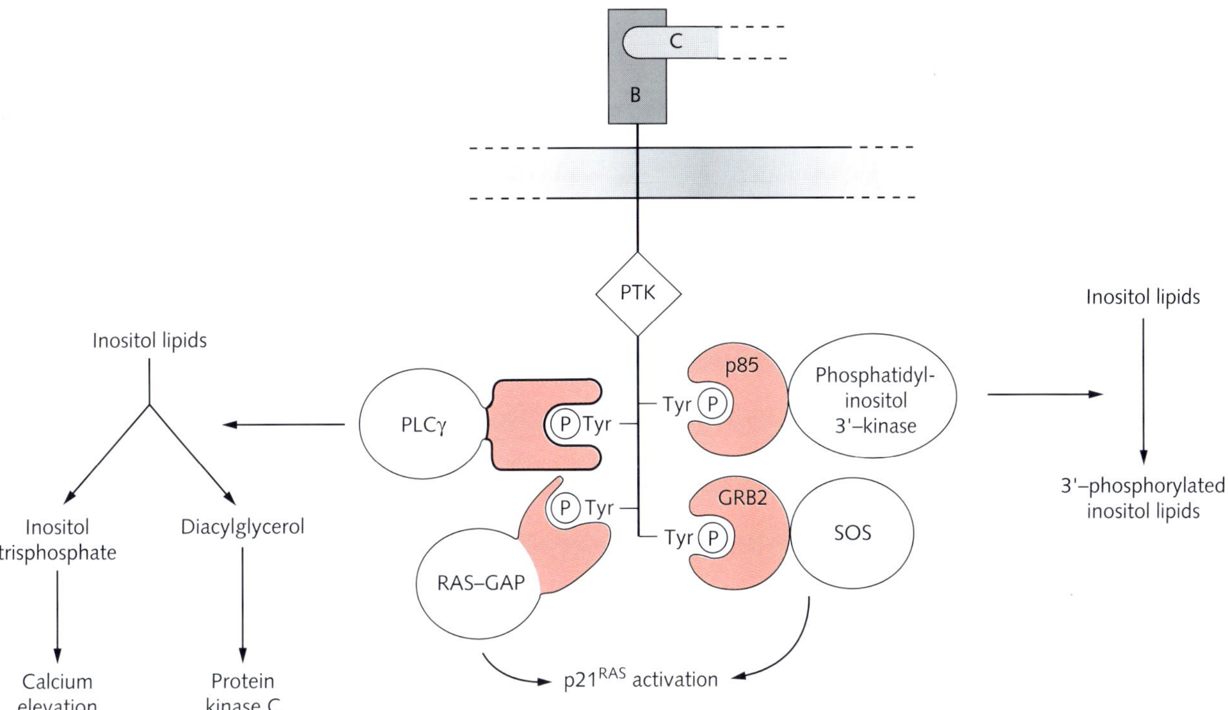

Fig. 3.2 Activation of multiple signal transduction pathways consequent to tyrosine phosphorylation of growth factor receptors

For clarity, only one member of the receptor dimer is shown. SH2 domains are shown in red. PLCγ, phospholipase Cγ; RAS-GAP, RAS GTPase-activating protein; SOS, son-of-sevenless guanine nucleotide-exchange factor. The mechanism of activation of $p21^{RAS}$ following receptor binding of RAS-GAP and the GRB2-SOS complex is shown in detail in Figure 3.3.

expression via the regulation of transcription factors (*see below*).

Phosphatidylinositol 3′-kinase

The catalytic subunit of phosphatidylinositol 3′-kinase is translocated to activated receptors via binding of an 85 kDa SH2-containing adaptor (Figure 3.2). Translocation allows phosphorylation of membrane-localised inositol lipids on the 3′ position of the inositol ring. The 3′ phosphorylated lipids bind to and activate protein kinase B, a serine/threonine-specific enzyme (also known as AKT). Events mediated by protein kinase B block the induction of apoptosis and therefore play important roles in the promotion of cell survival by growth factors and cytokines (*see below*, Figure 3.9).

Regulation of $p21^{RAS}$ proteins

The three *RAS* genes (H-*RAS*, K-*RAS* and N-*RAS*) encode 21 kDa proteins ($p21^{RAS}$) which play crucial roles in signal transduction. In unstimulated cells, $p21^{RAS}$ is bound to the guanine nucleotide GDP and is inactive in signal transduction. Activated receptors bind GRB2, an SH2-containing adaptor which binds in turn the SOS (son-of-sevenless) protein (Figure 3.2). SOS is a guanine nucleotide-exchange factor which interacts specifically with the $p21^{RAS}$ proteins and catalyses the replacement of bound GDP with GTP (Figure 3.3). The resulting change in the conformation of $p21^{RAS}$ results in the activation of a cascade of protein kinases (*see below*).

The $p21^{RAS}$ proteins possess a weak intrinsic GTPase activity which hydrolyses bound GTP and returns the protein to the inactive GDP-bound form (Figure 3.3). The GTPase activity is augmented following binding of RAS-GAP to $p21^{RAS}$. In unstimulated cells, RAS-GAP maintains $p21^{RAS}$ in the inactive conformation by constitutively stimulating its GTPase activity. Following receptor activation, the intrinsic SH2 domain of RAS-GAP mediates its binding to phosphotyrosine residues. This binding abrogates interaction with $p21^{RAS}$ and therefore serves to increase the proportion of the RAS protein in

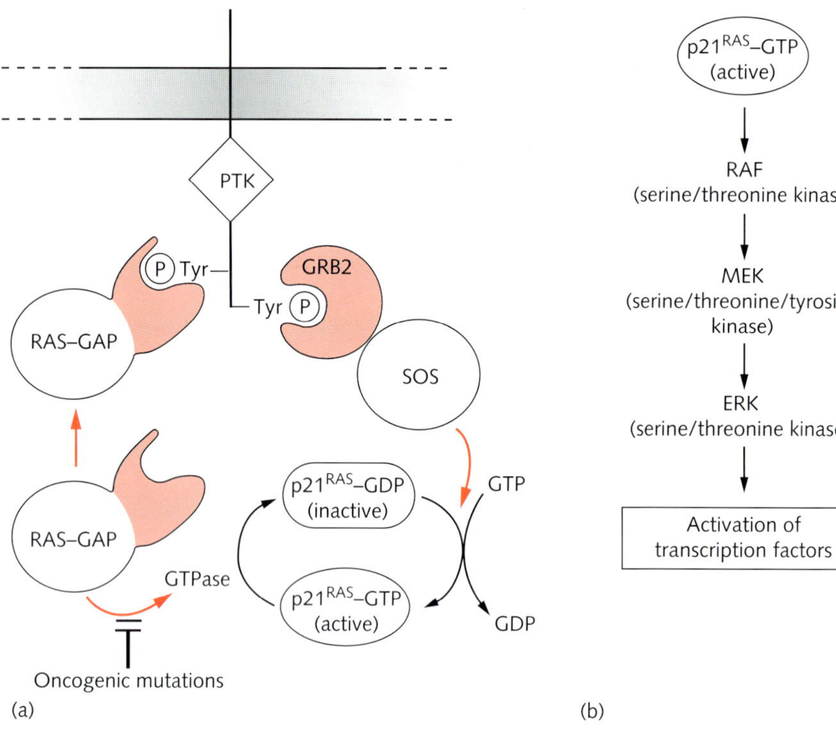

Fig. 3.3 Activation of the $p21^{RAS}$-initiated signalling cascade following tyrosine phosphorylation of growth factor receptors (a) The dynamic equilibrium between the inactive GDP-bound form and the active GTP-bound form of $p21^{RAS}$ is modulated by the binding of RAS-GAP and the GRB2-SOS complex to tyrosine-phosphorylated receptors. Note that GRB2-SOS is activated, whereas GAP activity is diminished following receptor binding. (b) GTP-bound $p21^{RAS}$ activates a protein kinase cascade which eventually modulates the activity or expression of nuclear transcription factors. MEK, MAP kinase/ERK kinase; ERK, extracellular signal regulated kinase.

the active GTP-bound form. Therefore, receptor binding of the GRB2-SOS complex and of RAS-GAP synergises in augmenting RAS-mediated signalling (Figure 3.3).

$p21^{RAS}$-activated protein kinase cascades

The active, GTP-bound form of $p21^{RAS}$ binds to and activates a serine/threonine-specific protein kinase, RAF (Figure 3.3). In turn, the RAF kinase phosphorylates and activates MEK (MAP kinase/ERK kinase). MEK exhibits an unusual specificity, since it can phosphorylate target proteins on serine, threonine or tyrosine residues. Tyrosine and serine phosphorylation of ERK (extracellular signal-regulated kinase) by MEK results in ERK activation, which triggers the expression of genes required for cell cycle transit. These gene activation events are mediated through the phosphorylation of specific transcription factors.

Transcription factor families involved in the regulation of cell proliferation and differentiation

Transcription factors are multi-domain proteins which regulate the expression of specific genes. The DNA-binding domain of a transcription factor binds to specific enhancer sequences located upstream of a structural gene (Figure 3.4). The transactivation domain of the factor binds RNA polymerase (in association with accessory factors) and augments its binding to a promoter DNA sequence (TATA) near the transcription start site of the gene. RNA polymerase now generates an RNA transcript of the gene. In this way, specific transcription factors trigger expression of specific genes via binding to specific enhancers.

The majority of transcription factors are dimers of identical or different protein subunits. Dimerisation generates a complete DNA-binding domain as a result of the juxtaposition of the subunits. Transcription factors important in gene regulation in the haematopoietic system are divided into families on the basis of the protein domains used in dimerisation and DNA binding. The key features of these families are summarised in Table 3.1.

Activation of transcription factors by the $p21^{RAS}$/protein kinase pathway

The *FOS* gene is an example of an 'immediate early' gene whose expression is triggered directly by the protein kinase cascade triggered consequent to $p21^{RAS}$ activation. The *FOS* gene product is itself a transcription factor of the leucine zipper family. Expression of *FOS* is regulated by a transcription factor complex consisting of the serum response factor (SRF) and the ELK-1 protein

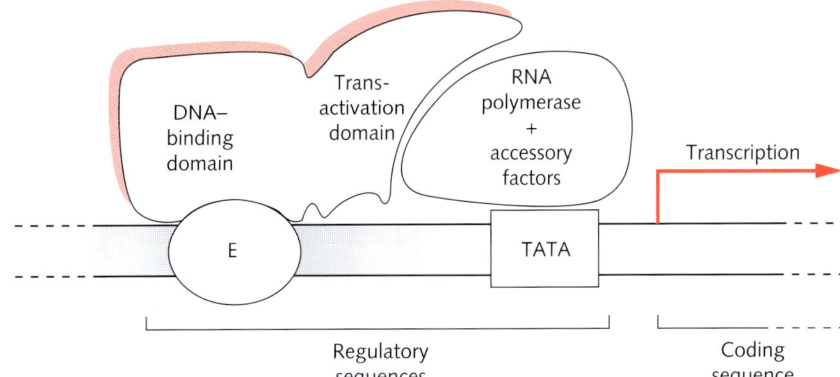

Fig. 3.4 Model of regulation of specific gene expression by a transcription factor
E, enhancer; TATA, promoter sequence.

Table 3.1 Transcription factor families involved in haematopoiesis and leukaemogenesis.

Family name	Characteristics	Examples
Leucine zipper	Regularly repeated leucine residues mediate dimerisation	FOS, JUN
Helix–loop–helix (HLH)	Helix–loop–helix dimerisation motif	MYC, MAX, E2A, TAL-1 (SCL), TEL, (ETV6)
Homeobox	Dimerisation domain homologous to *Drosophila* homeobox transcription factors	PBX-1, HOX 11
Zinc finger	DNA-binding 'fingers' generated by chelation of Zn^{2+} by four cysteine residues	PML, retinoic acid receptor α, ETO, MLL1 (ALL1)
LIM	Metal-binding domains similar to zinc fingers	Rhombotin 1 and 2
REL	Homology to retroviral v-REL. Activated consequent to dissociation from inhibitory subunits	NFκB, BCL-3
STAT	Dimerisation mediated by binding of SH2 domains to phosphotyrosine residues	STATs 1 to 6

(Figure 3.5). The complex is constitutively bound to a *FOS* upstream enhancer, the SRF. Phosphorylation of ELK-1 by activated ERK augments the transactivation capacity of the complex and therefore triggers FOS expression, resulting in an increase in the cellular level of FOS protein.

The leucine zipper dimerisation motif of the FOS protein consists of a regular repeat of leucine residues. This motif mediates dimerisation with pre-existing JUN molecules, which also contain leucine zippers (Figure 3.6). The resulting JUN/FOS dimer is a transcription factor of the AP-1 family which triggers the expression of genes required for cell cycle transit following binding to specific AP-1-responsive enhancer sites. In this way, biochemical signals initiated by binding of growth factors to cell-surface receptors are transduced into programmes of regulated gene expression.

Other 'immediate early' genes induced by growth factor signalling include the *MYC* gene, whose protein product forms a transcriptionally active dimer with the MAX protein (Table 3.1). The mechanism of *MYC* induction is unclear, but this factor plays an important role in triggering cell proliferation. However, MYC also induces apoptosis. Therefore, a net increase in cell number following growth factor stimulation requires that a separate signal which blocks the apoptotic programme (*see below*, Figure 3.9) is delivered at the same time as is the signal which upregulates *MYC* expression.

Signalling by cytokine receptors lacking an intrinsic protein tyrosine kinase domain

The receptors for the majority of cytokines are transmembrane proteins which lack an intrinsic PTK domain.

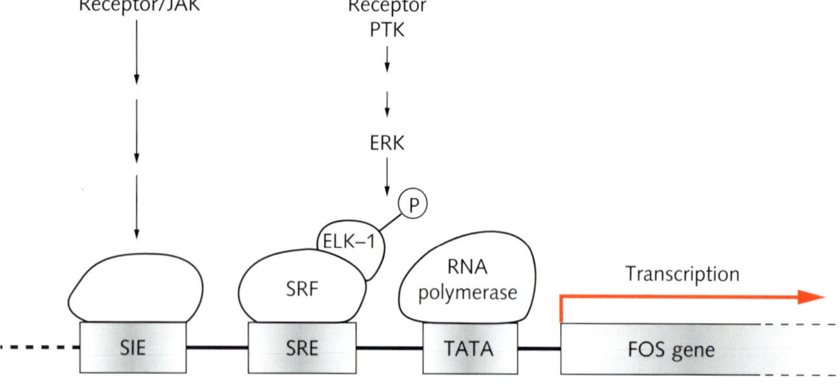

Fig. 3.5 Activation of *FOS* gene transcription by protein kinase cascades SRF, serum response factor; SRE, serum response element; SIE, sis-inducible element.

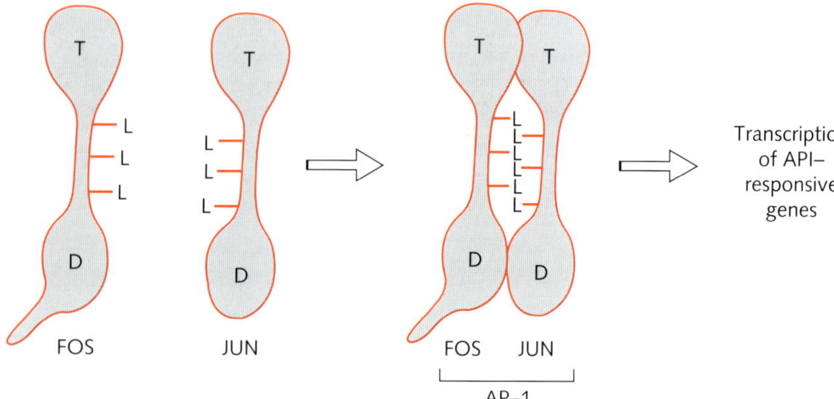

Fig. 3.6 Generation of AP-1 family transcription factors L, leucine residues; D, DNA-binding domain; T, transactivation domain.

Nevertheless, these receptors activate transcription factors via interaction with cytoplasmic PTKs belonging to the Janus kinase (JAK) family. For example, the α and γ subunits of the interleukin (IL)-4 receptor bind JAKs 1 and 3, respectively (Figure 3.7). Dimerisation of the receptor subunits following IL-4 binding results in the intermolecular tyrosine phosphorylation and consequent activation of the JAKs. In turn, the JAKs phosphorylate members of the STAT (signal transducer and activator of transcription) family of transcription factors (Table 3.1). The STATs contain SH2 domains, which mediate dimer formation between phosphorylated STAT monomers (Figure 3.7). The dimers now bind specific STAT-responsive enhancers and trigger transcription of specific genes.

In addition to STAT activation, cytokine receptors without an intrinsic PTK domain also trigger some biochemical pathways activated by PTK-containing growth factor receptors. For example, the IL-4 receptor-associated JAK1 phosphorylates the insulin receptor substrate (IRS) molecule, thereby generating phosphotyrosine sites which recruit and activate phosphatidylinositol 3′-kinase. Some cytokines, for example IL-6, trigger cell proliferation by upregulated expression of *FOS*. Cytokine induction of FOS is mediated by a sis-inducible element (SIE) located upstream of the SRF (Figure 3.5).

The role of cyclins in the regulation of cell cycle checkpoints

The cyclin protein family plays an important role in mediating the transition of cells through checkpoints located at the boundaries of adjacent cell cycle phases. Cyclins A, B, D and E are synthesised and degraded in a periodic manner, such that peak concentrations of individual species are greatest at or near cell cycle checkpoints (Figure 3.8). Cyclins themselves possess no enzymatic activity. However, binding of these proteins to pre-existing cyclin-dependent protein kinases (CDKs) strongly activates the CDKs to phosphorylate critical protein substrates and consequently permit transit of the cell through a checkpoint. For example, the cyclin D1-CDK complex mediates the G_1 to S phase transition

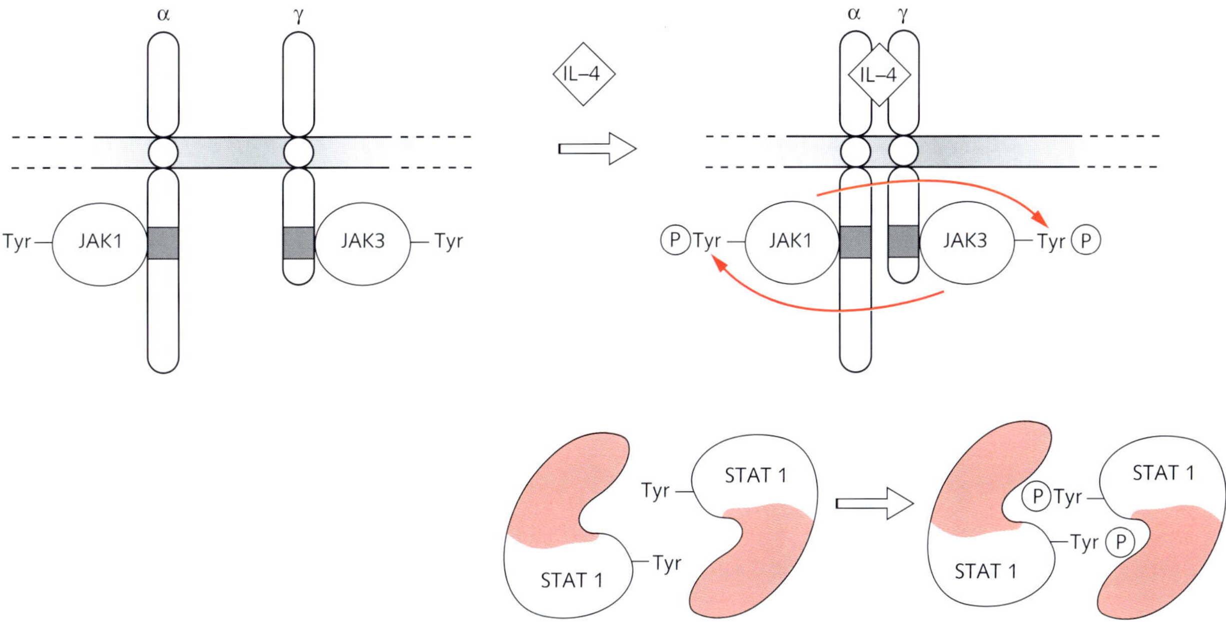

Fig. 3.7 Activation of specific gene transcription following binding of IL-4 to its receptor
STAT 1 SH2 domains are shown in red.

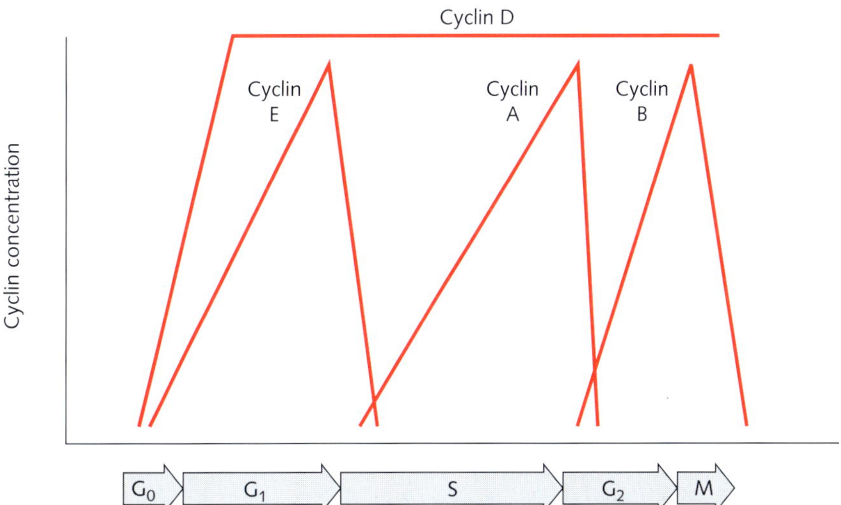

Fig. 3.8 Specific cyclins are synthesised and degraded at specific stages of the cell cycle

through phosphorylation of the product of the retinoblastoma tumour suppressor gene, as described in *Chapter 8* (Figure 8.4).

The cyclin-CDK complexes are also regulated by a set of polypeptide inhibitors which serve as negative regulators of cell proliferation. The 16 kDa product of the *INK4a* gene (also known as *CDKN2* or *MTS1*) and the 15 kDa product of the *INK4b* gene specifically inhibit complexes of cyclin D and CDKs 4 or 6.

The regulation of cell survival

Apoptosis is a form of physiological cell death characterised by internucleosomal DNA cleavage, chromatin condensation, cell shrinkage and engulfment by macrophages. This form of cell death is dependent on the cleavage and consequent activation of a family of cysteine proteases, the *caspases*. Some caspases can activate other family members, resulting in cascades of caspase

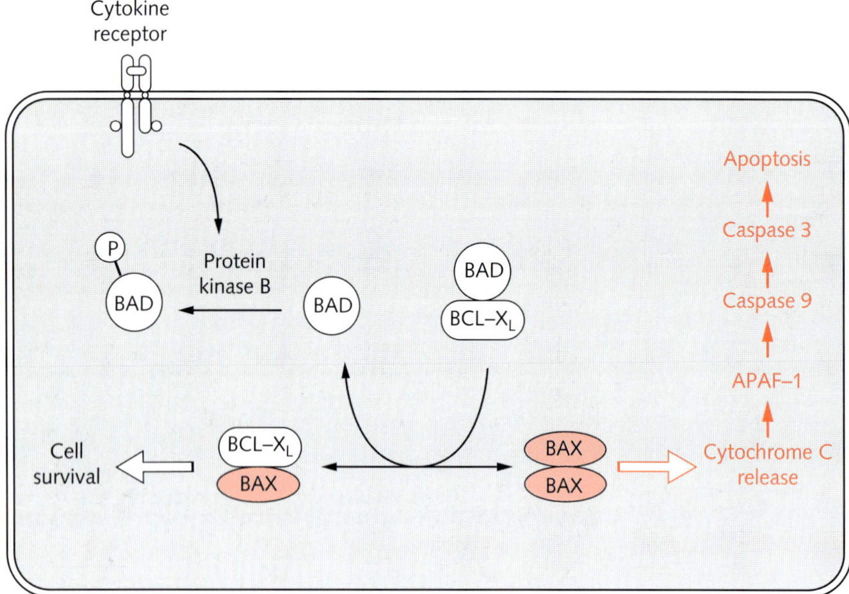

Fig. 3.9 Model for the regulation of apoptosis

activation steps. These cascades culminate in the cleavage of a subset of critical protein substrates including poly (ADP-ribose) polymerase, lamin and gelsolin, thus initiating the characteristic morphological events of apoptosis.

Caspase activation is mediated in part by the BCL-2 family of proteins. The BAX protein promotes apoptosis by triggering the release of cytochrome c from mitochondria. Within the cytosol, cytochrome c binds to the APAF 1 protein, unmasking its potential to bind and activate caspase 9 by autocatalytic cleavage. Subsequent activation of caspase 3 then initiates apoptosis (Figure 3.9). The anti-apoptotic functions of BCL-2 and BCL-X_L are dependent on their ability to form heterodimers with BAX, consequently blocking cytochrome c release (Figure 3.9).

The binding of cytokines to cell-surface receptors plays an important role in promoting cell survival by blocking apoptosis. The BCL-2 family member BAD binds and sequesters BCL-2 and BCL-X_L, thereby increasing the free concentration of the pro-apoptotic BAX protein. Activation of the phosphatidylinositol 3′-kinase/protein kinase B pathway (Figure 3.2) by some cytokines (e.g. IL-3, IL-4) results in phosphorylation of BAD. Phosphorylated BAD cannot bind BCL-2 or BCL-X_L. Therefore, the increase in the free concentration of these anti-apoptotic proteins results in enhanced cell survival via sequestration of BAX. The protein kinase B pathway modulates cell survival by other mechanisms in addition to the BAD phosphorylation pathway, including the direct phosphorylation and inactivation of caspase 9.

Maintenance of genomic integrity by the p53 pathway

Induction of DNA damage by cytotoxic drugs or by radiation results in the augmentation of cellular levels of the p53 protein through a post-transcriptional stabilisation mechanism. p53 is a transcription factor which contributes to the maintenance of genomic integrity by induction of a block at the G_1/S phase boundary, thereby allowing the repair of DNA damage. This block is mediated via augmented expression of the 21 kDa *WAF* gene product, an inhibitor of cyclin-CDK complexes (Figure 3.10). However, p53 also promotes the apoptotic destruction of cells with damaged DNA, thus safeguarding against the perpetuation of potentially harmful mutations. This aspect of p53 action is mediated in part by the induction of expression of the pro-apoptotic BAX gene (Figure 3.10).

The p53 gene is a tumour suppressor, and loss or functional inactivation of both alleles results in the simultaneous loss of a cell cycle checkpoint and of an important mechanism of apoptosis induction. p53 inactivation is a frequent event in more advanced stages of leukaemia (for example blast transformation in chronic myeloid leukaemia, CML) and is a bad prognostic feature, resulting in part from the decreased capacity of the leukaemia cells to undergo apoptosis in response to

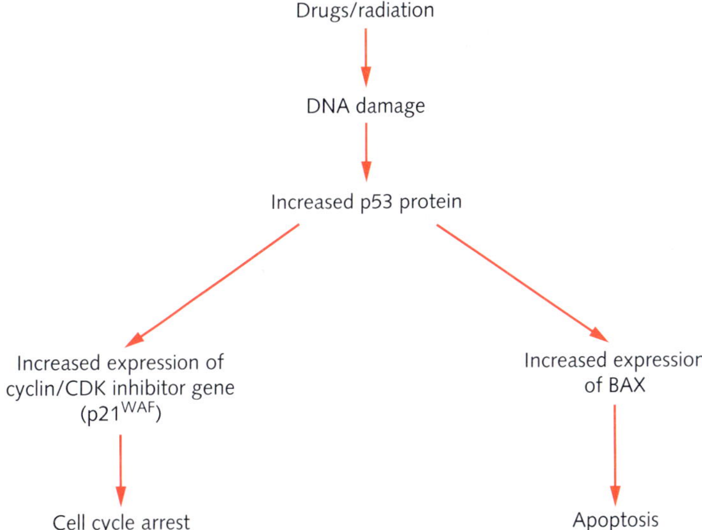

Fig. 3.10 Induction of p53-dependent cell cycle arrest and apoptosis following DNA damage

cytotoxic therapy. Loss of one p53 allele in families with Li–Fraumeni syndrome is responsible for the increased susceptibility to malignant transformation.

The ataxia telangiectasia gene (*ATM*) is located on chromosome 11q23. Its product shows strong homology to proteins involved in the control of cell cycle checkpoints in lower eukaryotes. The *ATM* gene product acts as a sensor of DNA damage and controls a G_1/S phase checkpoint by induction of the p53 protein. Ataxia telangiectasia is a recessive multisystem disease associated with mutations in the *ATM* gene. Homozygous loss of the *ATM* gene results in the loss of the G_1/S phase checkpoint. The consequent inability to repair DNA damage results in genetic instability and malignant transformation. Ataxia telangiectasia patients show an increased susceptibility to lymphoid leukaemias and to lymphomas, but not to myeloid malignancies.

The molecular basis of leukaemia and lymphoma

Malignant transformation is usually dependent on the cooperation between multiple genetic changes within a single cell. Chromosomal translocations involving genes whose products are involved in the regulation of cell proliferation, differentiation and apoptosis frequently underlie leukaemogenesis and lymphomagenesis. In some instances, these translocations result in a quantitative increase in expression of a critical regulatory protein as a result of juxtaposition of its gene to T-cell antigen receptor or immunoglobulin loci, both of which contain powerful cell type-specific enhancer elements. In other cases, fusion of sequences from two genes results in the expression of abnormal chimeric oncoproteins whose altered biochemical properties contribute to the disruption of normal signalling mechanisms. Gene amplification and mutation are less frequent in haematological malignancies than in solid tumours. Examples of the genetic and biochemical changes underlying malignant transformation of haematopoietic cells are discussed below.

Acute myeloid leukaemia (AML)

Translocations involving the PML and RARα genes in acute promyelocytic leukaemia

The t(15;17)(q21;q22) translocation in acute promyelocytic leukaemia (APML, FAB subtype M3) is associated with a favourable prognosis. APML responds to treatment with all-*trans* retinoic acid (ATRA). The translocation juxtaposes the retinoic acid receptor α (*RARα*) gene on chromosome 17 to the *PML* gene on chromosome 15. RARα is a transcription factor whose ability to bind specific DNA sequences and to activate transcription of adjacent genes is dependent on the binding of retinoic acid to a ligand-binding domain (Figure 3.11). The product of the *PML* gene also exhibits characteristics of a transcription factor, contains zinc finger DNA-binding motifs (Table 3.1) and is widely expressed in human tissues. The *PML-RARα* chimeric gene encodes a protein in which one of the two N-terminal transactivation domains of RARα is replaced by PML-encoded sequences (Figure 3.11). The breakpoints within the *RARα* gene are always located within intron 2. The nine exon *PML* gene is disrupted in either introns 3 or 6 with the consequent generation of short (S) or long (L) forms

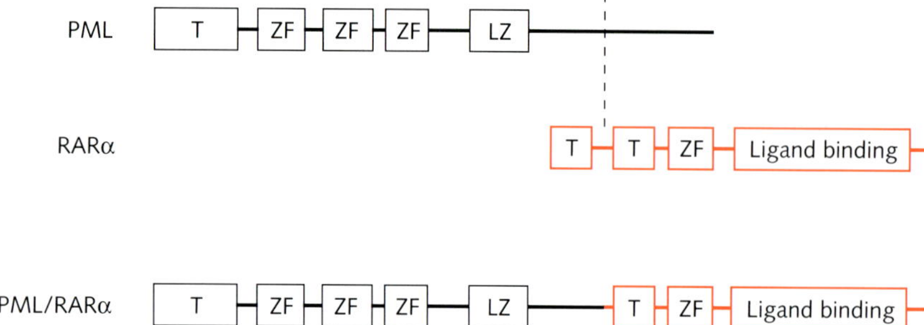

Fig. 3.11
Proteins encoded by the *PML* gene (chromosome 15), the *RARα* gene (chromosome 17) and by *PML-RARα* chimeric gene t(15;17). T, transactivation domains; ZF, zinc finger DNA-binding motifs; LZ, leucine zipper dimerisation motif.

of the chimeric oncoprotein. A 158 amino acid proline-rich domain found in the L form is absent in the S form. This domain contains several serine and threonine residues whose phosphorylation may modulate transactivation. In some studies, the S form translocation has been associated with a worse prognosis than the L form.

APML cells are blocked in differentiation at the promyelocyte stage and fail to undergo apoptosis normally. Expression of the PML-RARα oncoprotein may block the functions of both the normal PML and RARα proteins. It is unclear as to which aspect of the oncoprotein's actions is important in inducing the differentiation block. In normal cells, the PML protein is a component of large supramolecular nuclear structures, the nuclear bodies (also known as PML oncogenic domains). These structures may play a role in the regulation of gene expression via modulation of mRNA transport. The PML-RARα oncoprotein acts in a dominant negative manner and disrupts formation of nuclear bodies. It is plausible that the consequent perturbation of gene expression may result in the differentiation block. Treatment of APML cells with ATRA results in restoration of normal nuclear bodies and may underlie the ability of this agent to promote differentiation of the malignant cells *in vitro* and to induce remissions in APML patients. Restoration of nuclear body formation by ATRA treatment may be a consequence of the ability of the hormone to promote selective caspase-catalysed proteolytic degradation of the chimeric oncoprotein.

The PML-RARα oncoprotein may also block the expression of retinoic acid-responsive genes whose expression is required for normal myeloid differentiation. The RARα moiety of the chimeric protein binds a complex consisting of a nuclear co-repressor and histone deacetylase which blocks RARα-dependent transcription and cellular differentiation. ATRA may relieve this repression by binding to the RARα moiety and promoting the release of the co-repressor complex.

A minority of cases of APML harbour the t(11;17)(q13;q11) translocation which fuses the *RARα* gene to the *PLZF* gene, which encodes a zinc finger-containing transcription factor.

Genetic changes involving core binding factor genes in acute myeloid leukaemia

Core binding factor (CBF) is a heterodimeric transcription factor consisting of two subunits, CBFα (also known as AML1) and CBFβ (Figure 3.12). CBFβ stabilises binding of CBFα to specific enhancers. CBFα contains a domain with homology to the *Drosophila* developmental gene, *RUNT*. CBF upregulates transcription of the IL-3, granulocyte-macrophage colony-stimulating factor (GM-CSF), M-CSF receptor and T-cell antigen receptor genes, and is therefore thought to play important roles in normal haematopoiesis. Translocations involving the *CBFα* and *β* genes are associated with a good prognosis.

The translocation t(8;21)(q22;q22) is associated with 15% of AML, usually of the M2 subtype. This translocation results in the juxtaposition of the *CBFα* gene (chromosome 21) to the *ETO* gene (chromosome 8). The product of the *ETO* gene is also a transcription factor containing zinc finger DNA-binding motifs. The chimeric AML1/ETO protein (Figure 3.12) blocks transactivation by normal CBF, suggesting that malignant transformation by the chimera is the result of a block in haematopoietic maturation.

Inv(16)(p13;q22) is associated with AML M4 with eosinophilic differentiation and results in the fusion of the smooth muscle myosin heavy chain (*SMMHC*) gene to the *CBFβ* gene. The resulting chimeric oncoprotein contains those domains of CBFβ which are required for interaction with CBFα and an oligomerisation domain contributed by SMMHC (Figure 3.12). Studies on *CBFβ-SMMHC* 'knock-in' mice are consistent with the interpretation that the chimera contributes to leukaemogenesis via a dominant negative action on CBF-mediated transcription required for normal haematopoietic maturation.

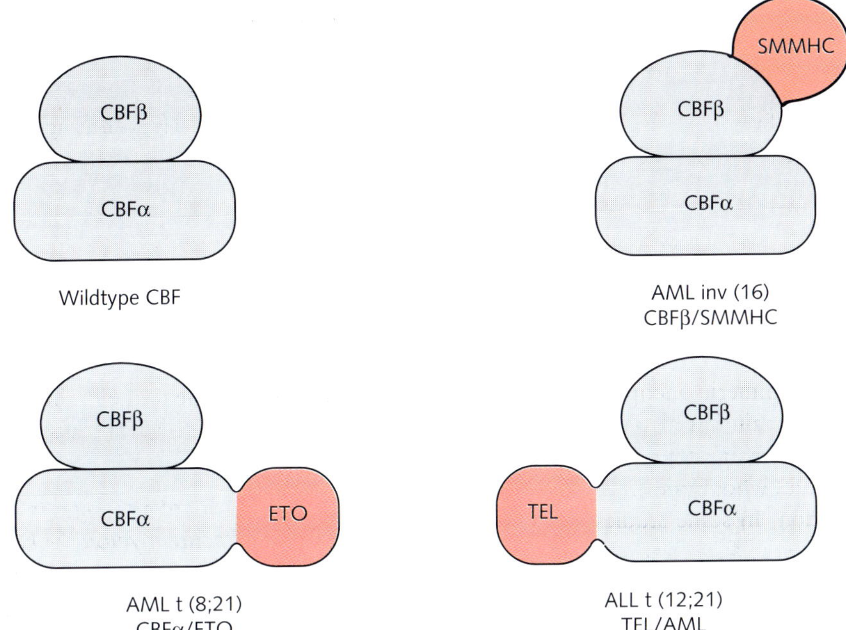

Fig. 3.12 Translocations involving core binding factor (*CBF*) genes in AML and ALL
The wild-type CBF is a heterodimer of the DNA-binding CBFα (AML1) protein and CBFβ, which stabilises DNA binding by CBFα.

Genetic changes involving the MLL1 gene in acute myeloid leukaemia

The *MLL1* gene located on chromosome 11q23 is homologous to the *Drosophila* developmental gene, *TRITHORAX*, and is involved in translocations with at least 15 different partners. *MLL1* translocations are particularly associated with infant and childhood leukaemias. The protein product of this gene, which is also known as *ALL1*, *HTRX* or *HRX*, contains several zinc finger DNA-binding motifs, a domain homologous to DNA methyltransferase and a DNA-binding AT-hook domain. Genetic studies in mice suggest that the *MLL1* gene plays an important role in normal haematopoiesis, possibly by upregulating expression of *HOX* genes, whose expression may be critical at specific stages of haematopoiesis. Transformation by *MLL1* fusion proteins may result from a block in downregulation of expression of specific *HOX* genes, therefore preventing terminal myeloid differentiation.

MLL1 rearrangements are frequently undetectable by conventional cytogenetic analysis but can be identified by Southern blotting, polymerase chain reaction (PCR) or fluorescence *in situ* hybridisation analysis. The t(4;11)(q21;q23) translocation (Table 3.2) which is frequently found in childhood pre-B acute lymphoblastic leukaemia (ALL) fuses *MLL1* to the *AF4* gene, whose product shows no homology to known proteins. The t(9;11)(p22;q23) translocation is associated with M5 myeloid leukaemia in adults and fuses *MLL1* to the *AF9* gene, which encodes a nuclear protein. Rearrangements involving *MLL1* are seen at high frequency in patients who have been treated with etoposide or teniposide and then developed secondary AML.

RAS mutations in acute myeloid leukaemia

Point mutations which result in substitution of amino acids at positions 12, 13, 59 or 61 of the $p21^{RAS}$ proteins abrogate the ability of RAS-GAP to stimulate their intrinsic GTPase activity (Figure 3.3). Therefore, these oncogenic RAS proteins accumulate in the active GTP-bound form and consequently trigger deregulated cell proliferation. Oncogenic mutations of the *RAS* gene (usually N-*RAS*) have been detected in 20–30% of AML. It is likely that these mutations have occurred after the initial leukaemogenic event since they are found in only a proportion of leukaemic cells. Therefore, *RAS* mutations may result in the evolution of more aggressive variants of the original leukaemic clone.

Translocations involving the BCR and ABL genes in chronic myeloid leukaemia

Almost all cases of CML are characterised by the presence of the Philadelphia translocation (t(9;22)(q34;q11)), which results in the translocation of the c-*ABL* PTK gene to the *BCR* locus, which encodes a multi-

Translocation	Genes involved	
T-ALL		
t(1;14)(p32;q11)*	TAL1	T-cell receptor δ
t(7;11)(q35;p13)	T-cell receptor β	Rhombotin 2
t(8;14)(q24;q11)	MYC	T-cell receptor α
t(10;14)(q24;q11)*	HOX11	T-cell receptor α
t(11;14)(p13;q11)	Rhombotin 2	T-cell receptor δ
t(11;14)(p15;q11)	Rhombotin 1	T-cell receptor δ
B-ALL		
t(1;19)(q23;p13)	PBX1	E2A
t(4;11)(q21;q23)	AF4	MLL1
t(8;14)(q24;q23)	MYC	Immunoglobulin heavy chain
t(12;21)(q22;p13)	TEL (ETV6)	CBFα (AML1)
t(17;19)(q22;p13)*	HLF (hepatic leukaemia factor)	E2A

Table 3.2 Translocations involving transcription factor genes in acute leukaemia
All rearrangements in T-ALL result in upregulated expression of transcription factor genes due to their juxtaposition to T-cell receptor loci. With the exception of t(8;14), translocations in B-ALL result in the generation of chimeric transcription factors with novel oncogenic properties. Translocations identified by an asterisk result in a block in apoptosis induction.

functional signalling protein (Figure 3.13). The chimeric gene encodes a 210 kDa chimeric protein, $p210^{BCR\text{-}ABL}$. Intramolecular interaction between the SH2-binding domain of the BCR moiety and the SH2 domain of the ABL moiety prevents binding of a cell-encoded polypeptide inhibitor to the SH3 domain. Therefore, $p210^{BCR\text{-}ABL}$ exhibits an increased PTK activity compared to $p145^{c\text{-}ABL}$, the product of the untranslocated c-*ABL* gene. This PTK activity is essential for malignant transformation by the chimeric protein. Furthermore, while $p145^{c\text{-}ABL}$ is located in the nucleus, $p210^{BCR\text{-}ABL}$ is associated with the cytoskeleton through interactions involving the C-terminal actin-binding domain. This altered subcellular localisation is also important in transformation, since it enables the chimeric oncoprotein to interact with different downstream targets compared to $p145^{c\text{-}ABL}$.

Transformation by $p210^{BCR\text{-}ABL}$ is dependent on the activation of multiple biochemical pathways. The activated PTK phosphorylates a tyrosine residue within the BCR moiety, thus providing a docking site for the GRB2/SOS complex (Figure 3.13). The resultant activation of $p21^{RAS}$, the RAF/MEK/ERK pathway and phosphorylation of the ELK-1 transcription factor contributes to deregulated cell proliferation.

Abrogation of apoptosis is also an important facet of transformation by $p210^{BCR\text{-}ABL}$. $p210^{BCR\text{-}ABL}$ activates phosphatidylinositol 3′-kinase via sequential binding of the SH2/SH3 domain-containing adaptor proteins CRKL, CBL and the p85 subunit of the kinase, resulting in the generation of 3′-phosphorylated inositol lipids and the consequent activation of protein kinase B-dependent survival pathways (Figure 3.13). Malignant cells expressing BCR-ABL oncoproteins are therefore characteristically resistant to apoptosis induction by cytotoxic drugs and ionising radiation.

Myelodysplastic syndromes

Chromosomal changes associated with myelodysplastic syndromes (MDS) are described in *Chapter 6*. Deletions of part or the whole of the long arms of chromosomes 5 or 7 are the most frequent aberrations. *RAS* gene mutations are associated with a bad prognosis and are detected in 15–20% of cases. p53 mutations are detected in advanced subtypes of MDS and may therefore be associated with the progression to leukaemia.

The interferon response factor 1 (IRF-1) gene encodes a transcription factor which upregulates expression of several growth suppressing genes. Hemizygous deletion of this gene has been reported in myelodysplasia with 5q deletions. However, not all patients with 5q– show deletion of IRF-1.

Acute lymphoblastic leukaemia

RAS mutations in acute lymphoblastic leukaemia

RAS gene mutations are seen in 20–30% of ALL. These oncogenic mutations frequently affect the N-*RAS* gene and are secondary events in transformation, associated with the evolution of more malignant variants of the original leukaemic clone.

p53 mutations and deletions in acute lymphoblastic leukaemia

p53 mutations are rare in ALL overall. Monosomy 17p results in the deletion of one p53 allele. The remaining allele is mutated in cases of ALL harbouring this abnormality, suggesting that loss of functional p53 may play a role in these ALL.

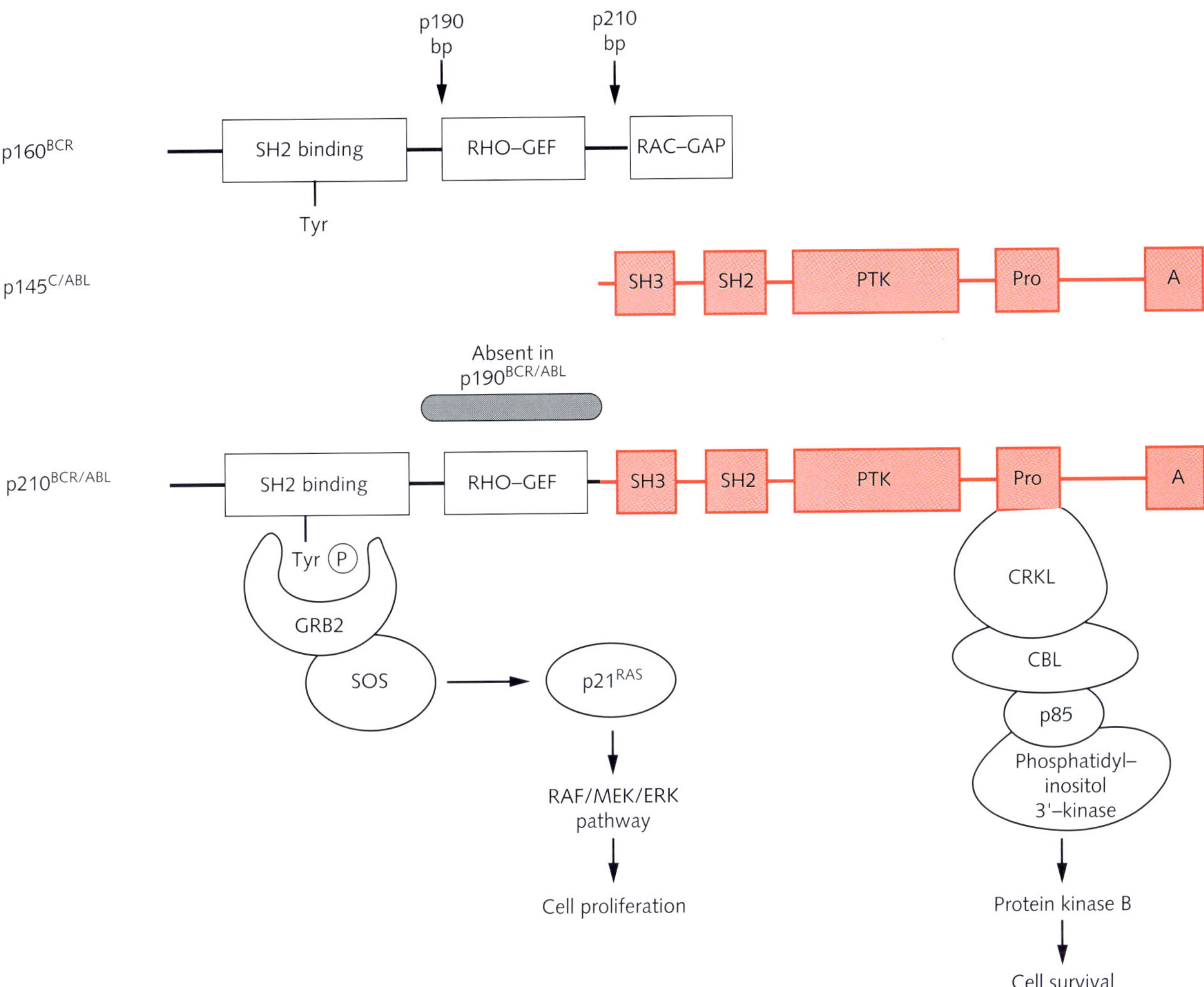

Fig. 3.13 Structure of the normal BCR and ABL gene products and the BCR-ABL chimeric oncoproteins
RHO-GEF, RHO G protein guanine nucleotide-exchange factor; RAC-GAP, activator of the GTPase of RAC G protein; Pro, proline-rich domain; PTK, protein tyrosine kinase; A, actin-binding domain; bp, breakpoint. SH3 domains mediate protein–protein interactions via binding to proline-rich sequences. Some of the biochemical pathways initiated by the BCR-ABL oncoproteins are shown.

Translocations involving the CBFα gene in B-lineage acute lymphoblastic leukaemia

The t(12;21)(q22;p13) translocation results in the fusion of the genes encoding the TEL(ETV6) and CBFα transcription factors. The fusion gene encodes a chimeric protein which contains the helix–loop–helix dimerisation domain of TEL and the DNA-binding and transactivation domains of CBFα (Figure 3.12). These translocations are detected by reverse transcriptase polymerase chain reaction analysis in 20–30% of paediatric ALL and therefore comprise the most frequent rearrangements in ALL. The *TEL/CBFα* fusion is associated with CD10+ B-lineage ALL and, in most studies, with a good prognosis. This rearrangement is invariably associated with loss of the remaining *TEL* allele, suggesting that loss of TEL function is important in malignant transformation of cells harbouring the translocation.

Translocations involving the BCR and ABL genes in acute lymphoblastic leukaemia

The Philadelphia translocation is found in about 25% of adults and 2% of children with ALL. Approximately half of these cases express p210$^{BCR\text{-}ABL}$ and may represent lymphoid blast transformations of previously undetected CML. The remaining cases express a variant translocation which results in the expression of a smaller chimeric protein, p190$^{BCR\text{-}ABL}$, which lacks the BCR-derived RHO-guanine nucleotide-exchange factor domain present in p210$^{BCR\text{-}ABL}$ (Figure 3.13). The Philadelphia chromosome is associated with a particularly bad prognosis in ALL.

Translocations involving the E2A and PBX1 genes in B-lineage acute lymphoblastic leukaemia

The t(1;19)(q23;p13) translocation seen in 5% of childhood acute pre-B-cell ALL results in the fusion of the *E2A* gene on chromosome 19 to the *PBX1* gene on chromosome 1. The *E2A* gene encodes a transcription factor of the helix–loop–helix family. The product of the *PBX1* gene is also a transcription factor which binds DNA via a homeodomain. The tissue-specific expression of PBX1 is suggestive of a role in the regulation of haematopoietic cell differentiation. It is not expressed by normal B lymphocytes. The chimeric oncoprotein encoded by the t(1;19) chromosome contains an N-terminal E2A-derived transactivation domain and a C-terminal DNA-binding homeodomain derived from PBX1. The chimeric oncoprotein therefore incorporates the transactivation properties of E2A and the DNA-binding specificity of PBX1. The mechanism of transformation by the E2A/PBX1 chimera is unclear, but is likely to be the result of abnormal transcriptional regulation by the oncoprotein. In transgenic mice, *E2A/PBX1* triggers increased cell proliferation but also induces apoptosis. Therefore, it is likely that transformation by the fusion protein requires co-operation with additional genetic changes which abrogate apoptosis.

Other chromosomal translocations in B-lineage acute lymphoblastic leukaemia

Other chromosomal translocations associated with B-lineage ALL usually result in the expression of chimeric transcription factors (Table 3.2). These translocations also result in the disruption of transcriptional regulation and consequently of normal differentiation. In contrast, translocation of the *IL-3* gene to the immunoglobulin (Ig) heavy chain locus in B-lineage ALL harbouring the t(5;14) translocation results in IL-3 overexpression driven by the powerful B lymphoid-specific enhancer of the Ig locus. IL-3 overproduction results in autocrine or paracrine growth of the leukaemia cells as well as protection from apoptosis. The t(8;14) translocation found in mature B-ALL (FAB L3) juxtaposes the *MYC* gene to the Ig heavy chain locus. The resulting deregulated expression of the *MYC* gene contributes to malignant transformation by driving excessive cell proliferation.

Translocations involving T-cell receptor genes in T-ALL

The majority of chromosomal translocations associated with T-ALL result in the overexpression of transcription factor genes resulting from their juxtaposition to one of the four T-cell antigen receptor loci, which contain powerful T lymphoid-specific enhancers (Table 3.2). The *TAL-1* (*SCL*) gene encodes a helix–loop–helix family transcription factor. Deregulated expression of *TAL-1*, which is not normally expressed in T cells, may contribute to leukaemogenesis in those T-ALL cases showing *TAL-1* abnormalities. In about 3% of T-ALL, the *TAL-1* gene, which is normally located on chromosome 1p32, is juxtaposed to the T-cell receptor δ locus (chromosome 14q11). However, deletions upstream of TAL-1, which are not detectable by conventional cytogenetics, are more frequently observed.

The *TAN-1* gene encodes a cell-surface receptor and is homologous to the *Drosophila* gene *NOTCH*, whose product is involved in the regulation of differentiation. *TAN-1* is translocated to the T-cell receptor β locus in T-ALL harbouring the t(7;9) translocation. The portion of the *TAN-1* gene which encodes the extracellular ligand-binding domain is deleted as a consequence of the translocation. The resulting truncation of the TAN-1 protein may result in the generation of a receptor with altered signalling properties. The p56^{LCK} gene encodes a PTK which plays an important role in triggering of T-cell proliferation following ligation of the antigen receptor. The t(1;7) translocation juxtaposes this gene to the T-cell receptor β locus, resulting in its overexpression.

Deletion of INK4 genes in acute lymphoblastic leukaemia

The genes encoding the cyclin-dependent protein kinase inhibitors INK4a and INK4b are tandemly linked on chromosome 9p21. Deletion of these tumour suppressor genes results in the loss of an important negative regulatory mechanism in cell cycle control. The 9p21 locus is frequently deleted in leukaemia. Deletions are far more frequent in lymphoid than in myeloid malignancies. Ten per cent of cases of childhood B-ALL and a smaller proportion of adult cases show homozygous loss of *INK4a* and *INK4b* genes. Eighty per cent of T-ALL patients show deletion of the *INK4a* gene, suggesting an important role as a tumour suppressor.

B-chronic lymphocytic leukaemia

Trisomy 12 and deletions involving chromosome 13q14 are common genetic events in B-chronic lymphocytic leukaemia (B-CLL) and are discussed in *Chapter 8*. The biochemical consequences of these aberrations are unknown.

The cytokine IL-4, the interferons α or γ, the CD40 ligand or growth on bone marrow stromal layers promotes extended survival of B-CLL cells *in vitro* and may also do this *in vivo*. The ability of these agents to promote survival is, in some cases, linked to their ability to maintain elevated expression of the anti-apoptotic *BCL-2* gene. In 10–20% of cases of B-CLL, *in vitro* maintenance of *BCL-2* expression and extended survival are independent of added cytokines, suggesting that an unidentified genetic change may contribute to the malignant phenotype in this subset of B-CLL through the abnormal regulation of *BCL-2* expression and hence of cell survival. The ability of cytokines to abrogate apoptosis induction may also contribute to the failure of chemotherapy, since IL-4 addition *in vitro* blocks the induction of apoptosis by cytotoxic drugs. Rare cases of B-CLL harbour translocations which juxtapose the *BCL-2* gene to the immunoglobulin κ or λ light chain genes on chromosomes 2 or 22, respectively. In contrast to the translocations of *BCL-2* in follicular lymphoma (*see below*), the breakpoints in B-CLL are located on the 5′ side of the *BCL-2* gene.

The malignant cells of 35% of B-CLL patients show decreased expression of the *ATM* gene product. These patients show a shorter survival time compared to patients with normal expression of *ATM*. The role of the *ATM*-encoded protein in regulating apoptosis via the p53 pathway suggests that loss of its expression in some B-CLL may play a role in the resistance to apoptosis characteristic of this malignancy. Homozygous loss of *ATM* genes is also detected in approximately 60% of cases of T-prolymphocytic leukaemia.

In a subset of B-CLL harbouring the t(14;19) translocation, the *BCL-3* gene is placed under the control of the Ig heavy chain enhancer. The resulting overexpression of the BCL-3 protein results in enhanced expression of genes responsive to the NF-κB transcription factor. Some of these NF-κB-responsive genes encode proteins which protect cells from the induction of apoptosis.

Oncogenic mutations involving the *RAS* genes have not been detected in B-CLL. Mutations of p53 are detected in 15% of B-CLL, are associated with prolymphocytic morphology, a poor prognosis and are frequent in Richter's transformation.

Genetic changes in non-Hodgkin's lymphoma

Burkitt's lymphoma

The translocations of the *MYC* gene to Ig loci, which result in overexpression of the MYC protein in Burkitt's lymphoma, are described in *Chapter 8*. One-third of Burkitt's lymphoma cases and half of L3 B-ALL harbour mutations in p53. These observations may reflect the ability of overexpressed *MYC* to trigger both proliferation and apoptosis. Therefore, malignant transformation as a result of *MYC* overexpression requires a second genetic event which abrogates apoptosis induction, for example loss of functional p53.

Follicular lymphoma

The translocation of the anti-apoptotic *BCL-2* gene to the Ig heavy chain locus in follicular lymphoma is described in *Chapter 8*. The consequent overexpression of BCL-2 is partly the result of juxtaposition to the Ig enhancer. However, splicing out of the very large intron of the *BCL-2* gene is also enhanced by the presence of Ig gene-derived sequences in the primary fusion transcript of the *Ig/BCL-2* locus. Thus, the generation of spliced mRNA and hence of BCL-2 protein is augmented in cells harbouring the translocation compared to cells containing normal *BCL-2* genes.

Transformation of follicular lymphoma to higher grade disease is associated with p53 mutation in 30% of cases. Therefore, detection of these mutations by polymerase chain reaction may be useful as an early warning of a more aggressive stage of the disease. Homozygous deletion of the *INK4a* gene is also associated with transformation of low-grade non-Hodgkin's lymphoma to a more aggressive stage.

Mantle cell lymphoma

Translocation of the cyclin D1 gene to the immunoglobulin locus in mantle cell lymphoma is described in *Chapter 8*.

Diagnostic and therapeutic applications of molecular information

The detailed information now available on the genetic and biochemical basis of some haematological malignancies has resulted in novel approaches to the diagnosis and treatment of these diseases. The presence of a specific genetic abnormality, for example the *BCR-ABL* translocations in CML or ALL and the *PML-RARα* translocation in APML, confirm the diagnosis of these leukaemias and are relevant to prognosis. In several instances, molecular techniques are useful in the detection of abnormalities that cannot be detected by conventional cytogenetics, for example the t(12;21) translocation in B-lineage ALL. The monitoring of patients for minimal residual disease based on detection of fusion genes or analysis of clone-specific rearrangements of the immunoglobulin or T-cell receptor loci is described in *Chapter 4*.

APML patients whose malignant cells harbour the t(15;17) translocation respond well to ATRA, which induces differentiation of the malignant cells. However, long-term survival is improved when ATRA therapy is followed by conventional chemotherapy.

The ability of cytotoxic drugs or radiation to kill malignant cells is compromised in leukaemias or lymphomas which harbour genetic changes resulting in the abrogation of apoptosis, for example expression of the BCR-ABL oncoprotein in CML or the overexpression of *BCL-2* in follicular lymphoma. Strategies designed to specifically decrease expression of these oncoproteins may therefore be of value in enhancing the actions of cytotoxic regimes. Antisense oligonucleotides are short DNA molecules complementary to selected sequences of specific mRNAs and which interfere selectively with the expression of proteins encoded by these RNA species. For example, antisense oligonucleotides which span the breakpoint of the *BCR-ABL* mRNA form a stable hybrid with the chimeric transcript but not with the normal ABL or BCR transcripts. However, the cytotoxic actions of antisense oligonucleotides have, in some instances, been shown to be mediated by non-specific effects. Hammerhead ribozymes are enzymatically active RNA species whose catalytic centre is flanked by sequences which target the ribozyme to specific mRNAs. A *BCR-ABL*-specific ribozyme selectively degrades the chimeric transcript when introduced into a cell line derived from a Philadelphia-positive CML patient and consequently inhibits its proliferation.

Selective inhibitors of the biochemical actions of oncoproteins may also have therapeutic potential. Herbimycin A, a selective inhibitor of the protein tyrosine kinase activity of the BCR-ABL oncoprotein, enhances the ability of etoposide or of radiation to induce apoptosis in cell lines derived from Philadelphia-positive CML and ALL patients. Protein tyrosine kinase inhibitors which target JAK-mediated signalling limit the proliferation of ALL cells *in vitro*.

The p53 protein blocks the lytic infection of human cells by adenoviruses. The adenovirus genome encodes a protein, E2B, which binds p53 and consequently permits viral replication and host cell lysis. Mutant adenoviruses which lack the *E2B* gene are therefore unable to replicate in normal human cells but establish lytic infections in malignant cells lacking functional p53, consequently triggering their selective destruction.

Conclusions

Here we have summarised the biochemical pathways involved in the regulation of proliferation, survival and differentiation of normal cells. Examples of the genetic changes which underlie the generation of leukaemias and lymphomas have been described. The impacts of these genetic changes on normal regulatory mechanisms are the result of overexpression of critical regulatory proteins, the generation of mutant or chimeric proteins with altered biochemical properties or the loss of expression of proteins which negatively regulate an increase in cell number. It is anticipated that ongoing studies on the molecular basis of leukaemia and lymphoma will result in the introduction of novel diagnostic and therapeutic strategies.

Further reading

Signal transduction

Darnell JE. (1997) STATs and gene regulation. *Science*, **277**, 1630–1635.

Ihle JN. (1995) Cytokine receptor signalling. *Nature*, **377**, 591–594.

Karin M, Hunter T. (1995) Transcriptional control by protein phosphorylation: signal transmission from the cell surface to the nucleus. *Current Biology*, **5**, 573–580.

Pawson T, Scott JD. (1997) Signaling through scaffold, anchoring and adaptor proteins. *Science*, **278**, 2075–2080.

Sherr CJ. (1996) Cancer cell cycles. *Science*, **274**, 1672–1677.

Regulation of apoptosis

Green DR, Reed JC. (1998) Mitochondria and apoptosis. *Science*, **281**, 1309–1312.

Hemmings BA. (1997) Akt signaling: linking membrane events to life and death decisions. *Science*, **275**, 665–668.

Thornberry NA, Lazebnik Y. (1998) Caspases: enemies within. *Science*, **281**, 1312–1316.

Wickremasinghe RG, Hoffbrand AV. (1999) Biochemical and genetic control of apoptosis: relevance to hematological malignancies. *Blood*, **93**, 3587–3600.

Yang E, Korsmeyer SJ. (1996) Molecular thanatopsis: a discourse on the BCL2 family and cell death. *Blood*, **88**, 386–401.

Tumour suppressor genes

Levine AJ. (1997) p53, the cellular gatekeeper for growth and division. *Cell*, **88**, 323–331.

Meyn MS. (1995) Ataxia telangiectasia and cellular responses to DNA damage. *Cancer Research*, **55**, 5991–6001.

Prokocimer M, Rotter V. (1994) Structure and function of p53 and their aberrations in cancer cells: projection on the hematologic cell lineages. *Blood*, **84**, 2391–2411.

Taylor AM, Metcalfe JA, Thick J, Mak YF. (1996) Leukemia and lymphoma in ataxia telangiectasia. *Blood*, **87**, 423–438.

Genetics of leukaemia: general

Rabbitts TH. (1994) Chromosomal translocations in human cancer. *Nature*, **372**, 143–149.

APML

Dyck JA, Maul GD, Miller WH *et al.* (1994) A novel macromolecular structure is a target of the promyelocyte-retinoic acid receptor oncoprotein. *Cell*, **76**, 333–343.

Grignani F, De Matteis S, Nervi C *et al.* (1998) Fusion proteins of the retinoic acid receptor-alpha recruit histone deacetylase in promyelocytic leukaemia. *Nature*, **391**, 815–818.

Pandolfi PP, Alcalay M, Fagioli M *et al.* (1992) Genomic variability and alternative splicing generate multiple PML/RAR α isoforms in acute promyelocytic leukemia. *EMBO Journal*, **11**, 1397–1407.

Fusions involving core binding factor genes

Golub TR, Barker GF, Boghlander SK *et al.* (1995) Fusion of the TEL gene on chromosome 12p13 to the AML1 gene on 21q22 in acute lymphoblastic leukemia. *Proceedings of the National Academy of Sciences (USA)*, **92**, 4917–4921.

Liu PP, Hajra A, Wijmenga C, Collins FS. (1995) Molecular pathogenesis of the chromosome 16 inversion in the M4Eo subtype of acute myeloid leukemia. *Blood*, **85**, 2289–2302.

Meyers S, Lenny N, Hiebert SW. (1995) The t(8;21) fusion protein interferes with AML-1B-dependent transcriptional activation. *Molecular and Cellular Biology*, **15**, 1974–1982.

Romana SP, Poirel H, Leconiat M *et al.* (1995) High frequency of t(12;21) in childhood B-cell precursor acute lymphoblastic leukemia. *Blood*, **86**, 4263–4269.

Fusions involving MLL1

Corral J, Lavenir I, Impey H *et al.* (1996) An MLL-AF9 fusion gene made by homologous recombination causes acute leukemia in chimeric mice: a method to create fusion oncogenes. *Cell*, **85**, 853–861.

Domer PH, Fakharzadeh SS, Chen S-S. (1993) Acute mixed-lineage leukemia t(4;11)(q21;q23) generates an MLL-AF4 fusion product. *Proceedings of the National Academy of Sciences (USA)*, **90**, 7884–7888.

Hilden JM, Frestedt JL, Moore RO *et al.* (1995) Molecular analysis of infant acute lymphoblastic leukemia: MLL gene rearrangement and reverse transcriptase-polymerase chain reaction for t(4;11)(q21;q23). *Blood*, **86**, 3876–3882.

Acute leukaemia

Look AT. (1997) Oncogenic transcription factors in the human acute leukemias. *Science*, **278**, 1059–1064.

Ogawa S, Hangaishi A, Miyakawa S *et al.* (1995) Loss of the cyclin-dependent kinase 4-inhibitor (p16;MTS1) gene is frequent and highly specific to lymphoid tumors in primary human hematopoietic malignancies. *Blood*, **86**, 1548–1556.

Secker-Walker LM. (1998) Cytogenetics. In: Hoffbrand AV, Lewis SM, Tuddenham EGD, eds. *Postgraduate Haematology*. Oxford: Butterworth-Heinemann.

Chronic myeloid leukaemia

Riordan FA, Wickremasinghe RG. (1998) Signal transduction by the Philadelphia chromosome-encoded BCR/ABL-oncoproteins: therapeutic implications for chronic myeloid leukemia and Philadelphia-positive acute lymphoblastic leukemia. *Hematology* **3**, 387–396.

Skorski T, Bellacosa A, Nieborowska-Skorska M *et al.* (1997) Transformation of hematopoietic cells by BCR/ABL requires activation of a PI-3 kinase/Akt-dependent pathway. *EMBO Journal*, **16**, 6151–6161.

B-CLL

Catovsky D. (1998) Chronic lymphoid leukaemias. In: Hoffbrand AV, Lewis SM, Tuddenham EGD, eds. *Postgraduate Haematology*. Oxford: Butterworth-Heinemann.

Stankovic T, Weber P, Stewart G *et al.* (1999) Inactivation of ataxia telangiectasia mutated gene in B-cell chronic lymphocytic leukaemia. *Lancet*, **353**, 26–29.

Starostik P, Manshouri T, O'Brien S *et al.* (1998) Deficiency of the ATM protein expression defines an aggressive subgroup of B-cell chronic lymphocytic leukemia. *Cancer Research*, **58**, 4552–4557.

Non-Hodgkin's lymphoma

Linch DC, Goldstone AH, Mason DY. (1998) Malignant lymphomas. In: Hoffbrand AV, Lewis SM, Tuddenham EGD, eds. *Postgraduate Haematology*. Oxford: Butterworth-Heinemann.

Petrovic AS, Young RL, Hilgarth B *et al.* (1998) The Ig heavy chain 3′ end confers a post-transcriptional processing advantage to bcl-2 IgH fusion RNA in t(14;18) lymphoma. *Blood*, **91**, 3952–3961.

Therapeutic strategies

Bischoff JR, Kirn DH, Williams A *et al.* (1996) An adenovirus mutant that replicates selectively in p53-deficient human cells. *Science*, **274**, 342–376.

Druker BJ, Tamura S, Buchdunger E *et al.* (1996) Effects of a selective inhibitor of the abl tyrosine kinase on the growth of Bcr/Abl-positive cells. *Nature Medicine*, **2**, 561–566.

Leopold LH, Shore SK, Reddy EP. (1996) Multi-unit anti-BCR-ABL ribozyme therapy in chronic myelogenous leukemia. *Leukemia and Lymphoma*, **22**, 365–373.

Meydan N, Greenberger T, Dadi H *et al.* (1996) Inhibition of acute lymphoblastic leukaemia by a Jak-2 inhibitor. *Nature*, **379**, 645–648.

O'Brien SG, Kirkland MA, Melo JV *et al.* (1994) Antisense BCR-ABL oligomers cause non-specific inhibition of chronic myeloid leukemia cell lines. *Leukemia*, **8**, 2156–2162.

Riordan FA, Bravery CA, Mengubas K *et al.* (1998) Herbimycin A accelerates the induction of apoptosis following etoposide treatment or γ-irradiation of bcr/abl-positive leukemia cells. *Oncogene*, **16**, 1533–1542.

Tallman MS, Andersen JW, Schiffer CA *et al.* (1997) All-trans retinoic acid in acute promyelocytic leukemia. *New England Journal of Medicine*, **337**, 1021–1028.

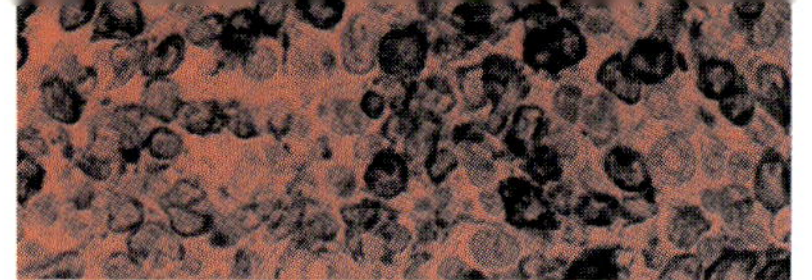

Chapter 4

Detection of minimal residual disease in haematological malignancies

Drew Provan & John G Gribben

Introduction

Despite advances in the treatment of human haematological malignancies, a significant proportion of patients relapse, usually with the same malignant clone found at diagnosis. Until recently, detection of residual leukaemia or lymphoma cells in marrow, blood or lymph nodes relied on light microscopy and flow cytometry. However, these techniques are not sensitive for detection of small numbers of malignant cells. Other, more sensitive, methods are now available to assess whether early detection of residual tumour might allow intervention and prevent relapse of disease. Molecular techniques, such as polymerase chain reaction (PCR), seem to offer highly sensitive detection of malignant DNA sequences and this technique has been applied to a wide variety of diseases.

Many studies have now been carried out in a variety of disorders, and whilst it is true that for many haematological cancers persistence of PCR detectable disease predicts patients who will do less well, this does not hold true for all diseases studied. It appears that patients with some malignancies may harbour residual tumour cells for many years without ever showing any evidence of clinical relapse. This will be discussed in detail later in this chapter.

This chapter outlines the methods available, with particular emphasis on PCR amplification, and their clinical application to a variety of haematological malignancies including lymphomas and leukaemias. The molecular basis of leukaemia and lymphoma is discussed in detail in *Chapter 3*.

What is minimal residual disease?

Minimal residual disease (MRD) describes the *lowest level of disease detectable using available methods*. Previously, light microscopy, cytogenetic analysis and flow cytometry were standard techniques used for detection of residual malignant cells in blood and marrow of patients following treatment. However, the sensitivities of these methods do not allow identification of low levels of disease, nor do they allow accurate quantitation of malignant cell numbers. Since these residual malignant cells may be the source of ultimate relapse, there has been great interest in developing molecular techniques for detection of residual tumour. For many years Southern blot hybridisation has been the 'gold standard' for detection of DNA sequence alterations at specific genetic loci, but this has largely been superseded by PCR amplification of DNA sequences. Due to the power of PCR technology we are now able to detect one residual malignant cell in a background of one million normal cells. Molecular targets for PCR-based approaches include chromosomal translocations and antigen receptor (immunoglobulin and T-cell receptor) gene rearrangements.

Methods available for the detection of residual disease

To date, several methods have been used to determine the presence of residual neoplastic cells in blood, bone marrow or other tissue following therapy (Figure 4.1).

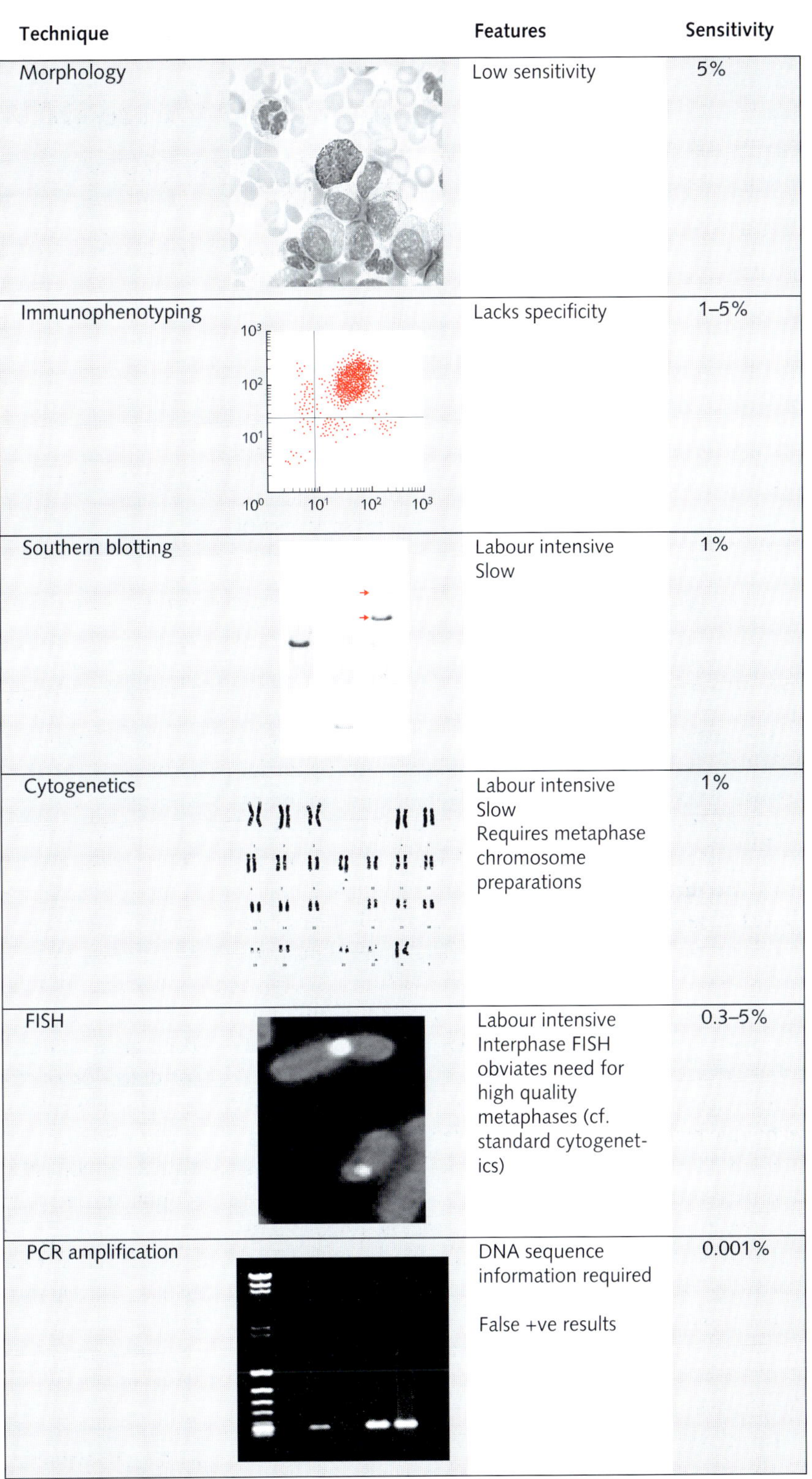

Technique	Features	Sensitivity
Morphology	Low sensitivity	5%
Immunophenotyping	Lacks specificity	1–5%
Southern blotting	Labour intensive Slow	1%
Cytogenetics	Labour intensive Slow Requires metaphase chromosome preparations	1%
FISH	Labour intensive Interphase FISH obviates need for high quality metaphases (cf. standard cytogenetics)	0.3–5%
PCR amplification	DNA sequence information required False +ve results	0.001%

Fig. 4.1 Methods of detection of marrow infiltration in non-Hodgkin's lymphoma, showing the sensitivities of each

The ideal assay system for detection of small numbers of malignant cells in a marrow or blood sample should fulfil the following criteria: the methodology should be applicable in most cases of the disease under investigation; the method should be specific for the neoplastic cell type; the method should be sensitive; the method should allow quantitation of tumour burden for prognostic purposes.

Methods include

- Morphology.
- Flow cytometry and immunophenotypic analyses.
- Cell culture assays.
- Karyotypic analysis.
- Fluorescence *in situ* hybridisation techniques.
- Molecular analyses including Southern blotting and PCR.

Morphology

In acute leukaemia, remission is the term used to describe a bone marrow containing less than 5% blast (i.e. leukaemic) cells using conventional light microscopy, but this may still represent a considerable tumour burden since, at diagnosis, the leukaemic cell number may be 10^{12} and, following therapy, the neoplastic cell number may drop only by 2 logs to 10^{10} even in the presence of fewer than 5% marrow blasts. Standard morphology alone is not a sensitive method for determining low levels of disease and is a poor indicator to attempt to predict impending relapse (Table 4.1).

Flow cytometry and immunophenotyping

Immunophenotypic analysis using single monoclonal antibodies to cell membrane or cytoplasmic proteins lacks absolute specificity for leukaemia or lymphoma cells and is therefore of limited value. Combining monoclonal antibodies allows for more specific detection of residual disease and quantitation is possible, although the tumour cell burden may be underestimated. The technique is further hampered by the lack of true 'tumour-specific' surface determinants and tumour-associated antigens are normal differentiation antigens present on developing haematopoietic progenitor cells. Using combinations of monoclonal antibodies and multicolour flow cytometric analysis, the sensitivity of this technique can be greatly enhanced. Except in the most expert hands, this technique is limited to a sensitivity of around 10^{-4} (i.e. 1 malignant cell in 10,000 normal cells).

Table 4.1 Sensitivity of methods for MRD detection.

Method	Sensitivity
Standard morphology	1–5%
Cytogenetics	5%
Fluorescence *in situ*	0.3–5%
Immunophenotyping	10^{-4}
Translocations	
PCR	10^{-6}
Gene rearrangements	
Southern blotting	1–5%
PCR	10^{-4}–10^{-6}

Cell culture assays

This involves growing T-cell depleted marrow in culture after the patient undergoes treatment, followed by subsequent morphological, immunophenotypic and karyotypic analyses on the colonies produced. Due to the variability of culture techniques between and within laboratories, this method has proved unreliable and insensitive for detecting persisting blasts. In addition, culture techniques do not provide any estimate of cell number and hence provide little information about tumour cell burden.

Karyotypic analysis

Detection of non-random chromosomal translocations is of great value in the diagnosis of leukaemias and lymphomas. Chromosomal abnormalities are present in at least 70% of patients with acute lymphoblastic leukaemia (ALL) and 50% of patients with chronic lymphocytic leukaemia (CLL). However, karyotypic analysis is of limited value following therapy with a sensitivity level of around 5% making it little better than standard morphological analysis. In addition, cytogenetics relies on obtaining adequate numbers of suitable metaphases for analysis, which is difficult in some malignancies.

Fluorescence in situ hybridisation (FISH)

FISH can detect smaller chromosomal abnormalities than standard karyotyping and allows analysis of interphase nuclei (cf. metaphase preparations in standard karyotyping). The method involves the binding of a nucleic acid probe to a specific chromosomal region. Preparations are counterstained with fluorescent dye allowing the chromosomal region of interest to be detected. The technique is useful in the diagnosis of trisomies and monosomies. The sensitivity of the technique is around 1% making it considerably more useful than

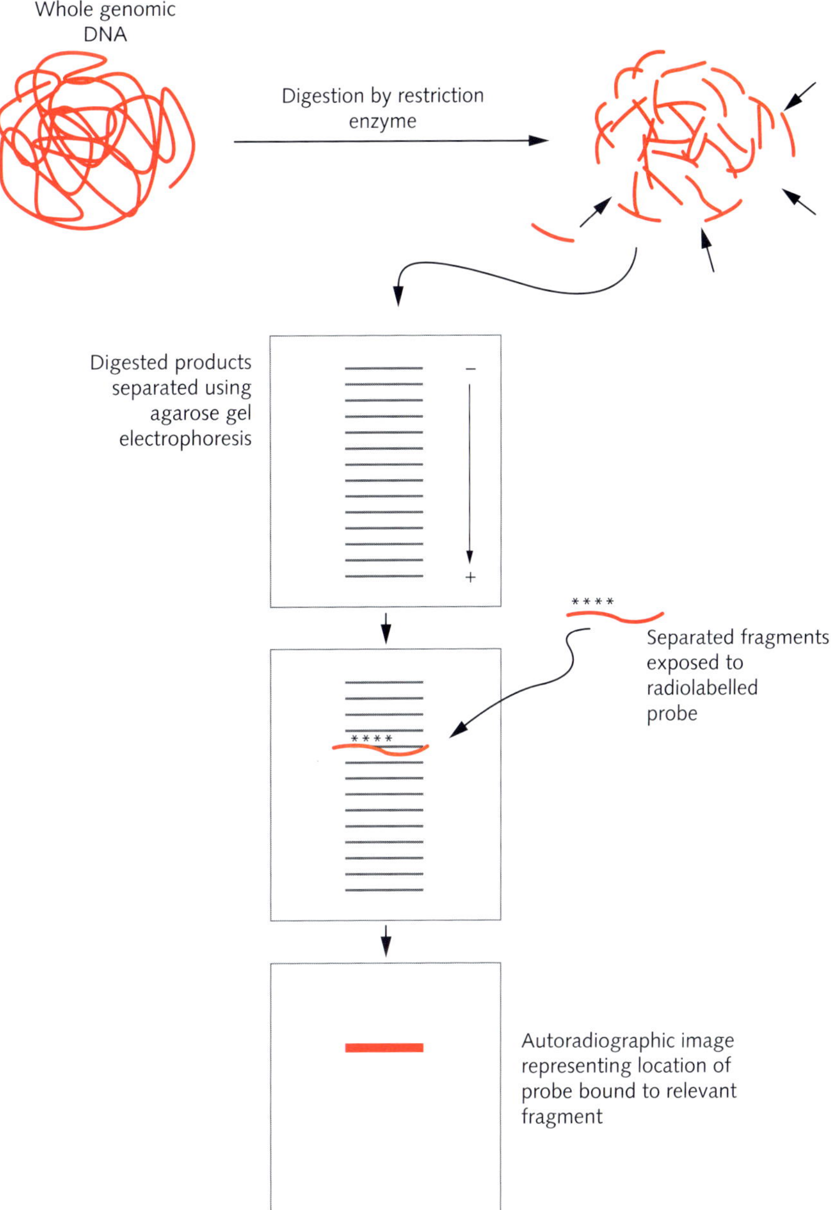

Fig. 4.2 Principle of Southern blotting
Genomic DNA is digested using restriction enzyme following which the fragments are separated on the basis of size using agarose gel electrophoresis and finally transferred to a nylon membrane. Radiolabelled probe for the gene of interest is hybridised to the DNA on the membrane and, after removal of the non-specifically hybridised probe, the location and size of the fragment are determined using autoradiography.

standard karyotyping for follow-up marrows in patients with leukaemias or lymphomas, but is still of limited value for MRD detection.

Molecular techniques—Southern blot hybridisation

Initially described by its inventor, Professor Ed Southern in the 1970s, Southern blotting involves digestion of chromosomal DNA using bacterial restriction enzymes, with size separation of the DNA fragments using electric current and gel electrophoresis before transferring these to a nylon support membrane. A labelled probe for the gene of interest is applied which binds to its complementary sequence on the membrane and visualisation of the gene is by autoradiography (Figure 4.2).

Southern blotting is useful for initial diagnosis of leukaemia and lymphoma using probes specific for translocations or gene rearrangements. With Southern blotting, a non-germline or rearranged gene pattern may be seen in DNA from a population of cells where more than 1% of the total population is made up by a clone of malignant lymphoid cells. In other words, Southern blotting will detect a rearranged gene providing the cells containing the rearranged gene exceed 1 in 100 normal cells. The downside of Southern blotting is that the technique is not sufficiently sensitive for the detection of small numbers of malignant cells that persist following therapy and which give rise to disease relapse. For this reason, Southern blotting has largely been replaced by PCR for detection of MRD.

Polymerase chain reaction amplification of DNA

As described above, Southern blotting is a useful technique for assessing whether there is a clone of abnormal cells in blood, marrow or other tissue but is not useful if these cells are present in only very small amounts. In this case, techniques that involve amplification of specific DNA sequences are required. PCR has filled the void in this respect and has found a place in diagnostic laboratories investigating oncogenes, haematological malignancies, single gene disorders and infectious diseases. Part of the attraction of a PCR-based approach is its extreme simplicity and the speed with which results are obtained.

What is PCR amplification?

In essence, two short oligonucleotide DNA primers are synthesised that are complementary to the DNA sequence on either side of the translocation or gene of interest. The region between the primers is filled in using a heat-stable bacterial DNA polymerase (Taq) from the hot-spring bacterium *Thermus aquaticus*. After a single round of amplification has been performed, the whole process is repeated (Figure 4.3). This takes place 30 times (i.e. through 30 cycles of amplification) and leads to a million-fold increase in the amount of specific sequence. After the 30 cycles are complete, a sample of the PCR is electrophoresed on agarose or polyacrylamide gel. Information about the presence or absence of the region or mutation of interest is obtained by assessing the size and number of different PCR products obtained after 30 cycles of amplification.

The specificity of PCR can be further increased by the use of nested PCR which involves re-amplification of a small amount of the amplified product (obtained using outside, external, primers) using internal oligonucleotide primers.

PCR has the advantage that very little tissue sample is required for analysis and the technique can be applied to a variety of different sample types, for example fresh, unfixed, cryopreserved, formalin fixed paraffin embedded tissue as well as haematoxylin and eosin stained and formalin fixed tissue.

PCR may be used to detect the presence of chromosomal translocations. The most commonly investigated rearrangements include the t(9;22) chromosomal translocation in chronic myeloid leukaemia (CML), t(1;19) found in a subset of pre-B-cell ALL, the t(14;18) found in 85% of follicular and 15% diffuse large cell lymphoma, and several others. Alternatively, in the lymphoid malignancies, if the tumour being investigated does not carry a translocation marker, PCR may be used to amplify rearranged antigen receptor (Ig or TCR) genes.

Molecular targets

Chromosomal translocations

Translocations, involving transfer of DNA between chromosomes, are found in many of the haematological malignancies. Other chromosomal abnormalities include chromosomal deletions and inversions. Table 4.2 shows some of the translocations described in myeloid and lymphoid malignancies. As a result of chromosomal translocation a gene from one chromosome ends up adjacent to a gene on the chromosome to which the DNA has been translocated, and this may have important consequences for the cell (and the patient). If a potentially cancerous gene (proto-oncogene), which is generally not transcriptionally active, abuts onto a gene that is being actively transcribed, this may result in upregulation of expression of that proto-oncogene. This is exactly the situation in many translocations described to date. In some cases, such as the translocation between chromosomes 14 and 18 found in many cases of follicular lymphoma, the *BCL-2* gene is moved to chromosome 14 and comes under the transcriptional control of the immunoglobulin heavy chain (IgH) gene, which is transcribed actively. The increase in BCL-2 protein prevents apoptosis (programmed cell death) and this may explain, in part, the underlying pathogenesis of some lymphomas.

The first non-random chromosome translocation described was the Philadelphia chromosome, in which reciprocal translocation of DNA between chromosomes 9 and 22 takes place. In the t(9;22), the distal ends of 9 and 22 are exchanged in a so-called reciprocal translocation, i.e. there is no overall net loss or gain of genetic material. The C-*ABL* proto-oncogene from chromosome 9 becomes joined to *BCR* (breakpoint cluster region) on chromosome 22 resulting in a chimeric fusion protein which has tyrosine kinase properties,

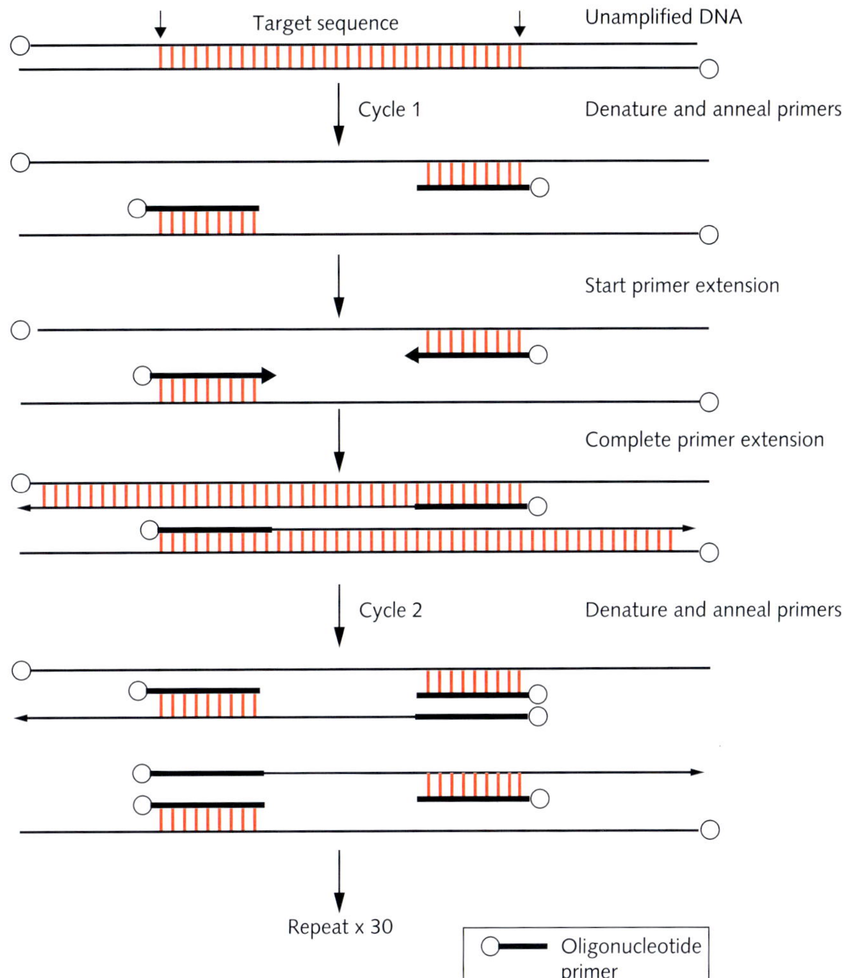

Fig. 4.3 Simplified PCR schema
Double-stranded DNA is denatured to allow binding of specific oligonucleotides on either side of the region of interest. Taq DNA polymerase extends the oligonucleotides before the double-stranded molecules are denatured and the process repeated.

and through some unknown mechanism leads to the typical CML phenotype (*discussed in detail in Chapter 5*).

Detecting the presence of translocations (Table 4.3)

Some translocations are disease-specific

Follicular lymphoma is characterised by the t(14;18) which is found in almost 90% of cases. However, this translocation is found in other types of non-Hodgkin's lymphoma (NHL) and at very low copy number in virtually every healthy individual, so that the t(14;18) is not, in itself, diagnostic of one particular malignancy. In contrast, acute promyelocytic leukaemia (AML M3) is characterised by a reciprocal translocation between chromosomes 15 and 17 which is found in the majority of cases, but unlike t(14;18) the t(15;17) is not found in any other neoplasm or in health and so serves as a diagnostic marker for this disease (although its absence does not exclude the diagnosis).

Translocations may be used for detecting residual disease

Translocations serve as useful diagnostic disease markers at presentation for a variety of leukaemias and lymphomas. For detection of MRD, standard cytogenetic analysis for detection of translocations is not sufficiently sensitive for follow-up but other techniques can be applied, including FISH and PCR. FISH techniques are constantly being improved (*see Chapter 2*) and may be of value for MRD detection. However, more sensitive MRD detection is possible using PCR in cases where the translocations are well characterised and DNA on either side of the breakpoints has been sequenced. MRD using the chromosomal translocations t(14;18) and t(9;22) is described later.

Disease	Translocation	Genes involved
Acute myeloid leukaemia		
M2	t (8;21)	*ETO–AML1*
M2 or M4	t (6;9)	*DEK–CAN*
M3	t (15;17)	*PML–RARα*
M4	inv (16)	*CBFβ–MYH11*
Acute lymphoblastic leukaemia		
B-lineage	t (9;22)	*BCR–ABL*
	t (1;19)	*E2A–PBX1*
	t (17;19)	*HLF–E2A*
	t (12;21)	*TEL–AML-1*
	t (4;11)	*AF4–MLL*
	t (8;14)	*MYC–IgH*
T-lineage	TAL interstitial deletion	*TAL*
	t (1;14)	*TAL-1–TCRδ*
	t (10;14)	*HOX11–TCRα*
	t (11;14)	*11p13–TCRδ*
Lymphomas		
Follicular and diffuse NHL	t (14;18)	*BCL-2–IgH*
Mantle cell lymphoma	t (11;14)	*BCL-1–IgH*
Burkitt's lymphoma	t (8;14)	*MYC–IgH*
Anaplastic lymphoma	t (2;5)	*ALK–NPM*
Gene rearrangements		
Immunoglobulin heavy chain	B-cell lymphoma/leukaemia	
T-cell receptors	T-cell lymphoma/leukaemia	

Table 4.2 PCR amplifiable chromosomal translocations and gene rearrangements in human haematological disorders.

Table 4.3 Detecting the presence of translocations.

Standard cytogenetics
If the translocation alters the appearance of banded chromosomes using standard cytogenetic analysis.
Fluorescence *in situ* hybridisation (FISH)
Using metaphase or interphase techniques.
Polymerase chain reaction
Requires the DNA on either side of the breakpoint to be sequenced to allow oligonucleotide primers to be constructed.

Antigen receptor gene rearrangements—immunoglobulin and TCR genes as molecular markers

Many haematopoietic malignancies have no detectable translocation suitable for PCR amplification, and in these cases an alternative strategy is required. In the lymphoid malignancies there is rearrangement of the antigen receptor at the IgH or TCR genes. Immunoglobulin (Ig) and TCR molecules belong to a group of related proteins termed the immunoglobulin superfamily. Other members include CD8, N-CAM and MHC molecules. Both Ig and TCR molecules have many similarities and have been shown to share common amino acid motifs. It is estimated that the immune system requires in excess of 10^{10} specific antibodies to respond to antigenic determinants encountered in the environment. If each Ig molecule were encoded separately in the germline most of our genome would consist simply of Ig genes. Elegant work by Tonegawa has shown that Ig and TCR genes exist in the germline state as non-contiguous DNA segments that are rearranged during lymphocyte development (Table 4.4). Gene rearrangement involves recombination of germline gene segments resulting in a permanently altered non-germline configuration (Figure 4.4). The process of Ig and TCR gene assembly ensures almost limitless variation of Ig and TCR molecules using only a limited amount of chromosomal DNA. Other features that ensure Ig and TCR variability include imprecise joining of individual V, D and J segments, duplication and inversion of segments, and somatic mutation (in Ig genes) of V, D and J.

The immunoglobulin heavy chain locus

During normal lymphoid development, both B and T

Table 4.4 Immunoglobulin and T-cell receptor diversity is achieved through rearrangement of separate germline segments.

Diversity of immunoglobulin and TCR genes	Immunoglobulin			T-cell receptor			
	H	κ	λ	α	β	γ	δ
V segments	250	100	100	60	80	8	6
D segments	15	0	0	0	2	0	3
J segments	6	5	4	50	13	5	3
VDJ recombination	104	500	400	3000	2000	40	18
N regions	2	0	0	1	2	1	4
N region additions	V–D, D–J	none	none	V–J	V–D, D–J	V–J	V–D1, D1–D2, D1–J
V domains	10^{10}	10^4	10^4	10^6	10^9	10^4	10^{13}
V domain pairs	10^{14}			10^{15}		10^{17}	

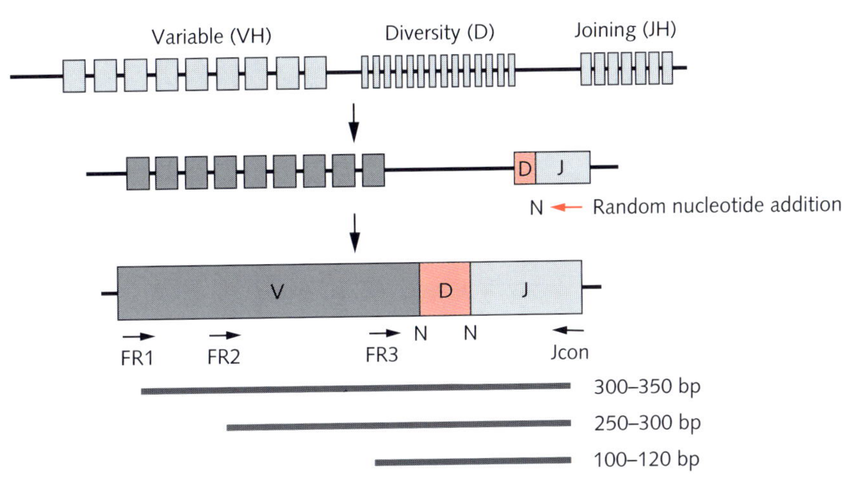

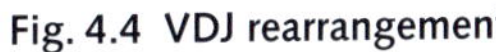

Fig. 4.4 VDJ rearrangement
Rearrangement of non-contiguous germline V, D and J region segments generates a complete V–D–J complex which serves as a useful marker of malignancy. FR1, 2 and 3 refer to framework regions 1, 2 and 3, respectively; N = random N nucleotides; Jcon = JH consensus primer. The sizes of the various PCR products are shown (FR1 + Jcon generates a fragment of 300–350 bp, and so on).

lymphocytes undergo rearrangement of their antigen receptor genes, i.e. Ig genes in B-cells and TCR genes in T-cells, and their clonal progeny bear this identical antigen receptor rearrangement. B-cell neoplasms including NHL, ALL, myeloma and CLL undergo irreversible somatic rearrangement of the IgH locus providing a useful marker of clonality and stage of differentiation in these tumours.

The IgH locus is located on chromosome 14q32.3. Unlike the light chain (IgL) locus IgH contains diversity segments in addition to V, J and C segments. In humans there are around 250 heavy chain variable region (VH) segments of which one-third are probably pseudogenes, representing ancestral gene remnants (denoted by ψ). The VH elements fall into seven families (VH1, VH2, VH3, VH4a, VH4b, VH5 and VH6). Unlike TCR and IgL loci, the IgH locus contains multiple heavy chain constant region (CH) segments (Figure 4.5), some 11 in total, including two pseudogenes (Cμ, Cδ, Cγ3, Cγ1, Cψε, Cα1, Cψγ, Cγ2, Cγ4, Cε and Cα2). Each C segment contains multiple exons corresponding to the functional domains in the heavy chain protein (CH1, CH2, CH3, etc.). The multiple C elements correspond to the different classes of heavy chain encountered during class switching. Cμ generates IgM, Cα generates IgA, and so on. This mechanism ensures that, although the heavy chains are of varying class, they will all bear identical V–D–J sequences.

Third complementarity determining region (CDR3)

The CDR3 region of the IgH gene is generated early in B-cell development and is the result of rearrangement of germline sequences on chromosome 14. One diversity segment is joined to a joining region (D → J). The resulting D–J segment then joins one variable region sequence

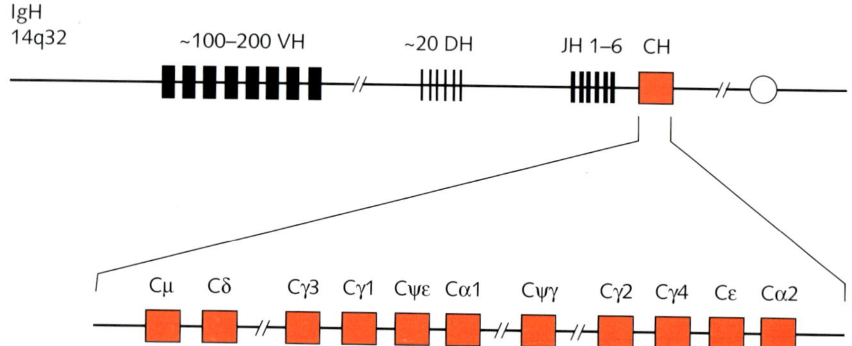

Fig. 4.5 Genetic map of region 14q32 The CH segments are shown towards the 3′ end of the region.

(V → DJ) producing a V–D–J complex (Figure 4.4). The enzyme terminal deoxynucleotide transferase (TdT) inserts random nucleotides at two sites: the V–D and D–J junctions. At the same time random deoxynucleotides are removed by exonucleases. Antibody diversity is further increased by somatic mutation, a process which is not found in TCR genes. The final V–N–D–N–J sequence (CDR3) is unique to that cell, and if the cell multiplies to form a clone then this region will act as a unique marker for that malignant clone. The V(D)J product corresponds to part of the variable region of the antibody molecule.

TCR genes undergo a similar process of rearranging their germline segments to produce complete TCR genes

Junctional region diversity

Imprecise recombination involving V(D)J region DNA enhances the number of possible different antibody molecule polypeptides due to loss or gain of addi2tional nucleotides during the recombination event. The resultant V(D)J product may be functional, i.e. generate antibody molecules or, if the reading frame is lost, non-functional. Whether functional or not, the CDR3 remains a unique marker for the malignant clone.

N region nucleotides are inserted into the CDR3 by TdT

N region nucleotide insertion is seen at the boundary of V, D or J coding segments and is template-independent. These N regions contain between 1 and 12 nucleotides and are more often guanine or cytosine rather than adenine or thymine, reflecting the role played by the enzyme TdT in this process.

Combinatorial association

T-cell receptor molecules are dimeric proteins, usually α + β (TCR α : β), although 5% of circulating T-cells bear the γ : δ T-cell receptor. The random combination of subunits in the TCR dimers further enhances the generation of diversity. The recombination events on one chromosome leading to production of a functional molecule such as TCR α : β result in the inhibition of recombination at that locus on the other chromosome. This so-called allelic exclusion ensures any given lymphocyte will express only one type of receptor molecule.

Somatic mutation

This describes the random introduction of mutations within the V, D and J segments and is well documented in immunoglobulin genes but does not contribute to diversity in the TCR genes. Rearranged V region sequences in B-cells have been analysed and found to differ from those of the germline V sequences from which they were generated. Most of these mutated V regions are found in the secondary immune response on rechallenge of B-cells with antigen. During this process the antibody of the primary response (IgM) is switched to IgG or IgA. The somatic mutation rate has been estimated to be as high as 10^{-3} per base pair per cell generation and the process occurs predominantly in variable regions of the molecule.

The clinical utility of the CDR3 DNA sequence

The description of V–D–J recombination may appear arcane with no obvious relevance in clinical terms, but it is the formation of this unique recombination product that generates a powerful tumour-specific marker which we can use for detection of malignant clones and MRD.

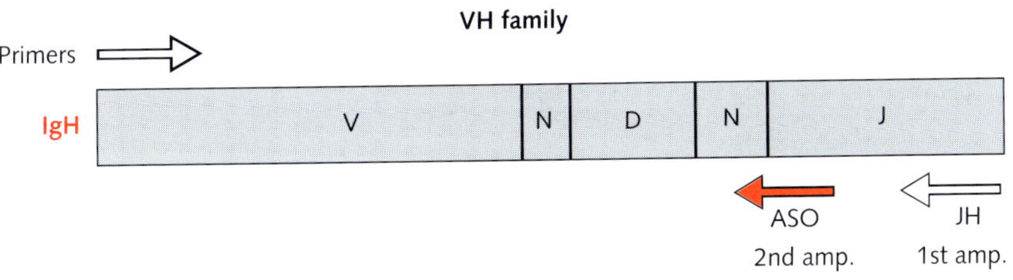

Fig. 4.6 Semi-nested PCR of IgH region in patient with B-cell tumour
V and J region primers are used to generate the initial PCR product. Using DNA sequence information an allele-specific oligonucleotide (ASO) primer unique to that patient is constructed and used with the V region primer to amplify an aliquot of the first round PCR product.

The DNA sequence within the V–D–J is determined by sequencing following which the individual V, D and J segments are delineated. This allows accurate identification of the N region nucleotides (which are generated randomly by the enzyme TdT) which form the basis of the unique clone-specific (patient-specific) probe (Figure 4.6).

There are two sites available for design of the customised probe—the DNA of the V–N–D sequence and that of the D–N–J sequence. Does it matter which one we use to make the probes? The V–N–D sequence generally has a larger N region with more random nucleotides inserted, but the D–N–J site appears preferable to use as a clone-specific probe since there is less base deletion of the 3′ end of the framework region 3 (FR3) than 5′ end of the J region. In addition, the D–J segments appear to be inherently more stable than V–D segments; and finally, where there is V → V switching as happens in some diseases like ALL, the D–J segment remains unchanged and the probe will still detect the clone even if the V regions alter. The consensus view at present is that the D–N–J is probably the best DNA sequence to use to make probes for MRD detection.

Quantitation of the neoplastic cells using PCR

Until fairly recently, PCR amplification simply confirmed the presence (+) or absence (–) of tumour DNA sequences with little scope for quantifying the tumour bulk, particularly when using DNA as the PCR template. A band on agarose gel may represent the DNA from one cell—or many millions of cells. Clearly this is of clinical importance if the information obtained is to be of value in determining the need for further chemotherapy, which underpins the main rationale for attempting to detect MRD in the first place.

In the early years of PCR detection of MRD the starting template was usually DNA, but more recently PCR amplification of reverse transcribed mRNA (termed complementary DNA or cDNA) has been used. This refinement in PCR amplification has evolved where analysis of translocations such as t(9;22) or t(15;17) is impossible using a DNA template, simply because of the enormous size of the target being amplified. In these translocations the primer binding sites are so far apart on the DNA template that amplification is virtually impossible. However, the mRNA transcribed from these translocations undergoes considerable modification with excision of introns making the mRNA counterpart of the translocation much smaller than the DNA.

Quantitation using competitive PCR templates has been possible for RNA-based PCR, and so we are able to quantitate the tumour cell burden in those diseases where RNA is the nucleic acid used for the PCR assays. Diseases in which reverse transcriptase PCR (RT-PCR) is possible, with quantitation of tumour burden, include CML (with t(9;22)), AML M3 (t(15;17)) and AML M2 (t(8;21)).

DNA templates are more difficult to quantitate, although competitive PCR templates may be of value here also. Recent technologies such as the TaqMan® real-time PCR machines may allow true quantitation using DNA as starting material. This system uses an internal oligonucleotide probe with added reporter and quenching activities (Figure 4.7). After primer and probe annealing, the reporter dye is cleaved off by the 5′-3′ nuclease activity of Taq DNA polymerase during primer extension (Figure 4.8). This cleavage of the probe separates the reporter from quencher dye, greatly increasing the reporter dye signal. The sequence detector is able to detect the fluorescent signal during thermal cycling. The advantages of this system are the elimination of post-PCR processing and the ability to examine the entire PCR process—not simply the endpoint of amplification. Moreover, since the probe is designed to be sequence

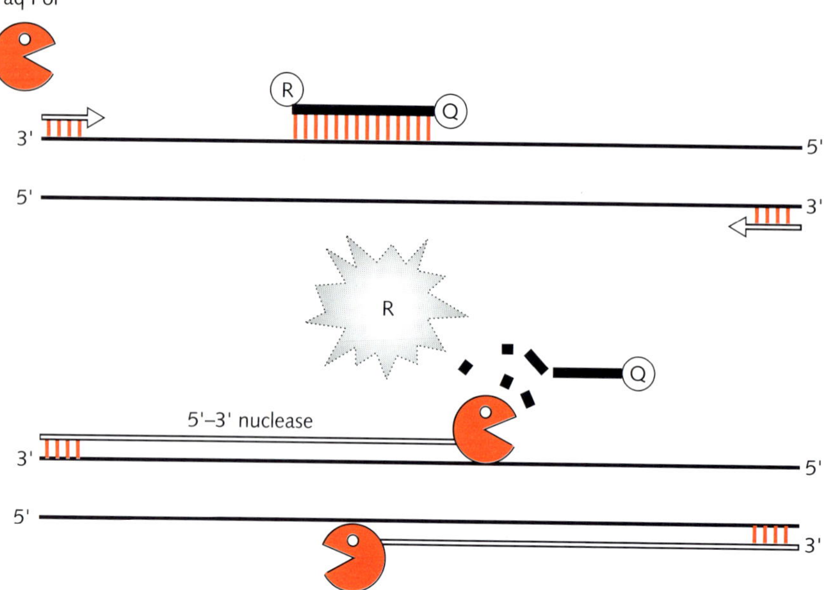

Fig. 4.7 Real-time PCR amplification
See text for details.

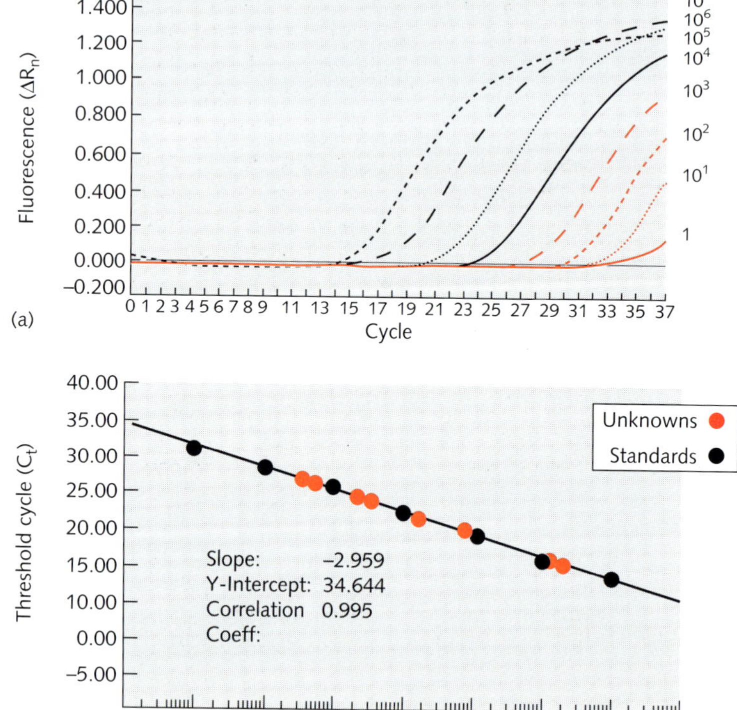

Fig. 4.8 Standard curves generated for accurate quantitation of leukaemic cell burden
Quantitation by real-time PCR requires generation of a standard curve. A known amount of template DNA is diluted into genomic DNA and PCR amplified. The 'threshold cycle' is the cycle number at which reported fluorescence is first detected above background and is proportional to the amount of starting template DNA. The threshold cycle number is then plotted against the known amounts and a standard curve can be generated. The 'threshold' cycle of the unknown samples can then be quantified by reading off the standard curve.

specific, non-specific amplification products are not detected.

Application of PCR for residual disease detection in non-Hodgkin's lymphoma

The standard technique used for the diagnosis of NHL is light microscopy of stained sections of lymph node or other tissue. This allows accurate classification of lymphoma subtype. In terms of detecting MRD, this technique has the limitation of detecting lymphoma cells only when they comprise approximately 5% or greater of all cells (i.e. 1 malignant cell in 20 normal cells). Application of flow cytometric analysis for the detection of NHL has been hampered by the lack of lymphoma-specific monoclonal antibodies (mAbs) since all the cell surface antigens identified to date on the surface of lymphoma cells are also present on normal B-cell or B-cell precursor cells (Table 4.5).

Table 4.5 Clinical utility of PCR-based studies in patients with non-Hodgkin's lymphoma.

- Detection of bone marrow infiltration as part of staging procedure.
- Detection of circulating lymphoma cells in peripheral blood.
- Detection of minimal residual disease following therapy.
- Assessing contribution of reinfused lymphoma cells to relapse in patients undergoing autologous bone marrow transplantation.
- Assessing ability of purging techniques to eradicate residual malignant cells in marrow.

Chromosomal translocations

As shown in Table 4.2, a number of chromosomal translocations and gene rearrangements associated with NHL have been identified, the breakpoints sequenced and are applicable for PCR amplification.

t(14;18) translocation

One of the most widely studied non-random chromosomal translocations in NHL is the t(14;18) occurring in 85% of patients with follicular lymphoma and 30% of patients with diffuse large cell lymphoma. In the t(14;18) the *BCL-2* proto-oncogene on chromosome 18 is juxtaposed with the IgH locus on chromosome 14 (Figure 4.9). The breakpoints have been cloned and sequenced, and have been shown to cluster at two main regions 3′ to the *BCL-2* coding region: the major breakpoint region (*MBR*) within the 3′ untranslated region of the *BCL-2* gene, and the minor breakpoint cluster region (m-*BCR*) located 20 kb downstream. Juxtaposition of the transcriptionally active IgH with the *BCL-2* gene results in upregulation of the *BCL-2* gene product and subsequent resistance to programmed cell death by apoptosis.

The clustering of the breakpoints at these two main regions at the *BCL-2* gene and the availability of consensus regions of the IgH joining (J) regions make this an ideal candidate for PCR amplification to detect lymphoma cells containing the t(14;18) translocation. A major advantage in the detection of lymphoma cells bearing the *BCL-2*/IgH translocation is that DNA rather than RNA can be used to detect the translocation. In addition, since there is a variation at the site of the break-

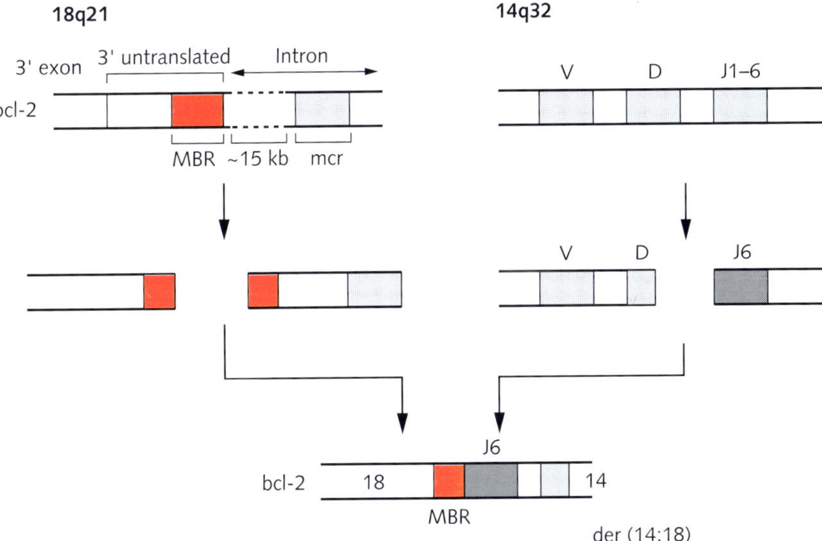

Fig. 4.9 t(14;18) translocation In the t(14;18) the *BCL-2* locus on chromosome 18 is juxtaposed to the IgH locus on chromosome 14. The breakpoints on chromosome 18 cluster at two main regions, the major breakpoint region (*MBR*) in the 5′ untranslated region of the *BCL-2* gene, and the minor cluster region (mcr) downstream in the intron. The chimeric gene product provides a unique tumour marker that can be PCR amplified using primers upstream of the *MBR* or mcr region with consensus primers within the J region of the IgH gene.

point at the *BCL-2* gene, the PCR products for individual patients differ in size and have unique sequences. The size of the PCR product can be assessed by gel electrophoresis and used as confirmation that the expected size fragment is amplified from a specific patient.

Other translocations in non-Hodgkin's lymphoma

t(11;14)(q13;q32) is associated with a number of B-cell malignancies including B-cell CLL, myeloma and more than 50% of mantle cell lymphomas (MCL). In this translocation the proto-oncogene *BCL-1* (also called *PRAD-1*) on chromosome 11 is juxtaposed to the IgH chain locus on chromosome 14.

One-third of anaplastic lymphomas express the chromosomal translocation t(2;5)(p23;q35) which involves a novel protein tyrosine kinase and nucleophosmin, resulting in a p80 fusion protein. This translocation is detected by RT-PCR where the mRNA sequence is converted into cDNA before PCR amplification.

Utility of molecular techniques for MRD detection

Lymphoma

Over the past decade a number of methods capable of detecting MRD have been developed. These techniques have clearly illustrated that patients in clinical complete remission (CR) often harbour malignant cells in low numbers. The clinical significance of the detection of such MRD is still being evaluated and remains unclear. The results of these studies will likely have great impact on the clinical management of patients as we understand more about the contribution of minimal disease to subsequent relapse. The prognostic significance of the achievement of a molecular CR remains elusive, and few studies to date have demonstrated the importance of eradicating MRD in the patient to achieve cure.

PCR detection of bone marrow (BM) infiltration as a staging procedure

Lymphomas generally originate in lymphoid tissue, but as the disease progresses there may be spread to other sites such as bone marrow and blood. At initial presentation all patients undergo staging investigations to determine the extent of disease as a means of planning treatment. A number of studies have examined the use of PCR detection of t(14;18) as a staging procedure to detect lymphoma cells in the bone marrow and peripheral blood at the time of initial presentation. However, PCR analysis cannot replace morphological assessment of BM since not all patients have translocations detectable by PCR, and these techniques are essentially complementary. These PCR studies have all detected lymphoma cells in the BM in a number of patients who had no overt evidence of marrow infiltration by morphology. Of great interest are those studies that have evaluated the clinical utility of MRD detection in those patients presenting with localised disease. Although the patient numbers studied are small, a significant number of patients can be found who would be upstaged from early stage to advanced stage disease by the results of PCR analysis. Whether PCR detection of minimal marrow infiltration will eventually lead to modifications in therapy in those patients currently treated with localised radiotherapy remains to be determined.

PCR detection of MRD following chemotherapy

In follicular lymphoma long-term analysis of patients after completion of conventional chemotherapy has shown that conventional dose chemotherapy does not eradicate PCR detectable disease, but this may not be associated with poor outcome. One study has shown no association between the presence or absence of PCR detectable lymphoma cells and clinical outcome. Moreover, this confirms the previous observation that some patients can indeed remain in long-term continuous complete remission despite the presence of PCR detectable lymphoma cells, strongly suggesting that the detection of residual lymphoma cells has no prognostic significance. Cells containing t(14;18) might not always represent residual lymphoma cells, but may be cells with this translocation but without the additional necessary cellular changes required for malignant transformation. However, an alternative explanation is that conventional chemotherapy might not cure any patients with advanced stage follicular lymphoma and that all patients with persistent lymphoma cells are destined to relapse. The long-term remission status of these small numbers of patients might therefore represent merely the very long tempo of their disease course.

These studies suggest that conventional dose chemotherapy does not result in a molecular remission. More novel treatment approaches including the use of bone marrow transplantation, more aggressive induction therapy and combinations of monoclonal antibody therapy with chemotherapy have all been reported to be capable of eradicating PCR detectable disease, achieving so-called 'molecular CR'. In all of these circumstances, eradication of PCR detectable disease has been shown to be associated with improved outcome in follicular lymphoma, strongly suggestive that eradication of MRD may be required for cure. With longer follow-up this question should be answered.

Detection of circulating lymphoma cells in peripheral blood (PB)

Blood is less frequently involved than marrow at presentation, but becomes more frequent as disease progresses. Recent studies of patients at the time of presentation have suggested a high level of concordance between the detection of lymphoma cells in the PB and BM when assessed by PCR. However, other studies have found that the BM is more likely than PB to contain infiltrating lymphoma cells in previously untreated patients. The presence of residual lymphoma in the BM but not in the PB argues strongly that the marrow is indeed infiltrated with lymphoma in these patients and does not simply represent contamination from the PB. The findings of PB contamination with NHL when assessed by PCR are likely to have profound implications since increasing interest is now being placed in the use of PB stem cells, rather than BM, as a source of haematopoietic progenitors. A number of studies have demonstrated that PB stem cell collections may also be contaminated with lymphoma cells when assessed by PCR techniques. In addition, much work is being performed to monitor the effects of chemotherapy and growth factors that are used to mobilise haematopoietic progenitor cells, to ensure that these agents do not also mobilise lymphoma cells.

Contribution of re-infused lymphoma cells to relapse after autologous bone marrow transplantation (ABMT)

In low-grade NHL there has been increasing interest in the use of high-dose therapy as salvage therapy for patients who have failed conventional dose chemotherapy regimens. The resulting myeloablation (ablation of patient's marrow) after high-dose therapy can be rescued by infusion of allogeneic or autologous BM. Autologous BM has several potential advantages over allogeneic BM for marrow rescue: there is no need for a histocompatible donor and there is no risk of graft-versus-host disease. Autologous stem cell transplantation (ASCT) can therefore be performed more safely and in older patients, and has become a major treatment option for an increasing number of patients with haematological malignancies.

The major obstacle to the use of ASCT is that the re-infusion of occult tumour cells harboured within the marrow may result in more rapid relapse of disease. To minimise the effects of the infusion of significant numbers of malignant cells, most centres obtain marrow for ABMT when the patient is either in CR or when there is no evidence by histological examination of BM infiltration of disease. A variety of methods have therefore been developed to *purge* malignant cells from the marrow in order to eliminate any contaminating malignant cells and leave intact the haematopoietic stem cells that are necessary for engraftment. The development of purging techniques has led subsequently to a number of studies of ASCT in patients with either a previous history of BM infiltration or even overt marrow infiltration at the time of BM harvest. Because of their specificity, mAbs are ideal agents for selective elimination of malignant cells. Clinical studies have demonstrated that immunologic purging can deplete malignant cells *in vitro* without significantly impairing haematologic engraftment.

Assessing purging efficacy by PCR

PCR has been used to assess the efficacy of immunological purging in models using lymphoma cell lines, demonstrating that PCR is a highly sensitive and efficient method to determine the efficacy of purging residual lymphoma cells. The efficacy of purging varies between the cell lines studied, making it likely that there would also be variability between patient samples.

PCR amplifications of the t(14;18), t(11;14) and IgH rearrangements have all been used to detect residual lymphoma cells in the BM before and after purging in patients undergoing ABMT to assess whether the efficiency of purging had any impact on disease-free survival. In one study, 114 patients with B-cell NHL and the *BCL-2* translocation were studied. Residual lymphoma cells were detected by PCR analysis in the harvested autologous BM of all patients. Following three cycles of immunologic purging using the anti-B-cell mAbs J5 (anti-CD10), B1 (anti-CD20) and B5 and complement mediated lysis, PCR amplification detected residual lymphoma cells in 50% of these patients. The incidence of relapse was significantly increased in the patients who had residual detectable lymphoma cells compared to those in whom no lymphoma cells were detectable after purging.

The majority of patients who relapse do so at sites of previous disease, suggesting that the major contribution to subsequent relapse came from endogenous disease and not from the infused marrow. However, there was an association between the detection of residual lymphoma cells in the circulation and the detection of residual lymphoma cells within the re-infused BM. Since follicular lymphoma cells use the same adhesion receptors as normal B-cells to bind to the germinal centre, circulating lymphoma cells may therefore be capable of homing back to the sites of previous disease and it is these sites that provide the microenvironmental conditions conducive for cell growth.

Detection of residual lymphoma cells in the marrow after transplantation is associated with increased incidence of subsequent relapse

Since PCR analysis detected residual lymphoma cells after conventional dose chemotherapy in the majority of patients studied, it is not surprising that it has not been possible to determine any prognostic significance for the persistence of PCR detectable lymphoma cells. At the Dana-Farber Cancer Institute, PCR analysis was performed on serial BM samples obtained after ASCT to assess whether high-dose therapy might be capable of depleting PCR detectable lymphoma cells. The persistence or re-appearance of residual detectable lymphoma cells greatly adversely influenced the disease-free survival of patients in this study after high-dose therapy. In contrast to previous findings that all patients had BM infiltration following conventional dose therapy, no PCR detectable lymphoma cells could be detected in the most recent BM sample obtained from more than 50% of patients following high-dose chemo-radiotherapy and ASCT, and none of these patients relapsed. All patients who relapsed had PCR detectable lymphoma cells in the BM prior to relapse, irrespective of the site of relapse. The results of this study suggest that detection of MRD by PCR following ASCT in patients with lymphoma identifies those patients who require additional treatment for cure, and also suggest that our therapeutic goal should be to eradicate all PCR detectable lymphoma cells.

Acute leukaemias

Acute lymphoblastic leukaemia

Childhood ALL has been one of the great success stories of modern chemotherapy and cure rates approaching 80% have been achieved in recently reported series. ALL cells usually rearrange either the IgH or TCR genes or both and these provide markers that can be used to assess the clinical significance of MRD detection in a disease with such a high likelihood of cure. Despite near uniformity in approaches of management of newly diagnosed ALL, the issue of whether eradication of PCR detectable MRD is necessary for cure remains highly controversial in this disease. The majority of studies have suggested that modern aggressive induction regimens are often associated with rapid elimination of PCR detectable disease. Additional studies have suggested an association between the rate of decrease of detectable disease and subsequent prognosis. However, a significant number of patients have persistence of PCR detectable disease and yet have not relapsed. One study suggested that, using the most sensitive PCR analysis, it is possible to detect persistent cells bearing the tumour-associated antigen receptor rearrangement in the majority of patients, indicating that it is neither possible nor necessary to eradicate PCR detectable disease for cure. For this reason, many current studies are addressing whether the quantitative assessment of MRD may be required to predict which patients are ultimately fated to relapse. Most studies addressing this issue have suggested that a quantitative increase in tumour burden is almost invariably associated with impending relapse.

t(12;21)

The *TEL/AML-1* gene rearrangement results from the cryptic reciprocal translocation t(12;21). This is the most common gene rearrangement found in childhood ALL and accounts for 25% of pre-B-cell ALL in children, but is rarely found in adult ALL. Some data are suggestive that the presence of this rearrangement is associated with a good prognosis.

APML—acute promyelocytic leukaemia (AML M3)

AML M3 is associated with a balanced chromosomal translocation between chromosomes 15 and 17 resulting in t(15;17)(q22;q21), leading to rearrangement of the *RARα* gene (also termed *RARA*) on chromosome 17 and *PML* on chromosome 15 (Figure 4.10). With rearrangement of DNA, the chromosomal translocation produces two novel fusion genes involving *PML* and *RARα* namely *PML/RARα* and *RARα/PML*. It is believed that the *PML/RARα* is responsible for the development of aberrant haematopoiesis. There are two isoforms of the *PML/RARα* fusion gene—long and short. Patients who possess the short isoform have a poorer clinical outcome than those in whom the long isoform is found, but the exact mechanism involved is unclear at present.

The resultant fusion protein (*PML/RARα*) contains functional domains in both *PML* and *RARα*, and binds all-*trans* retinoic acid (ATRA) to which the leukaemic cells in AML M3 are exquisitely sensitive. In fact ATRA,

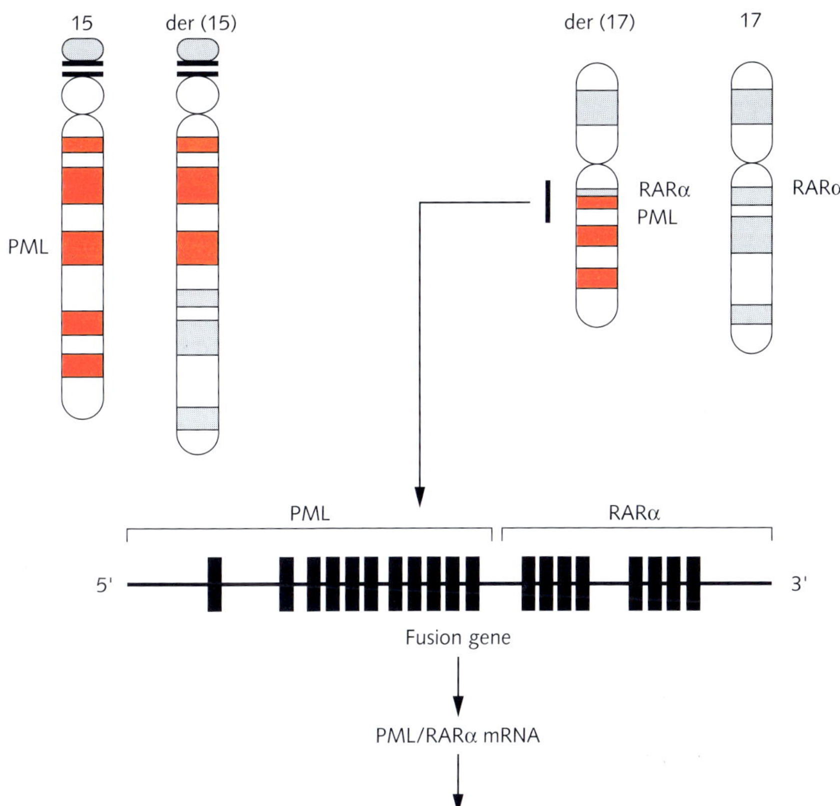

Fig. 4.10 t(15;17)(q22;q21) translocation
Balanced translocation involving *RARα* gene (at 17q21) and *PML* gene (15q22) found in AML M3 (APML) in >90% of cases. The chimeric PML/RARα protein plays a role in the differentiation block characteristic of APML.

which induces differentiation of the leukaemic cells, may alone achieve remission in 80% of *de novo* cases of AML M3. The effects of retinoids are mediated by two classes of retinoic acid receptor: RAR and RXR, both of which are members of a superfamily of related ligand-inducible transcriptional regulatory factors. RAR (α, β and γ) are activated by ATRA and 9-*cis* retinoic acid. RXR (α, β and γ) are activated by 9-*cis* retinoic acid only.

Patients with APML and t(15;17) who achieve remission are now regarded as 'good-risk' patients with a 60% chance of achieving long-term remission. The presence of the fusion gene may be inferred from cytogenetic analysis (i.e. the presence of typical translocation) or, more recently, by a RT-PCR method. In this, the *PML/RARα* mRNA is reverse transcribed into cDNA, which is then used for PCR detection of the abnormal transcript. The RT-PCR assay has been used to quantitate residual leukaemic cells in patients with M3 undergoing chemotherapy.

Trial data suggest that persistence of t(15;17) determined by the PCR approach predicts outcome; those patients who fail to become PCR negative or who become PCR positive following a period of PCR negativity subsequently suffer overt clinical relapse. This appears to be one leukaemia where attainment of 'molecular CR' does matter.

t(8;21)

Translocation t(8;21) occurs in up to 10% of *de novo* AML cases. It is more common in AML with features of maturation. This gene fuses the *AML* gene on 21q22 with the *ETO* gene on 8q22. The breakpoints in this translocation invariably occur within defined regions in the *AML* and *ETO* genes, resulting in a fairly uniform fusion product. Early studies of this translocation suggested that there was persistence of this transcript in almost all cases studied, even in patients in long-term remission. This is suggestive that the *AML1/ETO* translocation may be necessary, but in itself insufficient, for leukaemic transformation. Of note, more recent studies using quantitative PCR analysis have suggested, however, that a quantitative increase in the fusion transcript is predictive of subsequent relapse.

Chronic leukaemias

Chronic myeloid leukaemia

Detection of t(9;22) by PCR amplification

The t(9;22), termed the Philadelphia chromosome, was described in 1960 by Nowell and Hungerford, and represented the first non-random chromosomal abnormality shown to be associated with a specific neoplasm, namely CML (although it is found in other disorders). The t(9;22) is formed by the fusion of the *BCR* gene on chromosome 22 with the *ABL* proto-oncogene on chromosome 9 and occurs in the vast majority of patients with CML and in up to 20% of adult patients with ALL. The chronic myeloid leukaemic cells transcribe an 8.5 kb chimeric mRNA that is translated into a 210 kDa protein (p210) with tyrosine kinase activity. The breakpoints at the *ABL* gene can occur at any point up to 200 kb upstream in the intron and therefore cannot easily be amplified by PCR using genomic DNA as described earlier in this chapter. In contrast, the chimeric mRNA will usually be of two possible types. It is therefore possible to amplify the chimeric mRNA by first reverse transcribing to cDNA. Using this technique it is possible to detect one leukaemic cell in up to 10^6 normal cells (*see Chapter 5*).

Detection of MRD after bone marrow transplant (BMT) in chronic myeloid leukaemia

CML is incurable using standard chemotherapy and currently allogeneic BMT remains the treatment of choice for suitable patients. However, 20% of patients transplanted in chronic phase and more than 50% of patients transplanted in accelerated phase or blast crisis will relapse. Considerable effort has been made to establish whether persistence of MRD after allogeneic BMT is predictive of relapse. Early studies yielded conflicting results as to the clinical implications of persistence of PCR detectable disease. However, a recent large study from Seattle, including analysis from 346 patients, showed a clear association between relapse and persistence of PCR detectable disease. Detection of MRD early after BMT does not necessarily suggest a poor prognosis and a PCR-positive sample at 3 months post-BMT was not informative for clinical outcome. In contrast, a PCR-positive BM or peripheral blood sample at or after 6 months post-BMT was closely associated with subsequent relapse. Statistical analysis of the data revealed that the PCR assay for the *BCR-ABL* fusion transcript 6 to 12 months post-BMT is an independent predictor of subsequent relapse. In contrast, no clear prediction of clinical outcome could be made in patients who tested PCR-positive more than 3 years after BMT. This study and others have clearly demonstrated that most patients are PCR-positive at 3 months after BMT, indicating that BMT preparative regimens alone do not eradicate CML cells effectively. Nevertheless, since this treatment leads to cure in more than 50% of patients, other mechanisms, for example immunological mechanisms, must be responsible for tumour eradication.

Chronic lymphocytic leukaemia

This is the commonest leukaemia in adults and affects the elderly predominantly. A full description of CLL and its molecular abnormalities is provided in *Chapter 8*. Most are B-cell neoplasms (95%), which demonstrate a variety of cytogenetic abnormalities that are of value for molecular diagnosis and residual disease detection. Karyotypic abnormalities include trisomy 12, deletions or translocations of chromosomes 11 and 13. Since these tumours are of B-cell origin, rearranged IgH genes may be used to confirm clonality and also detect residual tumour following chemotherapy and, in younger poor-risk patients, bone marrow transplantation.

Bone marrow transplantation is generally precluded in most patients with CLL due to the advanced age of the patients affected. However, recent studies of younger patients with aggressive disease who have undergone either autologous or allogeneic BMT have shown that PCR detectable disease is often present at, or shortly after, transplant, but this does not predict relapse. In the largest single centre study, the methods used for the analysis involved PCR amplification of the IgH locus with sequencing of the CDR3 products, before constructing patient-specific oligonucleotide probes which were then used to probe the PCR products from marrow or blood samples following the transplant. Data suggest that patients who remain PCR-positive in the months following transplant or become PCR-positive, having been PCR-negative initially, tend to relapse. Those that remain PCR-negative or become negative after a period of PCR positivity remain in clinical and morphological remission (Figure 4.11). Obviously, with an indolent slow growing disease like CLL, we must wait some years before the data can be interpreted fully, since it may be that ultimately all patients will relapse.

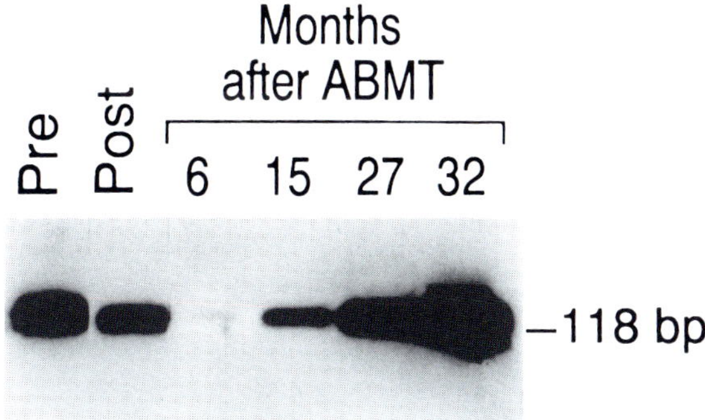

Fig 4.11 Detection of relapse of CLL in a patient undergoing autologous bone marrow transplantation using PCR
In the samples before (pre) and following (post) purging of the patient's marrow PCR positivity is clearly seen. Six months following ABMT no PCR detectable signal is seen. However, at 15, 27 and 32 months following the transplant PCR positivity is easily detected. These findings were confirmed clinically and using standard morphological examination of the patient's bone marrow.

Problems with PCR analysis for detection of minimal residual disease

The major concern with PCR-based disease detection will always be the fear of false positive results because of the ability of the technique to amplify even minute amounts of contaminating DNA. Unlike cell culture assays, it is not possible to determine whether cells detected by PCR are clonogenic (i.e. capable of division and causing relapse). Cells bearing a translocation may be committed progenitors incapable of further proliferation, or might have been sufficiently damaged by previous exposure to chemotherapy or radiotherapy to be already dead but will still be detectable by PCR analysis. A potential problem with the use of PCR of the *BCL-2*/IgH translocation is that this translocation may not be specific for lymphoma cells. Cells bearing the translocation have been detected in hyperplastic lymphoid tissue in healthy individuals with no evidence of lymphoma, and more recently have been shown to occur rarely in normal B-cells.

Conclusions

Methodologies have been developed for the sensitive detection of MRD in lymphoma and leukaemia that are applicable to many patients. The question that now remains to be answered is whether these techniques will have any clinical utility and will predict which patients will relapse. In NHL these studies are most advanced in patients with t(14;18). In these patients, conventional dose chemotherapy does not appear to be capable of depleting PCR detectable lymphoma cells although lymphoma cells were detectable in PB in only half of the patients studied. Following ASCT, the persistence or reappearance of PCR detectable lymphoma cells in the BM was associated with an increased likelihood of relapse. In lymphomas that do not express the t(14;18), it is not yet clear whether failure to detect MRD in PB and BM will predict which patients will relapse since other subtypes of lymphoma may relapse in nodal sites without detectable lymphoma cells in the circulation.

From available data there are clearly diseases in which persistence of PCR detectable disease following treatment predicts relapse, and others where it does not. The full relevance of these findings will become clearer as we understand more about the biology of the diseases and additional data are generated as part of ongoing major clinical trials.

Further reading

Polymerase chain reaction

Kwok S, Higuchi R. (1989) Avoiding false positives with PCR. *Nature*, **339**, 237–238.

Saiki RK, Gelfand DH, Stoffel S *et al.* (1988) Primer-directed enzymatic amplification of DNA with a thermostable DNA polymerase. *Science*, **239**, 487–491.

Antigen receptor genes

Aisenberg AC. (1993) Utility of gene rearrangements in lymphoid malignancies. *Annual Review of Medicine*, **44**, 75–84.

Griesser H, Tkachuk D, Reis MD, Mak TW. (1989) Gene rearrangements and translocations in lymphoproliferative diseases. *Blood*, **73**, 1402–1415.

Tonegawa S. (1983) Somatic generation of antibody diversity. *Nature*, **302**, 575–581.

Toyonaga B, Mak TW. (1987) Genes of the T-cell antigen receptor in normal and malignant T cells. *Annual Review of Immunology*, **5**, 585–620.

Acute leukaemias

Cave H, van der Werff ten Bosch J, Suciu S *et al.* (1998) Clinical significance of minimal residual disease in childhood acute lymphoblastic leukemia. European Organization for Research and Treatment of Cancer—Childhood Leukemia Cooperative Group. *New England Journal of Medicine*, **339**, 591–598.

Diverio D, Rossi V, Avvisati G *et al.* (1998) Early detection of relapse by prospective reverse transcriptase-polymerase chain reaction analysis of the PML/RARα fusion gene in patients with acute promyelocytic leukemia enrolled in the GIMEMA-AIEOP multicenter 'AIDA' trial. *Blood*, **92**, 784–789.

Mancini M, Nanni M, Cedrone M *et al.* (1995) Combined cytogenetic, FISH and molecular analysis in acute promyelocytic leukaemia at diagnosis and in complete remission. *British Journal of Haematology*, **91**, 878–884.

Marcucci G, Livak KJ, Bi W *et al.* (1998) Detection of minimal residual disease in patients with AML1/ETO-associated acute myeloid leukemia using a novel quantitative reverse transcription polymerase chain reaction assay. *Leukemia*, **12**, 1482–1489.

Sykes PJ, Brisco MJ, Hughes E *et al.* (1998) Minimal residual disease in childhood acute lymphoblastic leukaemia quantified by aspirate and trephine: is the disease multifocal? *British Journal of Haematology*, **103**, 60–65.

van Dongen JJ, Seriu T, Panzer-Grumayer ER *et al.* (1998) Prognostic value of minimal residual disease in acute lymphoblastic leukaemia in childhood. *Lancet*, **352**, 1731–1738.

Yamada M, Wasserman R, Lange B *et al.* (1990) Minimal residual disease in childhood B-lineage lymphoblastic leukemia. *New England Journal of Medicine*, **323**, 448–455.

Chronic leukaemias

Bose S, Deininger M, Gora-Tybor J, Goldman JM, Melo JV. (1998) The presence of typical and atypical BCR-ABL fusion genes in leukocytes of normal individuals: biologic significance and implications for the assessment of minimal residual disease. *Blood*, **92**, 3362–3367.

Khouri IF, Keating MJ, Vriesendorp HM *et al.* (1994) Autologous and allogeneic bone marrow transplantation for chronic lymphocytic leukemia: preliminary results. *Journal of Clinical Oncology*, **12**, 748–758.

Nowell PC, Hungerford DA. (1960) A minute chromosome in human granulocytic leukemia. *Science*, **132**, 125–132.

Provan D, Bartlett-Pandite L, Zwicky C *et al.* (1996) Eradication of polymerase chain reaction-detectable chronic leukemia cells is associated with improved outcome after bone marrow transplantation. *Blood*, **88**, 2228–2235.

Rabinowe SN, Soiffer RJ, Gribben JG *et al.* (1993) Autologous and allogeneic bone marrow transplantation for poor prognosis patients with B-cell chronic lymphocytic leukemia. *Blood*, **82**, 1366–1376.

Radich JP, Gehly G, Gooley T *et al.* (1995) Polymerase chain reaction detection of the BCR-ABL fusion transcript after allogeneic marrow transplantation for chronic myeloid leukemia: results and implications in 346 patients. *Blood*, **85**, 2632–2638.

Non-Hodgkin's lymphoma

Aisenberg AC, Wilkes BM, Jacobson JO. (1988) The bcl-2 gene is rearranged in many diffuse B-cell lymphomas. *Blood*, **71**, 969–972.

Crescenzi M, Seto M, Herzig GP *et al.* (1988) Thermostable DNA polymerase chain amplification of t(14;18) chromosome breakpoints and detection of minimal residual disease. *Proceedings of the National Academy of Sciences (USA)*, **85**, 4869–4873.

Davis TA, Maloney DG, Czerwinski DK, Liles TM, Levy R. (1998) Anti-idiotype antibodies can induce long-term complete remissions in non-Hodgkin's lymphoma without eradicating the malignant clone. *Blood*, **92**, 1184–1190.

Gribben JG. (1998) Molecular basis for stem cell transplantation in indolent lymphomas. *Cancer Journal of Scientific American*, **4**, Suppl. 2, S37–S45.

Gribben JG, Nadler LM. (1995) Detection of minimal residual disease. *Cancer Treatment Research*, **76**, 249–270.

Gribben JG, Neuberg D, Freedman AS *et al.* (1993) Detection by polymerase chain reaction of residual cells with the bcl-2 translocation is associated with increased risk of relapse after autologous bone marrow transplantation for B-cell lymphoma. *Blood*, **81**, 3449–3457.

Gribben JG, Neuberg DN, Barber M *et al.* (1994) Detection of residual lymphoma cells by polymerase chain reaction in peripheral blood is significantly less predictive for relapse than detection in bone marrow. *Blood*, **83**, 3800–3807.

Gribben JG, Saporito L, Barber M *et al.* (1992) Bone marrows of non-Hodgkin's lymphoma patients with a bcl-2 translocation can be purged of polymerase chain reaction-detectable lymphoma cells using monoclonal antibodies and immunomagnetic bead depletion. *Blood*, **80**, 1083–1089.

Lopez-Guillermo A, Cabanillas F, McLaughlin P *et al.* (1998) The clinical significance of molecular response in indolent follicular lymphomas. *Blood*, **91**, 2955–2960.

Sharp JG, Joshi SS, Armitage JO *et al.* (1992) Significance of detection of occult non-Hodgkin's lymphoma in histologically uninvolved bone marrow by culture technique. *Blood*, **79**, 1074–1080.

Taniwaki M, Nishida K, Ueda Y *et al.* (1995) Interphase and metaphase detection of the breakpoint of 14q32 translocations in B-cell malignancies by double-color fluorescence *in situ* hybridisation. *Blood*, **85**, 3223–3228.

Weiss LM, Warnke RA, Sklar J, Cleary ML. (1987) Molecular analysis of the t(14;18) chromosomal translocation in malignant lymphomas. *New England Journal of Medicine*, **317**, 1185–1189.

Yuan R, Dowling P, Zucca E, Diggelmann H, Cavalli F. (1993) Detection of bcl-2/JH rearrangement in follicular and diffuse lymphoma: concordant results of peripheral blood and bone marrow analysis at diagnosis. *British Journal of Cancer*, **67**, 922–925.

Zwicky CS, Maddocks AB, Andersen N, Gribben JG. (1996) Eradication of polymerase chain reaction detectable immunoglobulin gene rearrangement in non-Hodgkin's lymphoma is associated with decreased relapse after autologous bone marrow transplantation. *Blood*, **88**, 3314–3322.

Quantitation

Cross NC, Feng L, Chase A, Bungey J, Hughes TP *et al.* (1993) Competitive polymerase chain reaction to estimate the number of BCR-ABL transcripts in chronic myeloid leukemia patients after bone marrow transplantation. *Blood*, **82**, 1929–1936.

Mensink E, van de Locht A, Schattenberg A *et al.* (1998) Quantitation of minimal residual disease in Philadelphia chromosome positive chronic myeloid leukaemia patients using real-time quantitative RT-PCR. *British Journal of Haematology*, **102**, 768–774.

Pongers-Willemse MJ, Verhagen OJ, Tibbe GJ *et al.* (1998) Real-time quantitative PCR for the detection of minimal residual disease in acute lymphoblastic leukemia using junctional region specific TaqMan probes. *Leukemia*, **12**, 2006–2014.

Thompson JD, Brodsky I, Yunis JJ. (1992) Molecular quantification of residual disease in chronic myelogenous leukemia after bone marrow transplantation. *Blood*, **79**, 1629–1635.

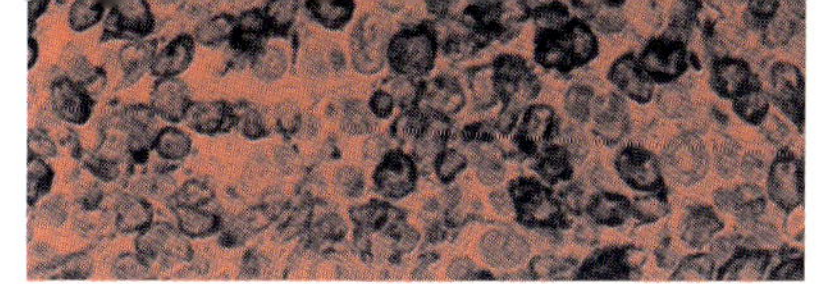

Chapter 5 Chronic myeloid leukaemia

Ian M Franklin & Ken Mills

Introduction

Chronic myeloid leukaemia (CML) was the first haematological malignancy to be associated with a *specific* chromosome abnormality. First recognised in 1960, the Philadelphia (Ph) chromosome was identified as being a balanced translocation between chromosomes 9 and 22 in 1973. These advances in cytogenetics were matched in the years following 1982 when the specific molecular translocation was elucidated. In this chapter, those aspects of CML in which the molecular findings have a particular bearing will be considered. In particular, the value of molecular detection in diagnosis, the assessment of prognosis, the response to therapy and the management of relapses following complete response will be discussed. In addition, the molecular characteristics of *BCR*, *ABL* and *BCR-ABL* will be discussed together with those signal transduction pathways related to the *BCR-ABL* fusion gene. In the past few years there have been major advances in the molecular methods of assessing the leukaemic cell burden and this, together with attempts to refine a graft-versus-leukaemia (GVL) effect, has led to the development of molecular therapeutic approaches.

Chronic myeloid leukaemia

Chronic myeloid leukaemia consists predominantly of a proliferation of the granulocyte compartment of the bone marrow. The disease divides into a number of convenient phases. Most patients present with non-specific symptoms with a white blood count usually in excess of 50×10^9/l. The haemoglobin may be normal or slightly reduced and platelets are more usually in the normal range but may be high or, rarely, low. Initial therapy is usually able to restore effective haematopoiesis rapidly such that haemoglobin and platelets will be in the normal range with the white count elevated. Splenomegaly is usual on presentation and may be gross, but initial therapy with, for example busulphan or hydroxyurea, will usually return the spleen to normal dimensions. This period of stable blood counts, absent or minimal splenomegaly and normal general health is known as *chronic phase* (CP). The duration of first chronic phase (CP1) is very variable and may be anything from a few months to many years. Depending on therapy the median duration of CP1 is 48–60 months.

Progression from CP1 can take one of two forms: more usually a gradual resistance to initial therapy, recurrence of symptoms and splenomegaly herald a requirement to change the initial therapy, which may act as the best marker of the end of CP1 and the onset of *accelerated phase*. Progression may or may not be associated with the occurrence of additional chromosome abnormalities including duplicate Ph chromosomes, entirely new translocations or deletions. As accelerated phase continues and the disease becomes more resistant to therapy, further aberrant clones may emerge, associated either with progressive bone marrow failure or, alternatively, a switch to an acute leukaemia-type picture known commonly as *blast crisis*. Transformation to blast crisis may occur at any time from the point of diagnosis and can occur directly from chronic phase or, rarely, from continuing complete remission following allogeneic bone marrow transplantation.

The median survival once the patient has progressed

from CP1 is usually measured in months rather than years. Hence, duration of CP1 has been seen as the most important measure of the effectiveness of therapeutic interventions in CML. Most therapies aim to prolong the duration of CP1, although allogeneic blood or marrow transplantation aims at cure of the disease with permanent eradication of the Ph chromosome-positive (Ph+) clone.

Cytogenetic and molecular characteristics of CML

The Ph chromosome, discovered in 1960, was later identified as the smaller of the two chromosomes derived from a reciprocal translocation involving chromosomes 9 and 22, i.e. t(9;22)(q34;q11) (Figure 5.1). Thus CML became the first disease in which the cytogenetic abnormality was defined on a molecular basis. The genes flanking the breakpoints involved in the reciprocal translocation between chromosomes 9 and 22 were shown to be *ABL* and *BCR*, respectively (Figure 5.2). In over 90% of CML patients, this translocation can be identified by conventional cytogenetics, although it may involve one or more additional chromosomes resulting in complex cytogenetic translocations. In general, the Ph chromosome is the only cytogenetic abnormality observed during chronic phase. However, as the disease progresses through accelerated phase and into the terminal blast crisis phase, additional cytogenetic abnormalities are frequently observed. The most common secondary abnormalities are the presence of an additional Ph chromosome, trisomy 8 and isochromosome 17q. These abnormalities may involve the *MYC* and p53 genes, but the exact molecular pathways of progression are not clearly defined. A frequent mechanism is the loss of p53 function, by mutation or deletion, which occurs in approximately 25–35% of patients in blast crisis. However, it would seem that the loss of p53 function is not in itself sufficient to induce blast crisis, but may act in concert with other genetic changes. One of these changes may be homozygous deletion of the p16 gene (*CDKN-2*) which inhibits CDK-4, a cell cycle checkpoint protein, that is acquired during the progression to blast crisis. Retinoblastoma (Rb) gene abnormalities or p21 alterations may also contribute to disease progression.

The breakpoint in the *ABL* genes usually occurs within the intron, either between the alternative first

Fig. 5.1 Schematic diagram of the structure of the Philadelphia chromosome

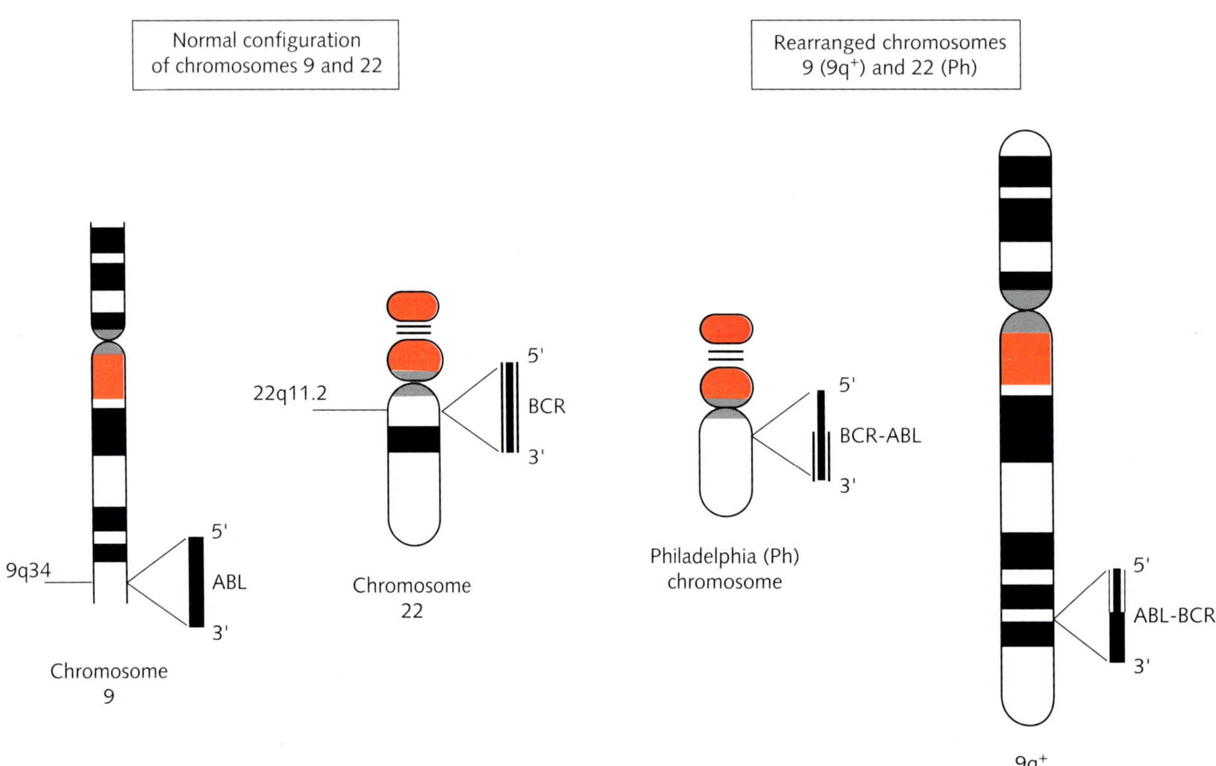

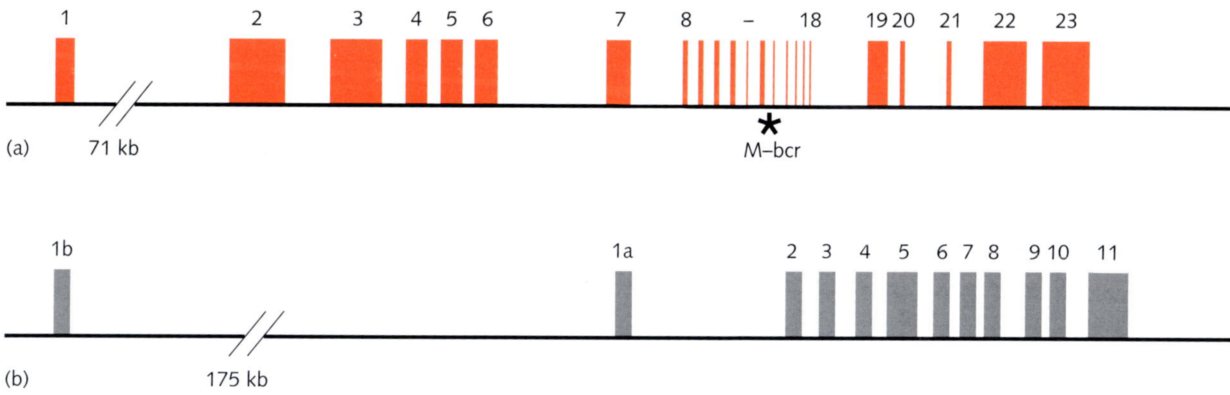

Fig. 5.2 Structure of the *ABL* (a) and *BCR* (b) genes showing locations of breakpoints

exons 1b and 1a, or between exons 1a and 2 (Figure 5.2a). This region is approximately 300 kb long. *ABL* exons 2–11 are moved from chromosome 9, to fuse with the 5′ portion of the *BCR* gene. The breakpoints on chromosome 22 are tightly clustered to a 5.8 kb or less region within the *BCR* gene, known as the major breakpoint cluster region (M-*BCR*) (Figure 5.2b). However, some degree of heterogeneity exists in the fusion *BCR-ABL* gene as the breakpoint in the M-*BCR* can occur either side of exon 14 (also known as exon b3). Therefore, two types of *BCR-ABL* mRNA are commonly formed, with either *BCR* exon b3 spliced to *ABL* exon a2 (a b3–a2 splice) or *BCR* exon 13 (b2) spliced to *ABL* exon a2, a b2–a2 splice junction (Figure 5.3). These mRNAs are transcribed into a novel *BCR-ABL* protein which has a molecular weight of 210 kDa ($p210^{BCR\text{-}ABL}$). A smaller BCR-ABL protein ($p190^{BCR\text{-}ABL}$) is associated with Ph-positive acute lymphoblastic leukaemias (ALL). This is formed from the fusion of *BCR* exon 1 directly with the *ABL* exon 2 involved in the CML variant. The 9q+ chromosome containing the reciprocal *ABL-BCR* gene fusion is expressed in about a half to two-thirds of CML patients, at a very low level, if at all. The *ABL-BCR* gene product may not have any significant role in the pathogenesis of CML, but if it is produced it may be involved in deregulating the GTPase activating protein (GAP) function of BCR.

The correlation between molecular phenotype and clinical characteristics has been investigated. It had been suggested that the site of the genomic breakpoint and/or the type of RNA splice site might be an important prognostic factor. Some studies have indicated a correlation with either of these molecular factors and the length of the chronic phase, platelet count at diagnosis or the patient's response to interferon. In these studies, the length of the chronic phase was longer in patients who had a 5′ M-*BCR* breakpoint, or who expressed a b2–a2 spliced mRNA. However, the majority of reports have not found any significant correlation. Similarly, the presence of a 5′ breakpoint or a b2–a2 mRNA has been correlated with a lower platelet count in a few cases. The response of patients to α-interferon has also been reported to correlate with the type of *BCR-ABL* and a correlation with *ABL-BCR* RNA expression has also been reported. However, in a large national study, *no* correlation with any clinical factor was observed. It is now generally accepted that there is no correlation between molecular phenotype and prognostic factors. Although given the different phenotypes of the p190 and p210 BCR-ABL proteins, it is possible that there may be differences in the pathology caused by the presence or absence of exon b3, but these are too subtle to be consistently observed.

Molecular characteristics of BCR, ABL and BCR-ABL

The *ABL* gene has a number of structural domains (Figure 5.3) which are involved in signal transduction. The structural elements include a tyrosine kinase domain, SH1 (*SRC* homology 1), two non-catalytic domains SH2 and SH3, as well as a DNA binding domain, an actin binding domain and a nuclear localisation signal. All these elements are present in the $p210^{BCR\text{-}ABL}$ protein. In the normal ABL protein, the SH3 element has been shown to be a negative regulator of transformation. The SH3 domain also binds to members of a family of nuclear proteins called the ABL interactor proteins (Abi-1 and Abi-2). The fusion of the *BCR* sequence in the *BCR-ABL* gene may lead to interference with the negative function of the SH3 domain, which could result in an active kinase.

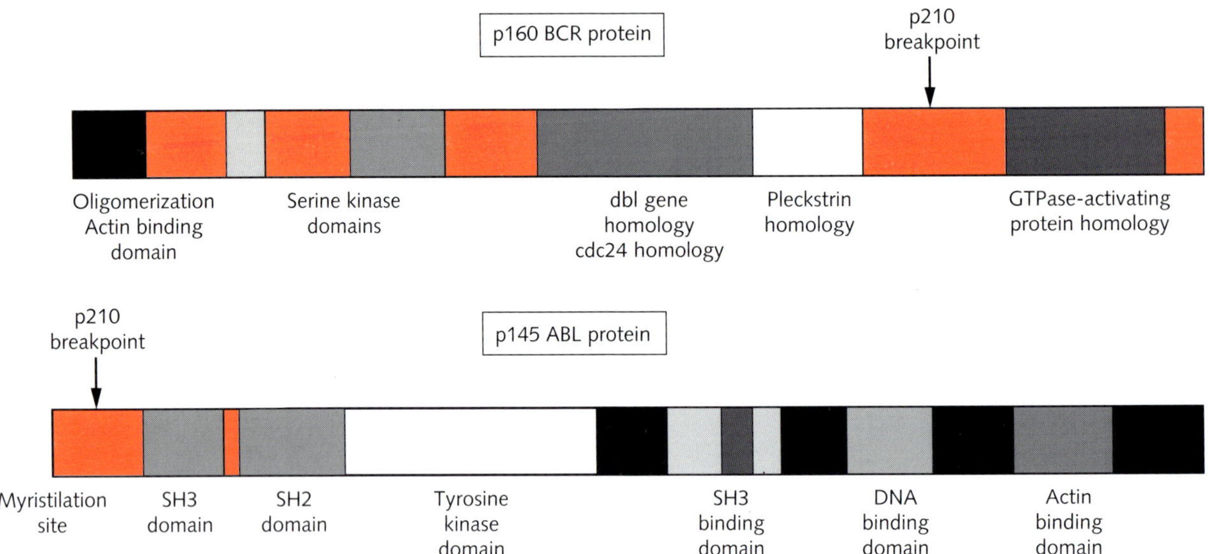

Fig. 5.3 RNA structure of *ABL* and *BCR* showing the location of the various domains

Conflicting evidence has been reported on the importance of mutations within the SH2 domain. Some studies have observed that mutations within the SH2 domain will remove the ability of BCR-ABL to transform fibroblasts or lymphocytes. However, no effect of SH2 mutations on the growth, tumorigenicity or apoptosis rates has been seen in haematopoietic cell lines. Within the SH1 domain, a mutation of the tyrosine autophosphorylation site, at Y1293, results in an impaired tumorigenicity whilst retaining its ability to induce growth factor-independent proliferation.

BCR sequences fused to the 5′ region of the *ABL* gene activate the tyrosine kinase activity. The *BCR* sequences also include an actin binding domain, a serine kinase domain, a region of homology to the guanine nucleotide dissociation stimulatory region of the oncogene dbl 45, and the pleckstrin homology (PH) domain. Mutations of the actin binding domain do not affect the kinase activity of BCR-ABL, although the association with F-actin or the ability to dimerise is eliminated. This results in an impaired ability of BCR to transform fibroblast and haematopoietic cells. The serine/threonine activity also is important in the transformation efficiency of BCR-ABL. The autophosphorylation site at Y177 of BCR becomes phosphorylated in the mBCR-ABL protein providing a binding site for the adaptor protein, Grb2. Deletion of the region containing Y177 results in the retention of the tyrosine kinase activity, but with a greatly decreased transformation ability. Three other BCR domains of interest are also present in the hybrid *BCR-ABL* gene product; however, none of these is involved in the translocation of the small BCR-ABL protein, $p190^{BCR\text{-}ABL}$, observed in ALL, although the two diseases, ALL and CML, exhibit different clinical phenotypes. One of these domains is the dbl homology domain which stimulates GTP binding to RhoA, Rac1 and Rac2 guanine exchange factors. A second domain, the PH domain, is found in a range of proteins, is approximately 100 amino acids long which form β strands and an α helix, and may be responsible for protein–protein interactions. The PH domains share a relatively low degree of homology, and may also allow the protein to interact with the cell surface via phosphatidyl-inositol(4,5)bisphosphate. A further domain is present within exons 19–23 of the *BCR* gene; this is a domain with GAP activity targeted to members of the Rho family. However, this domain is not present in the $p210^{BCR\text{-}ABL}$ protein, but if the reciprocal translocation product ABL-BCR is expressed, will form a part of that protein.

BCR-ABL signal transduction pathways

The biological consequences of the *BCR-ABL* translocation in haematopoietic cell lines result in the development of growth factor independence, altered apoptotic rates and altered adhesion properties. The various structural domains within the BCR and ABL regions indicate that the hybrid protein is capable of numerous protein–protein interactions. Many of these proteins

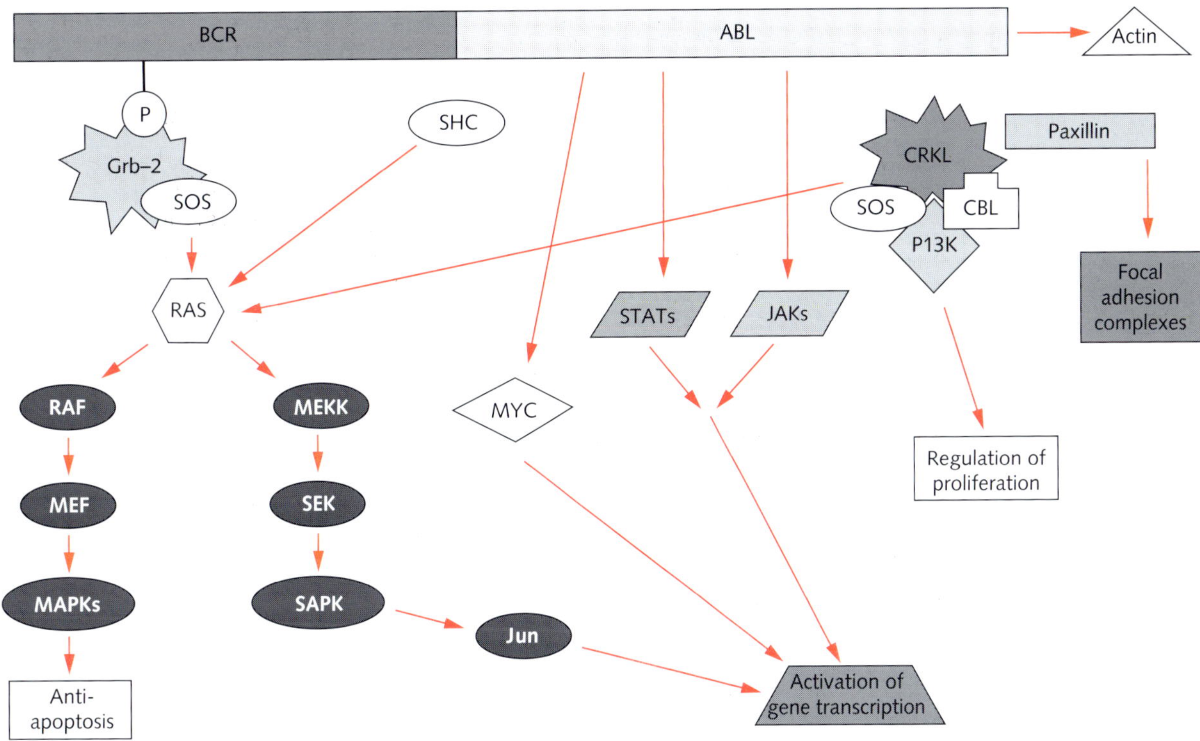

Fig. 5.4 BCR-ABL protein has been implicated in the activation of multiple signal transduction pathways

have been shown to be directly involved with several signal transduction pathways which lead to altered transformation, proliferation and adhesion characteristics (Figure 5.4). These pathways include activation of the RAS pathway along either of the MAPK or SAPK pathways, which represent parallel cascades of protein kinases that transmit regulatory signals to the nucleus. The pathways are both activated via the RAS protein. The mechanism of activation involves at least three adaptor proteins (Grb2, SHC and CRKL) each of which can complex with the BCR-ABL protein. Each adaptor can link to RAS through recruitment of guanine nucleotide exchange factors. The splice variants of the SHC protein (66, 52 and 46 kDa) possess an SH2 domain in their carboxy terminus, and it has been shown that, in cells transfected with a p210$^{BCR-ABL}$ expression vector, the p210$^{BCR-ABL}$ can bind several proteins, but specifically complexes with Grb2. However, as Grb2 can bind directly to BCR-ABL, the role of SHC may be to function through a separate, and independent, parallel pathway. Grb2, another adaptor protein, binds tyrosine phosphorylated proteins to its SH2 domain and a guanine nucleotide releasing factor protein, SOS1, to its SH3 domain. The BCR-ABL/Grb2/SOS1 complex can activate RAS GDP/GTP exchange with the biological consequences of increased transformation and altered adhesion characteristics. Although elevation of Grb2 expression alone has no effect on cell growth, co-expression with p210$^{BCR-ABL}$ enhances the transformation effect in fibroblasts or leukaemia model systems. From these studies it is clear that, although RAS mutations are uncommon in chronic phase CML, Grb2 and RAS co-activation are essential to development of BCR-ABL mediated transformation.

The adaptor protein CrkL (Crk-like) is a 39 kDa protein and is also located on chromosome 22. CrkL is homologous to the c-CRK protein (the human homologue of the chicken oncogene C-*SRC*) and contains a SH2 domain and two SH3 domains. It is also the major constitutively expressed tyrosine phosphorylated protein in CML cells, and forms complexes with BCR-ABL in cell lines and patient leukaemic cells. These proteins form part of a larger complex with the proto-oncogene C-*CBL* and the p85-phosphoinositol-3′-kinase (PI3K) subunit. PI3K has an increased kinase activity in BCR-ABL transformed cells, and downregulation of the p85 subunit inhibits proliferation of these cells. In addition to PI3K and CBL (the cellular homologue of the V-*CBL* proto-oncogene) in the BCR-ABL/CrkL complex, other focal adhesion proteins also form part of this complex, including paxillin and talin. The interaction of p120(C-*Cbl*) with paxillin is specific, since other focal adhesion proteins, such as p125(FAK), vinculin and α-actin, are not in this complex. The BCR-ABL oncogene may also alter the tyrosine phosphorylation status of p130(CAS) by disrupting the normal interaction of p130(CAS) with the focal adhesion protein tensin. These alterations in the structure of the p120(C-*Cbl*) and p130(CAS) signalling proteins in focal adhesion-like structures could contribute to the known adhesion abnormalities in CML cells.

Also implicated in the BCR-ABL induced pathogenesis of CML are the proto-oncogenes *MYC* and *BCL-2*. MYC protein is a nuclear transcription factor which, in a heterodimer with MAX, regulates the transcription of a spectrum of genes. A consequence of BCR-ABL transformation is that levels of *MYC* RNA are high. However, overexpression of dominant negative forms of *MYC* blocks transformation by BCR-ABL. Conversely, MYC–MAX dimers have also been implicated in mediating the apoptotic phenotype of BCR-ABL transformed cells, possibly by regulating the expression of cell cycle-dependent kinases, in particular cdc-25A. BCR-ABL transformed murine haematopoietic cells are growth factor independent; within these cells the *BCR-ABL* oncogene prevents apoptotic death by inducing a *BCL-2* expression pathway. Furthermore, if the *BCL-2* expression is suppressed, these cells revert to factor dependence and non-tumorigenicity. These results may help to explain the ability of the *BCR-ABL* oncogene to synergise with *MYC* in cell transformation and in the altered apoptotic phenotype. Data examining the effect of different levels of *BCR-ABL* expression have shown that high and low levels may activate distinct signalling. This is intriguing as the level of BCR-ABL protein has been shown to increase during progression from chronic to acute phase. Therefore, different signalling pathways may be activated in the early stages when compared to latter stages of the disease. For example, the activation of *MYC* via the RAS pathway may result in factor independence at low levels, whilst anti-apoptotic pathways, involving BCL-2 protein, may be important at higher levels of BCR-ABL protein.

Therapy of chronic myeloid leukaemia

Chemotherapy

For many years the mainstay of therapy was the alkylating agent busulphan. This is a convenient drug to use in CML, being administered orally, having a predictable and sustained effect against the leukaemia clone, and being very cheap. Unfortunately, it has a number of toxic effects which make it appropriate for use now only in the elderly. It causes early and permanent infertility, and prolonged use can lead to the 'Busulphan Syndrome' in which patients develop skin pigmentation and may go on to develop pulmonary fibrosis. In addition, the alkylating agent property has made busulphan prone to induce second malignancies.

During the 1980s busulphan came to be replaced by hydroxyurea which, it was hoped owing to it being an anti-metabolite, would not induce second malignancies. Although second malignancies appear to be infrequent in patients on hydroxyurea therapy, they do occur and patients receiving this agent should be advised of this. Recent studies from Germany have shown that, when used to achieve tight control of the blood count within the normal range, hydroxyurea therapy produces superior survival to busulphan.

The first concerted attempts to alter the prognosis in CML significantly were made in the late 1970s when a group at the Memorial Sloan-Kettering Hospital used intensive therapy, similar to that used in acute myeloid leukaemia, in an attempt to induce a transient Ph chromosome negativity. They achieved some success with an arduous regime but there were no long-term cytogenetic responders. What this strategy did show was that patients with CML do have residual haematopoiesis with normal Ph-negative status. Until that time it had been assumed that the Ph-positive clone had completely replaced the normal bone marrow.

These studies using intensive therapy were to be revisited over 10 years later when Carella and others began using intensive chemotherapy in order to induce the appearance, in the peripheral blood, of Ph-negative haematopoietic progenitors. These cells could then be collected and used in autologous transplants (*see below*).

α interferon therapy

α interferon has been used to control the peripheral white cell count in CML since the mid-1980s. When it was shown that a proportion of patients could achieve a significant reduction in the proportion of Ph+ cells in the bone marrow following responses to interferon, interest in this agent grew. A smaller proportion showed a complete cytogenetic response, although almost all of these have been shown to remain positive for the *BCR-ABL* translocation using more sensitive molecular techniques. Kantarjian *et al.* have shown that survival is

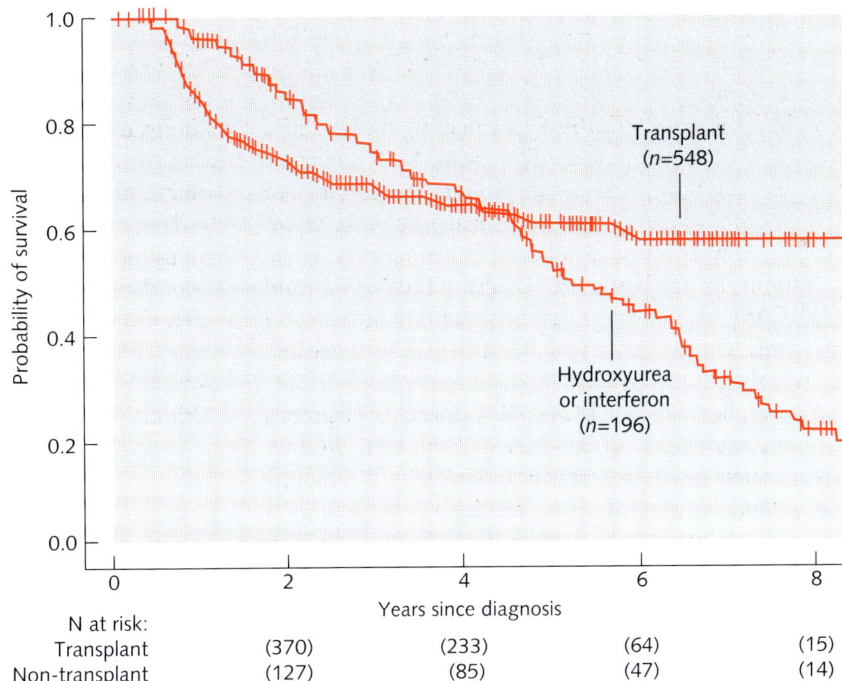

Fig. 5.5 Benefit of HLA identical sibling AlloBMT in CML is apparent after 4 years
Figure shows adjusted probabilities (from Cox regression model) of survival after diagnosis of CML in persons receiving BMT compared to hydroxyurea or α-interferon. Reproduced with kind permission of WB Saunders Co, FL, from Gale *et al.*, 1998.

prolonged in CML in those patients who enjoy a cytogenetic response. Certainly both the major Italian study group and the UK Medical Research Council (MRC) Trial showed approximately a 20-month improvement in survival for patients receiving interferon rather than hydroxyurea. In the Italian study this was correlated with response to interferon, but in the UK MRC Trial even interferon non-responders had an improved survival over those patients who received no interferon. Although cytogenetic analysis of bone marrow has been the usual method for monitoring response to treatment with α interferon in CML, it is also possible to monitor response using quantitative molecular techniques. The advantage of such a technique is that it allows for frequent follow-up and avoids repeated bone marrow aspirations required for cytogenetics, because the molecular techniques are applicable to peripheral blood. Periodic cytogenetic analysis will, however, continue to be essential since this is the only technique that can reliably detect additional chromosome aberrations which may be associated with incipient acceleration.

The French CML study group has explored the use of cytosine arabinoside (Ara-C) in combination with α interferon in CML. The CML protocol was developed in order to show the potential advantage of using the combination of interferon and Ara-C. This was published in 1997 and did indeed suggest that a significant advantage to the addition of Ara-C to interferon did exist. Though quality of life issues need to be taken into consideration, it does appear at present that this combination is the treatment of choice for new patients with CML in chronic phase who are not part of randomised controlled trials.

The previous Italian and UK studies did not show any disadvantage for patients receiving interferon therapy prior to proceeding to allogeneic bone marrow transplantation (AlloBMT). However, the recent data from the Seattle group suggested that there may be such a disadvantage. Further studies are required to resolve this issue, but in those patients under 30 years it would appear to be reasonable to search for a family donor for an AlloBMT prior to commencing interferon therapy. Any such patient who does have a sibling donor should proceed to AlloBMT without a trial of α interferon.

This view is supported by data from the International BMT Registry (IBMTR) in which 548 recipients of human leucocyte antigen (HLA) identical sibling transplants were compared with the outcome of 196 patients from a German CML study. The German patients were randomised to receive either hydroxyurea ($n = 121$) or α interferon ($n = 75$). Although the number of patients receiving interferon is relatively small in this study, what appears clear is that after 4 years from diagnosis there is a benefit for sibling AlloBMT (Figure 5.5). For transplants carried out within 1 year of diagnosis the benefits

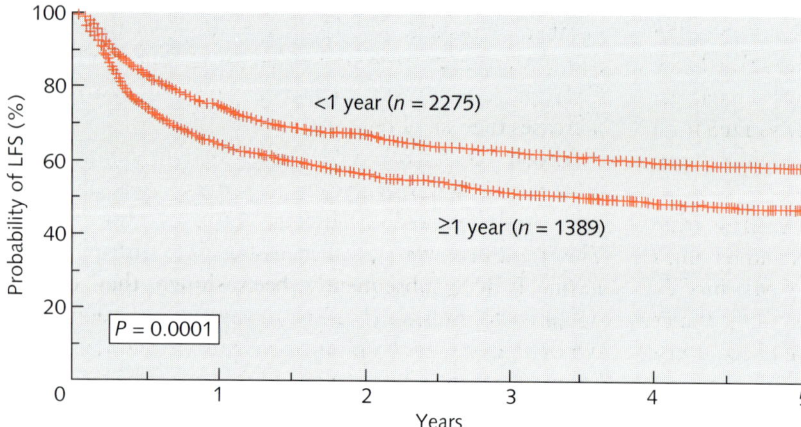

Fig. 5.6 International Bone Marrow Transplant Registry
Probability of leukaemia-free survival (LFS) after sibling donor BMT for CML in chronic phase, by time to transplant. Data from transplants performed 1990–1996 by 284 teams world-wide.

of transplantation were apparent earlier. Although there is a higher mortality in the immediate post-BMT period, the long-term survival advantage for HLA identical sibling transplants over conventional therapy with hydroxyurea or interferon appears compelling.

Allogeneic bone marrow transplantation

In the mid-1970s it had become apparent that AlloBMT was potentially curable for patients with acute myeloid leukaemia in first complete remission. Although CML was known to be incurable at that time, there was a natural reluctance to submit patients to a treatment that was experimental and had a high mortality, when many patients will enjoy several years of good quality life in CP1.

The presence of the Ph chromosome enabled post-transplant monitoring to be undertaken routinely for the first time after allografting, confirming that the malignant clone had indeed been eradicated. Since those early studies, results have improved significantly such that fully matched sibling transplants for CML in CP1 within 1 year of diagnosis should give long-term disease-free survival in excess of 70%. The current results from the IBMTR are shown in Figure 5.6. Attempts to reduce morbidity due to acute graft-versus-host disease by T-cell depletion of the graft were undertaken with some enthusiasm in the mid-1980s. Unfortunately, these showed that the loss of the graft-versus-host reaction was also associated with an increased risk of disease recurrence. *This issue will be discussed in more detail below under Graft-versus-leukaemia.*

The interval between diagnosis and transplantation also appears to be important. It is of interest that the increased mortality seen from transplantation beyond 1 year's duration of CP1 is not particularly related to an increased risk of relapse, but also to increased transplant related mortality. This suggests that the poorer outcome may not be due to the emergence of clones resistant to the transplant conditioning.

Unrelated and other alternative donors for allogeneic transplantation

Younger patients with CML make ideal candidates for allogeneic transplants from unrelated or partially mismatched donors. Firstly, this is because there is usually sufficient time to search donor registries to find the most appropriate donor, given the prolonged nature of the first chronic phase of CML in most cases. Secondly, patients with CML are known to be incurable other than by allogeneic transplant, although that small proportion of patients who have complete cytogenetic responses to α interferon may enjoy very prolonged survivals. Thirdly, most of the treatment strategies used to induce and maintain stable chronic phase are not unduly toxic and so most patients will be free of complications of prior therapy when they come for transplant. There has, however, been some recent concern about the potential effect of α interferon therapy in contributing to a worse outlook following AlloBMT, although not all series have found this effect. The results of matched unrelated donor (MUD) transplants in CP1 of CML vary between different studies as one might expect. There is considerable variation between the ages of patients included in particular studies, and over the last few years changes in the techniques of HLA matching mean that a degree of caution is required in interpreting data from studies which may have commenced several years ago. In general, disease-free survivals (DFS) vary between around 30 and 50%; for younger patients under 30 years with a full HLA matched donor a 43% DFS was obtained from donors provided by the

National Marrow Donor Panel (NMDP). Extending the choice of donors to those with a single HLA locus mismatch produced DFS of 31% for this younger age group, whereas older patients had only a 27% DFS for a fully matched donor and 14% with a single antigen mismatch.

Recently, mature data from Seattle suggest that younger patients, under the age of 50 years and having a fully matched unrelated donor graft for CML in CP1 within 1 year of diagnosis, should expect a 74% chance of DFS (Figure 5.7). Such data suggest that these transplants should be carried out only in major centres where there is considerable experience of both sibling and alternative donor transplants.

What of the opportunities for such transplant sources as cord blood? At present there are too few data, but it is clear that as confidence in the use of cord blood transplantation in adults increases over the next few years, the place of cord blood in the options for treatment of CML will become more clear.

Graft-versus-leukaemia in the management of relapse following AlloBMT

Since the early days of AlloBMT graft-versus-host disease (GVHD) has been the most serious complication occurring in up to two-thirds of patients even when their donor is a fully matched sibling. In an attempt to prevent acute GVHD, the T-cell depletion of donor grafts was undertaken in the mid-1980s using a variety of different techniques. Early studies showed clearly that acute GVHD could be virtually abrogated if a small enough number of residual T-cells was included in the transplant. Although there was a reduction in acute GVHD in CML patients transplanted in first chronic phase, this increases the risk of relapse.

Also, in 1995, Kolb and colleagues carried out the first infusions of donor leucocytes in order to treat patients who had relapsed following AlloBMT for CML. This treatment was given in association with α interferon. It has subsequently been shown that donor lymphocyte infusion (DLI) from the original allogeneic donor can be used on its own for the induction of immunotherapy. The benefits of DLI have to be balanced against the increased risk of GVHD.

Other toxicities related to DLI include bone marrow aplasia, particularly in those patients who have a substantial degree of CML present at the time of the infusions. However, in patients who are treated for progressive molecular or cytogenetic relapse, and yet who remain clinically normal, aplasia is unusual, although periods of pancytopenia may occur. Responses to DLI appear to be curative.

This success with adoptive immunotherapy has led to the desire to extend such treatment to patients who may be unsuitable for allogeneic transplantation in the first place and to use adoptive immunotherapy as a primary or secondary form of treatment for CML.

Other strategies are being introduced to utilise the GVL effect. Barrett and colleagues have reintroduced T-cell depleted BMT for first chronic phase of CML and have shown that, by giving specific doses of T-lymphocytes in the early post-transplant period, a effect can be

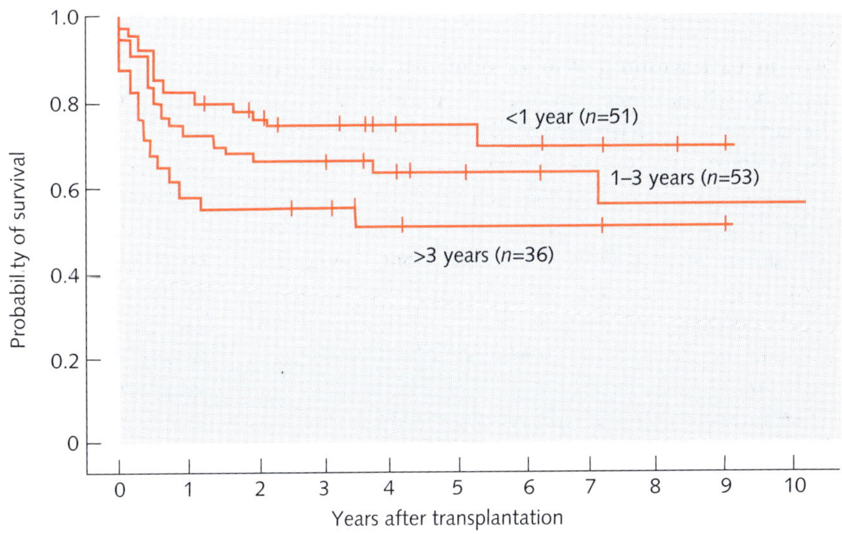

Fig. 5.7 Survival following unrelated donor BMT from CML
Seattle BMT Unit data for patients ≤50 years receiving a fully HLA-matched transplant according to the time from diagnosis.
From Hansen JA, Gooley TA, Martin PJ *et al.* (1998), Copyright© 1998 Massachusetts Medical Society. All rights reserved.

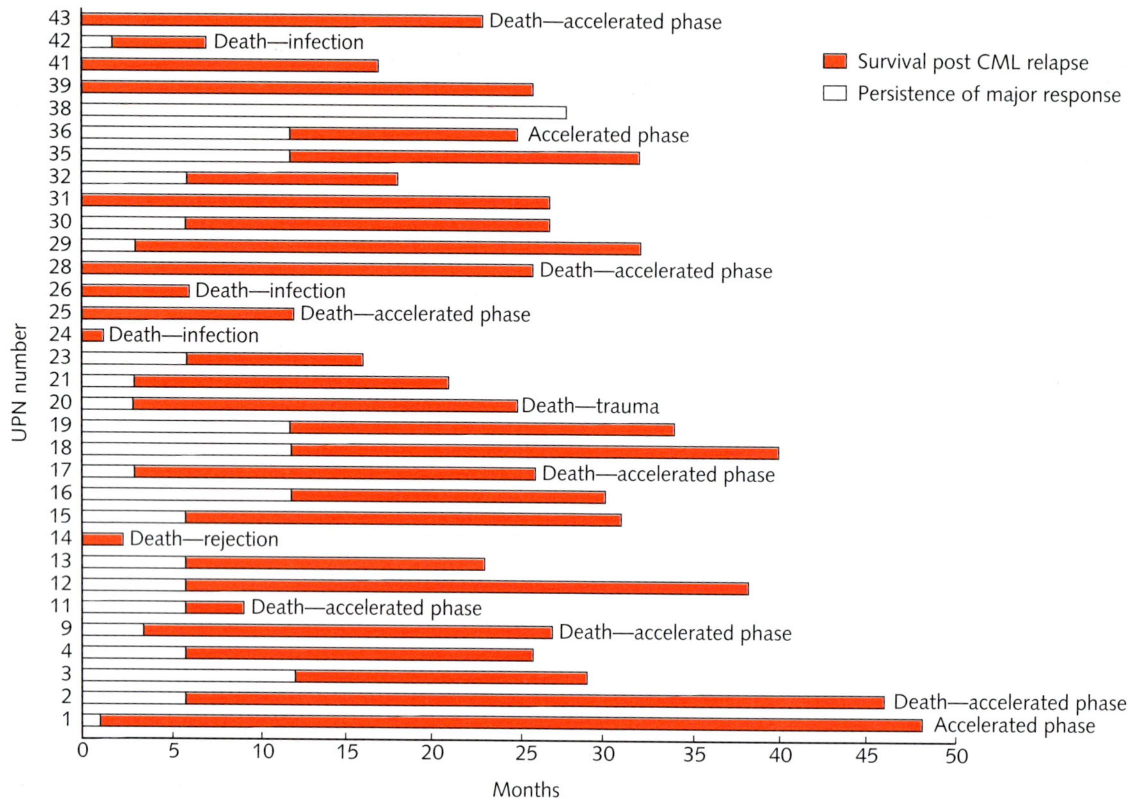

Fig. 5.8 Autologous blood and/or marrow transplants for CML
Survival and maintenance of Ph-negative status post-transplant in 33 patients.
From Singer & Franklin (1998) with kind permission of the BMJ Publishing Group.

conserved while maintaining a low risk of acute GVHD. It seems likely that over the next few years other strategies that utilise the retention of a GVL effect without acute or chronic GVHD will be developed using either *ex vivo* manipulated immune competent cells or infusions of specific T-cell subsets.

Autografting

Autologous BMT has a surprisingly long history in CML, dating from the late 1970s as a treatment for accelerated and blastic phases. After intensive chemotherapy there is a transient period of Ph-negative haematopoiesis during which it is possible to collect Ph-negative progenitor cells from the peripheral blood. Greater success in mobilising Ph-negative cells is obtained early in the course of the disease, and especially, as for AlloBMT, within 1 year of diagnosis.

Unfortunately, it appears likely that, although autografting may have potential to prolong survival in CML, a premise that requires testing in randomised controlled trials, the great majority of patients progress to Ph-positive haematopoiesis within 1 or 2 years of the autograft (Figure 5.8). However, if it were possible to exploit the period during which many autografted patients have only minimal residual disease by using an effective immunotherapeutic approach, autologous transplants in CML may remain of importance.

Immunotherapeutic strategies in CML

The awareness of the importance of the GVL effect in maintaining remission following AlloBMT for CML, and the experience gained using DLI to induce GVL and thereby reinstate remission, have taken place at a time when knowledge about the mechanisms of the immune response to cancer has increased substantially. In the normal state there is no immunological response to CML, possibly due to the lack of co-stimulatory molecules on the leukaemia cell surface. CML is, however, associated with a novel gene translocation, which produces a chimeric tyrosine kinase not found in the normal state. This, therefore, has potential to act as an antigen. A number of strategies have been proposed to stimulate an immune response against CML. One approach would be to enhance the immunogenicity of CML by upregulating the co-stimulatory molecules.

A more popular approach has been to use some form of *ex vivo* immunisation strategy using autologous T-cells from the patients. Bosch *et al.* have shown that it is possible to elicit responses in human CD4-positive T-cells to *BCR-ABL*-positive leukaemic cells following an *in vitro* immunisation protocol using a BCR-ABL breakpoint peptide. Since cytotoxic T-cell lines have been used successfully to treat post-AlloBMT lymphoproliferative disorders, this treatment strategy clearly has the potential to be effective. Another alternative, used by Barrett and colleagues, has been to take a proteinase III antigen, which is overexpressed in CML cells and is specific to myeloid lineages, and to generate cytotoxic T-lymphocytes specifically active against the proteinase III peptide. These workers have shown *in vitro* that CML colony growth can be inhibited by these cytotoxic T-cells.

Other ways in which immunological reactions may be stimulated include generating autologous dendritic cells and then pulsing these with leukaemic cells in the hope that they will process antigen. Such pulsed dendritic cells can then be used to transfer the processed antigen to cytotoxic T-cells which could be used therapeutically to mount a response against the leukaemia.

Finally, autologous natural killer cells have been generated that are capable of suppressing CML colony growth.

As yet all these approaches are *in vitro*, but it cannot be long before clinical data emerge as to the efficacy of such immunotherapeutic approaches in patients with CML. It is likely that such approaches would be carried out initially in patients relapsing following AlloBMT where the tumour burden is low. However, the real potential for these therapeutic manoeuvres exists in the treatment of patients prior to transplantation, i.e. abrogating the need for transplants altogether. Since it is known that most patients who present with CML have residual normal haematopoiesis, it would be helpful to attempt to harvest or mobilise normal stem cells to enable subsequent rescue following immunotherapeutic treatment of CML.

Molecular therapeutic approaches

The studies on dissecting the signal pathways activated during *BCR-ABL* induced transformation have indicated several potential targets for novel therapeutic approaches. One of the first molecular approaches attempted involved the use of antisense oligonucleotides to attempt to inhibit translation of the *BCR-ABL* or *MYC* transcripts. The *BCR-ABL* transcript is not found in normal cells, and the splice junction is unique to these transcripts making this an obvious target sequence for antisense therapy. Antisense oligonucleotides targeted to the splice junction inhibit the growth of BCR-ABL expressing cell lines *in vitro*. These studies have indicated that the decreased rate of apoptosis is one of the primary mechanisms by which BCR-ABL effects expansion of the leukaemic clone in CML. Mice treated with a *BCR-ABL* antisense oligonucleotide have an increased survival following injection of leukaemic cells compared with those mice injected with sense oligonucleotides, providing *in vivo* evidence for the effectiveness of a therapy based on antisense oligonucleotides. The combination of antisense and conventional chemotherapeutic agents is highly effective in killing leukaemic cells offering the prospect of a novel and more selective *ex vivo* treatment of CML.

The nuclear protein MYB is critical for haematopoietic cell proliferation and development and it has been argued that the effective disruption of MYB function may be a strategy for controlling cell growth. MYB antisense oligonucleotides have been utilised for this purpose *in vitro* and later *in vivo*. C-myb antisense oligonucleotides inhibit the growth of CML CFU-GM in a dose-dependent manner associated with a decrease in *BCR-ABL* expression. SCID mice injected with leukaemic cells show significantly increased survival times (between 3–8 times that of control, untreated mice) when injected with MYB oligonucleotides.

A variation on the theme of antisense technology is the use of ribozymes to inhibit gene transcription. Ribozymes are RNA molecules with enzymatic activity that can cleave RNA in a sequence-specific manner. They are targeted to the RNA by antisense arms, which flank the catalytic site. These arms can be designed to be homologous to the *BCR* and *ABL* portions of the hybrid mRNA. Ribozymes to the *BCR-ABL* mRNA have been shown to decrease cell proliferation, mRNA, protein levels and the tumorigenicity of BCR-ABL cells in mice. However, due to their structure, entry into the cells can be problematic, particularly as the molecules need to retain their catalytic activity. However, workers in the field remain confident that ribozymes and antisense technologies capable of blocking *BCR-ABL* mRNA will become a viable therapy for CML (*see also Chapter 16*).

A new class of compounds that specifically target the function or activity of components of the signalling path-

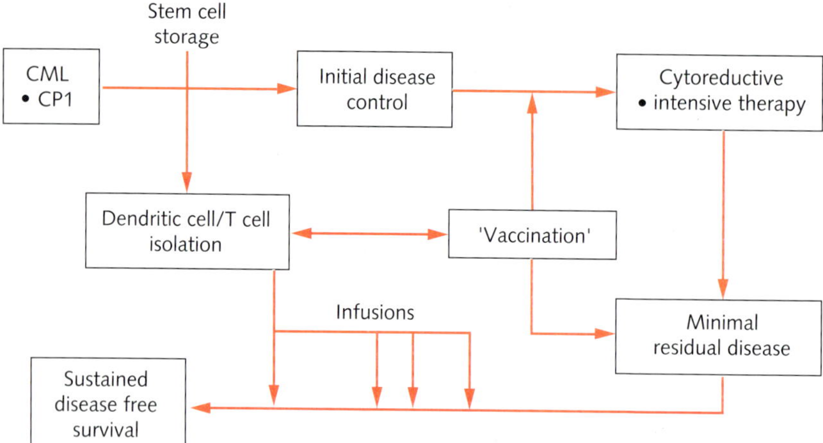

Fig. 5.9 Future management for CML? A theoretical schema that exploits residual Ph negative haematopoiesis, current knowledge of how to suppress the malignant clone transiently and the potential for immunotherapy. From Singer & Franklin (1998) with kind permission of the BMJ Publishing Group.

ways in *BCR-ABL* transformed cells has recently been described. One of these compounds is CGP 57148, a 2-phenylaminopyrimidine derivative, that selectively inhibits the tyrosine kinase activity of the BCR-ABL fusion protein and inhibits the cellular proliferation and tumour formation by BCR-ABL expressing cells. In colony-forming assays, there is a 95% decrease in the number of Ph-chromosome positive cells formed, but no inhibition of normal colony formation observed. V-*ABL* transformed cells treated with CGP 57148 have dramatically inhibited growth potential and loss of anchorage-independent growth. These findings suggest that compounds, such as CGP 57148, which, targeted against specific abnormal protein functions, may have a therapeutic potential for the treatment of CML.

Molecular methods of assessing leukaemic cell burden (Table 5.1)

The traditional method of diagnosing CML and monitoring disease status is the cytogenetic analysis of bone marrow-derived metaphases for the presence of the Ph chromosome. However, cytogenetics usually only detects approximately 90% of patients, the remaining 10% require other methods of detection. The majority of these patients can be identified by the use of fluorescence *in situ* hybridisation (FISH) or molecular techniques such as Southern blotting or reverse transcriptase polymerase chain reaction (RT-PCR). The level of sensitivity of cytogenetics or Southern blotting is about 1%, which means that in a patient in apparent cytogenetic remission more than 10^{10} leukaemic cells may still be present. The most sensitive method for the routine detection of residual leukaemic cells is by the use of RT-PCR, which can detect 1 cell in a background of 10^5 cells. However, this level of detection still means that, even with a negative result, a large number of malignant cells may still be available that could contribute to disease relapse.

FISH analyses can be performed on metaphase or interphase chromosomes, and relies on the co-localisation of large genomic probes specific to the *BCR* and *ABL* genes. The use of interphase FISH has several advantages over conventional cytogenetics. Firstly, due to the higher number of cells analysed than with conventional cytogenetics, a more accurate result can be obtained. In addition, it may be possible to identify variant translocations involving either the *BCR* or *ABL* genes. Secondly, it is possible to perform the analysis on both dividing and non-dividing cells. Thirdly, it can be performed on peripheral blood samples. One potential problem is the random co-localisation of the signals from the *BCR* and *ABL* probes, as this may give a significant false positive rate for interphase FISH.

Genomic DNA Southern blotting can be used to detect the breakpoint within the M-*BCR* region of the *BCR* gene. This is a small 5.8 kb region and contains approximately 98% of the breakpoints that occur in the *BCR* gene in CML. The technique involves restriction enzyme digestion, agarose gel electrophoresis, hybridisation with a radioactive probe and exposure to X-ray film, a process that can take several days, with a sensitivity of around 4–5%, although 1% can be achieved. Estimates of the number of Ph-positive cells obtained with Southern blotting are usually lower, and probably more accurate, than those obtained by cytogenetic analysis since Southern blotting allows analysis of all cell types

Table 5.1 Techniques for the detection of CML cells, indicating their relative sensitivity, advantages and disadvantages.

Method	Sensitivity	Target	Sample material	Comments
Conventional cytogenetics	1–10%	G-banded Ph chromosomes	BM	Low numbers of metaphase spreads (usually around 20–50) analysed means that the confidence interval is broad
Interphase FISH	1–5%	Ph chromosomes in interphase	PB, BM	Significantly higher false-positive rate than hypermetaphase FISH
Hypermetaphase FISH	0.3–2%	Ph chromosomes detected in large numbers of metaphase cells in which the translocation is detected by fluorescent probes	BM	Large number of metaphases analysed, increasing statistical confidence intervals
Southern blot	1–5%	Genomic rearrangement of the *M-BCR* region of *BCR* gene	PB, BM	Requires rearrangement to be detected by at least two restriction digests to eliminate rare polymorphisms. Rearrangement stable during the course of the disease
RT-PCR (nested)	0.0001%	Detects hybrid *BCR-ABL* mRNA	PB, BM	Very sensitive technique, although a single step PCR may not be sufficient to detect CML cells post-transplant or therapy
Western blot	1%	Detects hybrid BCR-ABL protein	PB, BM	Easily quantitative, although difficult to perform in a routine situation
Genomic PCR	0.001%	Uses primers flanking the *BCR* and *ABL* genomic breakpoints	PB, BM	Has potential to detect Ph cells even if they do not express the hybrid mRNA. However, requires cloning and sequencing of breakpoint from individual patients

BM = bone marrow, PB = peripheral blood.

in the sample, irrespective of whether or not they are dividing.

The usual method of choice for the detection of cells containing the *BCR-ABL* translocation is RT-PCR. This simple, rapid and sensitive technique allows the amplification of the region around the splice junction between *BCR* and *ABL*. The high sensitivity makes it the ideal technique for the detection of minimal residual disease following BMT or α interferon therapy. RT-PCR, and latterly quantitative RT-PCR, have been applied to detect residual CML cells following AlloBMT. These studies have shown that *BCR-ABL* transcripts can be detected for several months following transplantation. However, those patients who remain PCR positive after 6 months appear to have a higher risk of haematological or cytogenetic relapse. Quantitative RT-PCR analysis of CML patients after BMT has confirmed these results, and in addition has shown that a rising level of *BCR-ABL* mRNA in patients may indicate impending disease progression or relapse. In a similar manner, RT-PCR detection of residual *BCR-ABL* expressing cells following α interferon therapy has shown that quantitative analysis is a reliable and sensitive method of monitoring CML patients.

Conclusions

There is perhaps no other disease which has been so well characterised at the molecular level, and in which the knowledge of the molecular biology has been exploited in diagnosis, disease monitoring and therapy. Much remains to be discovered, however, from a detailed understanding of how the chromosome translocation leads to the CML phenotype to the best way to exploit the emerging data on immunotherapeutic strategies. While AlloBMT is becoming safer in CML, the majority of patients will continue to be too old or otherwise unsuitable for this procedure. However, knowledge gained from these allografts is already informing treatment protocols that will combine aspects of intensive therapy, vaccination and dendritic cell therapy, perhaps associated with the generation of cytotoxic T-cell clones. One such theoretical schema is shown in Figure 5.9. The next few years are likely to provide much new data in these and other areas which will in time lead to the successful treatment of more and more patients with CML.

Further reading

Molecular aspects of CML

de Klein A, van Kessel AG, Grosveld G *et al.* (1982) A cellular oncogene is translocated to the Philadelphia chromosome in chronic myelocytic leukaemia. *Nature*, **300**, 765–767.

Diekmann D, Brill S, Garrett MD *et al.* (1991) Bcr encodes a GTPase-activating protein for p21rac. *Nature*, **351**, 400–402.

Goga A, McLaughlin J, Afar DE, Saffran DC, Witte ON. (1995) Alternative signals to RAS for hematopoietic transformation by the BCR-ABL oncogene. *Cell*, **82**, 981–988.

Kurzrock R, Gutterman JU, Talpaz M. (1988) The molecular genetics of Philadelphia chromosome-positive leukemias. *New England Journal of Medicine*, **319**, 990–998.

LeMaistre A, Lee MS, Talpaz M *et al.* (1989) Ras oncogene mutations are rare late stage events in chronic myelogenous leukemia. *Blood*, **73**, 889–891.

Melo JV, Gordon DE, Cross NC, Goldman JM. (1993) The ABL-BCR fusion gene is expressed in chronic myeloid leukemia. *Blood*, **81**, 158–165.

Puil L, Liu J, Gish G *et al.* (1994) Bcr-Abl oncoproteins bind directly to activators of the Ras signalling pathway. *EMBO Journal*, **13**, 764–773.

Rowley JD. (1973) A new consistent chromosomal abnormality in chronic myelogenous leukemia identified by quinacrine fluoridate and Giemsa staining. *Nature*, **243**, 290–292.

Sattler M, Salgia R, Okuda K *et al.* (1996) The proto-oncogene product p120CBL and the adaptor proteins CRKL and c-CRK link c-ABL, p190BCR/ABL and p210BCR/ABL to the phosphatidylinositol-3′ kinase pathway. *Oncogene*, **12**, 839–846.

Sawyers CL. (1993) The role of myc in transformation by BCR-ABL. *Leukemia and Lymphoma*, **11** (Suppl. 1), 45–46.

Conventional and molecular therapeutics

Bosch GJ, Joosten AM, Kessler JH *et al.* (1996) Recognition of BCR-ABL positive leukemic blasts by human CD4+ T cells elicited by primary *in vitro* immunization with a BCR-ABL breakpoint peptide. *Blood*, **88**, 3522–3527.

Cross NC, Feng L, Chase A *et al.* (1993) Competitive polymerase chain reaction to estimate the number of BCR-ABL transcripts in chronic myeloid leukemia patients after bone marrow transplantation. *Blood*, **82**, 1929–1936.

Gale RP, Hehlmann R, Zhang MJ *et al.* (1998) Survival with bone marrow transplantation versus hydroxyurea or interferon for chronic myelogenous leukemia. The German CML Study Group. *Blood*, **91**, 1810–1819.

Hansen JA, Gooley TA, Martin PJ *et al.* (1998) Bone marrow transplants from unrelated donors for patients with chronic myeloid leukemia. *New England Journal of Medicine*, **338**, 962–968.

Kantarjian HM, Smith TL, O'Brien S *et al.* (1995) Prolonged survival in chronic myelogenous leukemia after cytogenetic response to interferon-alpha therapy. *Annals of Internal Medicine*, **122**, 254–261.

Lin F, van Rhee F, Goldman JM, Cross NC. (1996) Kinetics of increasing BCR-ABL transcript numbers in chronic myeloid leukemia patients who relapse after bone marrow transplantation. *Blood*, **87**, 4473–4478.

Singer IO, Franklin IM. (1998) Autografting as first line treatment for chronic myeloid leukaemia. *Journal of Clinical Pathology*, **51**, 92–95.

Szczylik C, Skorski T, Nicolaides NC *et al.* (1991) Selective inhibition of leukemia cell proliferation by BCR-ABL antisense oligodeoxynucleotides. *Science*, **253**, 562–565.

Graft-versus-leukaemia

Barrett AJ, Mavroudis D, Tisdale J *et al.* (1998) T cell-depleted bone marrow transplantation and T cell add-back to control GVHD and conserve a graft-versus-leukaemia effect. *Bone Marrow Transplantation*, **21**, 543–551.

Kolb HJ, Schattenberg A, Goldman JM *et al.* (1995) Graft-versus-leukemia effect of donor lymphocyte transfusions in marrow grafted patients. European Group for Blood and Marrow Transplantation Working Party Chronic Leukemia. *Blood*, **86**, 2041–2050.

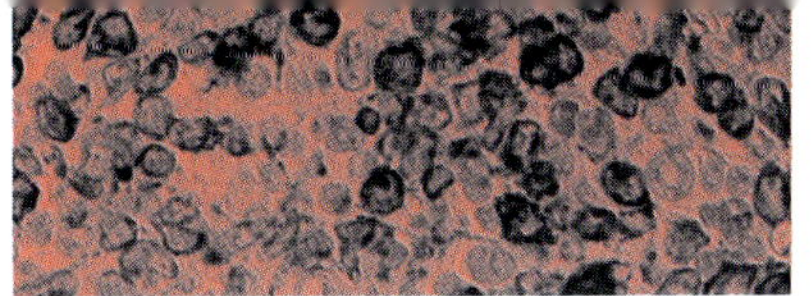

Chapter 6 Myelodysplastic syndromes

Thomas J Schuetz & Richard M Stone

Introduction

The term myelodysplastic syndrome (MDS) refers to a set of diseases characterised by primary bone marrow failure. These disorders share a common pathophysiology which involves clonal dysfunction of the haematopoietic stem cell (Figure 6.1). The pathognomonic manifestation of stem cell dysfunction is trilineage morphologic dysplasia in the bone marrow. The consequences of stem cell dysfunction result from the failure of stem cells to differentiate with subsequent development of refractory cytopenias, hypofunctional cells and a propensity for conversion of the MDS to overt acute myeloid leukaemia (AML).

Aetiology

MDS may be divided into *primary* (*de novo*) or *secondary* syndromes. Primary MDS occurs spontaneously without a known predisposing event. Speculation about aetiology includes genetic predisposition or even exposure to a viral agent. Secondary MDS is a term used to describe the disease that follows environmental toxins (e.g. industrial solvents such as benzene), chemotherapy or radiation exposure. Secondary MDS has been strongly associated with alkylating agent chemotherapy as well as therapy with topisomerase II inhibitors, especially the epipodophyllotoxins, although in the latter situation patients may develop AML without an MDS prodrome and display abnormalities of chromosome 11q23. Also, MDS is recognised as a complication of autologous bone marrow transplantation, especially following high-dose therapy for non-Hodgkin's lymphoma.

Classification and diagnosis

The diagnosis of a MDS relies on the morphologic examination of bone marrow aspirates and trephine bone marrow biopsy specimens. More recently, evaluation of cytogenetic abnormalities in the dysplastic clone has come to play an important role in the diagnosis.

The most widely used classification system is that proposed by the French–American–British (FAB) Cooperative Group in 1982. The FAB classification system outlines five subtypes of MDS which are defined based on bone marrow and peripheral blood morphology:

- Refractory anaemia (RA).
- Refractory anaemia with ringed sideroblasts (RARS).
- Refractory anaemia with excess blasts (RAEB).
- Refractory anaemia with excess blasts in transformation (RAEB-T).
- Chronic myelomonocytic leukaemia (CMML).

Table 6.1 outlines the original FAB criteria for the diagnosis of these syndromes. In addition to the commonly recognised criteria outlined in Table 6.1, the original FAB Cooperative Group also described other morphologic features which characterise the dysplastic morphologic findings in this disease (Table 6.2).

In addition to the examination of the morphologic features of the peripheral blood and bone marrow, evaluation of the chromosomal composition of the bone marrow is essential in any patient with suspected MDS. Cytogenetic analysis (Table 6.3) may be the most important prognostic variable in MDS.

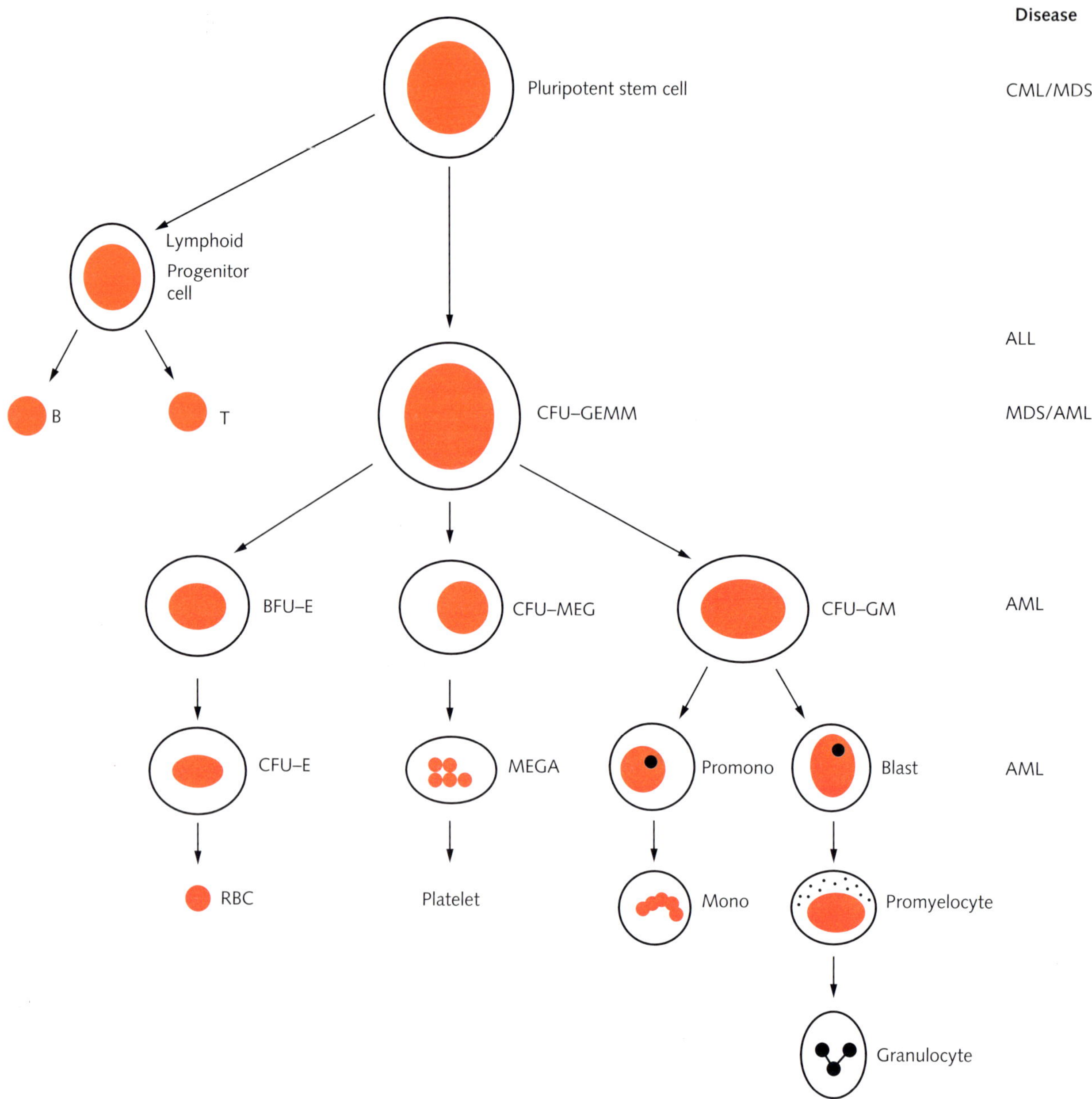

Fig. 6.1 Haematopoietic stem cell hierarchy
CML, chronic myeloid leukaemia; MDS, myelodysplastic syndrome; ALL, acute lymphoblastic leukaemia; AML, acute myeloid leukaemia; B, B-lymphocyte; T, T-lymphocyte; CFU-GEMM, granulocyte/erythroid/myeloid/megakaryocyte colony-forming unit; BFU-E, erythroid burst-forming unit; CFU-MEG, megakaryocyte colony-forming unit; CFU-GM, granulocyte/macrophage colony-forming unit; CFU-E, erythroid colony-forming unit; MEGA, megakaryocyte.

Clinical and laboratory features

MDS are characterised by the paradoxical combination of a hypercellular bone marrow and profound peripheral blood cytopenias. MDS occurs in younger people more often as a consequence of cytotoxic chemotherapy, but in general, MDS is a disease of the elderly with median age at diagnosis greater than 60 years. There is no difference in sex distribution, except in the 5q– syndrome which has a female predominance, and CMML which has a male predominance. There are approximately 15,000 new cases of MDS each year in the United States.

Table 6.1 MDS: FAB classification.

MDS subtype	Blast % Marrow	Blast % Peripheral blood	Other
Refractory anaemia (RA)	0–5%	0	
Refractory anaemia with ringed sideroblasts (RARS)	0–5%	0	>15% ringed sideroblasts
Refractory anaemia with excess blasts (RAEB)	6–19%	1–4%	
Refractory anaemia with excess blasts in transformation (RAEB-T)	20–29%	5–29%	
Chronic myelomonocytic leukaemia (CMML)	0–20%	0–29%	monocytes >1 × 10^9/l (>1000/μl) in peripheral blood

Table 6.2 Additional morphologic characteristics of myelodysplastic syndromes.

	Bone marrow	Peripheral blood
Erythroid cells	Ringed sideroblasts Abnormal nuclear shapes indentations irregular outline Multinuclear cells Abnormal cytoplasm unstained areas punctate basophilia	Nucleated red blood cells Abnormal morphology teardrop forms anisocytosis poikilocytosis macrocytosis
Granulocytic cells	Nuclear abnormalities hyposegmentation (Pelger–Hüet forms) Increased myeloblasts Abnormal granulation large granules hypogranulation lack of perinuclear granules peripheral rims of granules	Abnormal granulation hypogranular agranular
Megakaryocytes	Decreased numbers Micromegakaryocytes Nuclear abnormalities single nuclear forms multiple small and separated nuclei	Abnormal granules large platelets

However, based on ongoing demographic changes and on the increasing use of high-dose chemotherapy in the setting of autologous bone marrow transplant, which is clearly a risk factor for MDS, it is likely that the incidence will rise dramatically in the near future.

Except for cases of MDS associated with prior cytotoxic chemotherapy, most cases of MDS have no underlying identifiable aetiology. In rare cases, there is a prior exposure to radiation, industrial solvents or benzene.

Although patients may present with symptoms attributable to the consequences of anaemia, granulocytopenia or thrombocytopenia such as fatigue, infection and bleeding, respectively, the most common clinical presentation of MDS is the discovery of an abnormality in the 'routine' blood count of an elderly patient. Most patients are generally asymptomatic at presentation. Probably the most common clinical presentation is fatigue in an elderly patient due to mild anaemia. Physical examination findings are unusual and non-specific. The only exception is in CMML, where patients may be discovered to have consequences of extramedullary tumour involvement (splenomegaly, hepatomegaly, gum or skin involvement).

Laboratory abnormalities are as variable as the clinical presentations; granulocytopenia or thrombocytopenia as a single abnormality is uncommon at presentation. It is also uncommon for patients to have leucocytosis, except for CMML where patients may present with monocyte counts above 50,000/µl (50×10^9/l). An unusual presentation is thrombocytosis (associated with the 5q– syndrome). The most common laboratory feature on presentation is mild anaemia. In general, the anaemia is characterised by macrocytosis with normal or elevated vitamin B_{12} and folate levels. However, the anaemia may be normocytic, or even microcytic if there are bone marrow sideroblasts and an associated defect in iron mobilisation. Because of functional defects in granulocytes, red cells and platelets, patients may exhibit more profound clinical manifestations than those explained by the degree of cytopenia alone.

Table 6.3 Cytogenetic abnormalities in MDS.

Karyotype	Incidence
Complex (≥3 abnormalities)	15–50%
Monosomy 7*	10–50%
Deletion 5q*	20%
Trisomy 8	10–15%
Deletion 20q	3–4%
Monosomy Y (males)	3–4%

* Often noted in patients with alkylating agent-associated MDS. Interval between chemotherapy and MDS is approximately 3–7 years.

Multiple studies have addressed the prognosis in MDS. The initial FAB classification was an attempt to formulate potentially clinically useful prognostic subtypes. It has been known for at least 20 years that cytogenetic findings provide critical prognostic information. Recently, an international co-operative group combined seven previous studies on prognosis and used multivariate analysis to generate a system to predict the outcome in MDS patients. The International Prognostic Scoring System (IPSS) combines cytopenias, bone marrow blast percentages and cytogenetics into a weighted prognostic score for an individual patient (Table 6.4).

The clinical course of MDS in any given individual can vary greatly. The evaluation of a patient with suspected MDS now involves a combination of clinical and laboratory data that are synthesised into an assessment of a patient's prognosis. It is, as yet, unclear whether aggressive therapeutic interventions such as a bone marrow transplantation will be able to alter the prognosis of patients with high-risk disease.

Clinically, MDS are associated with a number of unusual autoimmune syndromes. Vasculitis, ulcerative colitis, Crohn's disease, haemolytic anaemia and seronegative arthritis are a few of the well-described

Table 6.4 International Prognostic Scoring System.

Blast % (marrow)	Score	
<5%	0.5	
5–10%	1	
11–20%	1.5	
21–30%	2.0	
Cytopenia*		
0–1	0.5	
2 or 3	1.5	
Karyotype		
Good (–Y, 5q–, 20q–)	0	
Intermediate (other)	0.5	
Poor (chromosome 7) or complex (≥3 abnormalities)	1.0	
Total score		**Median survival (yrs)**
0	Low risk	5.7
0.5–1.0	Low–intermediate risk	3.2
1.5–2.0	High–intermediate risk	1.2
≥2.5	High risk	0.4

* Cytopenia is defined as platelet count $<100 \times 10^9$/l, haemoglobin <10 g/dl, or neutrophil count $<1.5 \times 10^9$/l.

autoimmune diseases associated with MDS. If MDS is associated with excessive bone marrow apoptosis (programmed self-death), it is possible that self-antigens are continually exposed to the immune system; therefore, dysregulation of T-cell function may explain this unusual constellation of associated diseases. However, since MDS is clearly a disease of the multipotent haematopoietic stem cell, it is likely that defects in lymphopoiesis also contribute to the pathophysiology of these unusual phenomena. In addition, there is a small increase in the incidence of second tumours (independent of chemotherapy) in patients with MDS. Whether this reflects a general or an immunologically based predisposition to malignancy is unknown.

Pathogenesis, progression and evolution

MDS are clonal disorders of the haematopoietic stem cell. Isoenzyme analysis, restriction fragment length polymorphisms (Figure 6.2) and interphase cytogenetic analyses have all established the clonal nature of these diseases. The consequence of bone marrow stem cell dysfunction is the failure to produce peripheral blood cells. This may be secondary to either a lack of differentiation of the stem cell and/or an excess amount of apoptosis in the bone marrow.

As noted above, MDS are characterised by the paradox of peripheral blood cytopenias in the presence of a hypercellular bone marrow. The hypothesis that MDS is characterised by excessive apoptosis may provide an intriguing explanation for this apparent paradox. Part of the molecular pathology of apoptosis includes DNA fragmentation; the amount of 5′ DNA ends in a sample can be quantitated as a surrogate marker of the rate of apoptosis. Using this approach, kinetic studies of bone marrow turnover have been performed in patients with MDS. Patients are given infusions of labelled nucleotides, such as bromodeoxyuridine, and bone marrow samples are assayed for the quantity of 5′ DNA ends. Using such an assay, the majority of bone marrow samples from patients with MDS exhibit signs of excessive apoptosis. In addition, the same DNA labelling strategy can be used to measure cell turnover. Most bone marrow samples from patients

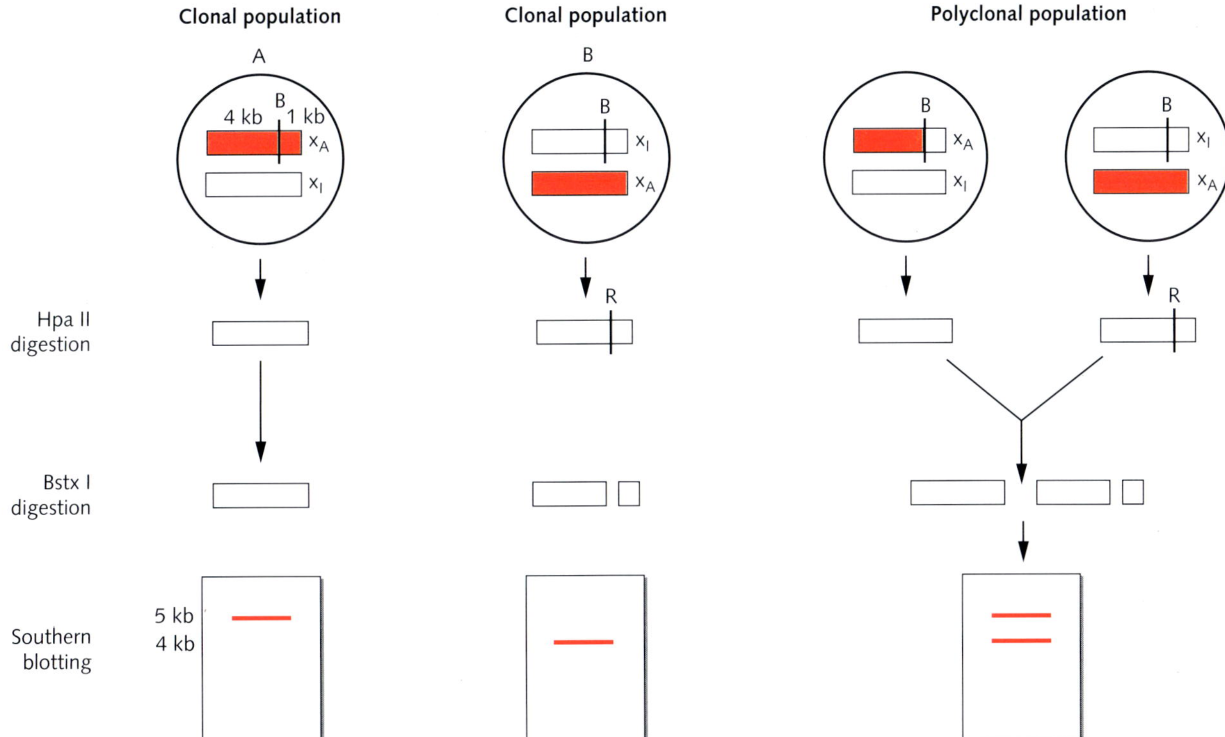

Fig. 6.2 Determining clonality by X-linked restriction fragment length polymorphism analysis
Hpa III digests the unmethylated active X chromosome (X_A).
Bstx I recognises a polymorphic site on the maternal chromosome, yielding 4 kb and 1 kb fragments.
Southern blotting, DNA fragments are separated electrophoretically by size and hybridised to the relevant probe.
(Courtesy of D. Gary Gilliland, MD PhD.)

with MDS also exhibit increased rates of cell growth. These data lead to the speculation that excess rates of growth lead to a hypercellular bone marrow, but increased rates of apoptosis render the hypercellular bone marrow ineffective with resultant peripheral blood cytopenias.

Cytokine dysregulation may also play an important role in the development of MDS. Some patients with MDS have low levels of haematopoietic cytokines. Approximately 20% of patients with MDS have inappropriately low levels of erythropoietin for the degree of anaemia. In addition, MDS patients have been found to have high levels of cytokines that could promote apoptosis, such as interleukin-1β (IL-1β), tumour necrosis factor-α (TNF-α) and transforming growth factor-β (TGF-β). Intriguingly, all of these cytokines probably share a common lipid-based intracellular signalling pathway which involves diacylglycerol metabolism.

Regardless of the imbalance between cell proliferation and apoptosis in MDS, a patient with this condition will probably succumb to the disease. In approximately 30–40% of patients with MDS, the bone marrow evolves to AML. Compared to *de novo* AML, these secondary forms of AML are more virulent; remission rates are lower and survival is short once a patient with MDS converts to AML. However, most patients do not convert to overt acute leukaemia. Approximately half of patients will die of the consequences of granulocytopenia and granulocyte dysfunction. Given the advanced age of the majority of patients with MDS, 10–20% of patients die of co-morbid disease rather than from progression of MDS.

Chromosomal abnormalities

As noted above, chromosomal analysis plays a critical role in the evaluation of the patient with suspected MDS. Approximately half of patients with MDS will have a bone marrow stem cell clone which contains a non-random clonal cytogenetic abnormality. Table 6.3 lists the more common cytogenetic abnormalities in MDS. One specific chromosomal abnormality, 5q–, is associated with a distinct syndrome. While it is the most common abnormality in MDS, approximately half of the time it is an isolated cytogenetic abnormality. When present as an isolated anomaly it is often associated with a well-described clinical entity, characterised by a marked female predominance, refractory anaemia FAB subtype and distinctive laboratory and bone marrow findings. Patients display thrombocytosis despite a relatively severe anaemia and concomitant transfusion requirement. The bone marrow analysis often reveals hypolobated megakaryocytes ('micromegakaryocytes'). In addition, conversion to AML in this syndrome is rare. In the acute leukaemias the study of genes disrupted by balanced translocations has yielded critical pathophysiological insight. The reader is referred to other sections of this book for discussions of disruptions of transcription factors, for example t(8;21) and inv(16) in AML leading to a failure of normal differentiation. Experiments have proven that the chimeric proteins cause the disease. However, such balanced translocations are rare in MDS. Defining which, if any, are the critical genes gained in cases of trisomy 8 MDS, or lost in cases of 5q– or 7q– MDS, has proven to be very challenging (*see next section*).

Genetic abnormalities associated with MDS

Like most human neoplasias, MDS, and certainly AML, most likely arise in the setting of multiple genetic lesions that accumulate in a stepwise fashion. Combinations of mutations in both classic dominant oncogenes and recessive tumour suppressor genes allow for the generation of the malignant phenotype. Since MDS is often characterised by large chromosomal deletions, much work has focused on the hypothesis that tumour suppressor genes may be involved in the pathogenesis of MDS. For example, the tumour suppressor p53 gene on chromosome 17q has been reportedly mutated in some patients with MDS.

The *RAS* oncogene was initially discovered as the transforming gene in rodent sarcoma viruses. It has become clear that the cellular homologues of the viral *RAS* genes are one of the most commonly mutated dominant oncogenes in human tumours. The RAS protein is involved in intracellular signalling at the cell membrane surface (Figure 6.3). RAS binds GTP and has GTPase activity. *RAS* mutations are found very commonly in AML, and therefore *RAS* involvement in MDS has been extensively studied.

RAS mutations are one of the most common oncogenic mutations in MDS. In some studies, as many as one-third of MDS specimens bear *RAS* gene mutations. *RAS* mutations are found in all morphologic subtypes of MDS, but of note, the most common MDS subtype to contain detectable *RAS* mutations is CMML, and in one study over 50% of CMML isolates studied had mutant *RAS* genes identified. It is intriguing since the monocytic subtypes of AML also have a significant incidence of *RAS* mutations. In general, the mutant *RAS* gene is the N-*RAS* gene, and unlike other tumour types, there does

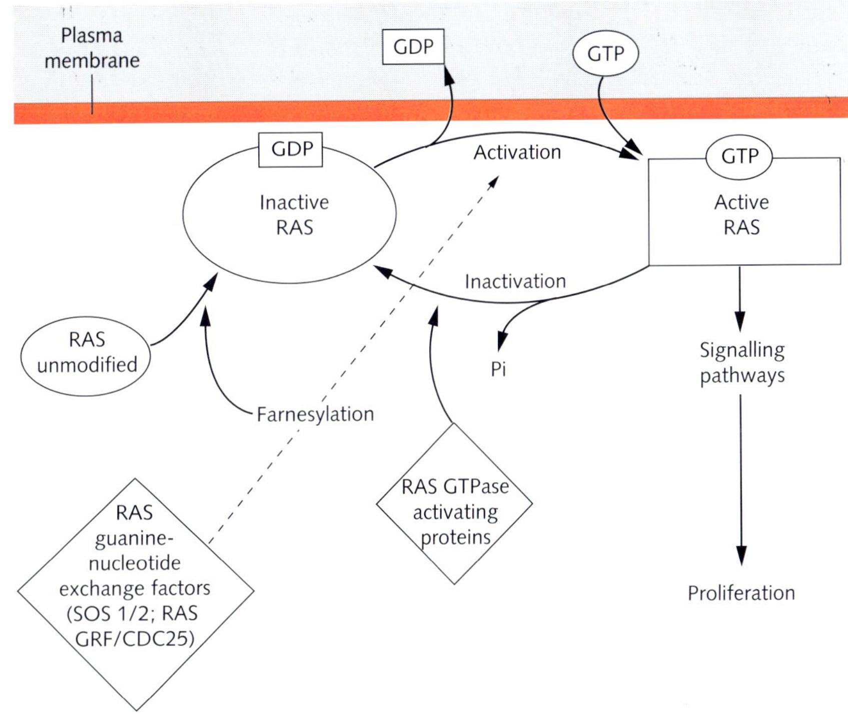

Fig. 6.3 RAS proteins in signal transduction
GDP, guanosine diphosphate; GTP, guanosine triphosphate; Pi, inorganic phosphate.

not appear to be a specific *RAS* mutant allele associated with MDS.

Changes involving chromosome 5 are very common in MDS, and especially in forms of MDS related to prior chemotherapy exposure. It is somewhat paradoxical that an isolated loss of the long arm of chromosome 5 which results in the 5q− syndrome carries a very favourable prognosis (5q− alone is in the good prognosis cytogenetic category in the IPSS), yet chromosome 5 changes related to chemotherapy portend a very poor prognosis.

Much work has focused on identifying the minimal region on chromosome 5q that is altered. There are a number of intriguing candidate genes at band 5q31 including interleukin-3, 4, 5 and 9, interferon response factor 1, granulocyte-macrophage colony-stimulating factor and the colony-stimulating factor 4 receptor.

Since this region is frequently lost completely in MDS and AML, it is interesting to speculate that a tumour suppressor locus might be found at 5q31. In this light, another gene in this region is *EGR1*, the early growth response gene. This gene is a putative transcription factor which contains a zinc finger motif. In addition, this gene is homologous to the Wilm's tumour suppressor gene. However, the remaining allele of this gene is not altered in most cases of the 5q− syndrome.

As mentioned earlier, the colony-stimulating factor 1 (also known as M-CSF: macrophage colony-stimulating factor) receptor gene is found on chromosome 5q, and it is near this region at band 5q33. This receptor is the cellular homologue of the *FMS* oncogene. Surprisingly, CMML is also the most common subtype of MDS to bear *FMS* mutations (Figure 6.4).

A similar approach has been taken to the analysis of the long arm of chromosome 7. Namely, the hypothesis has been presented that a putative leukaemogenic tumour suppressor gene exists at chromosome 7q. Studies of interstitial deletions of chromosome 7 have narrowed the region to long arm bands q22 to q33. Previously, it was believed that the genes for erythropoietin and plasminogen activator inhibitor 1, which map near band 7q22, might be involved in the 7q deletions. However, recent high resolution mapping studies have suggested that the minimal region involved in 7q deletions does not contain either of these two genes. The isolation of a yeast artificial chromosome (YAC) clone containing this region has been recently described and may contain the tumour suppressor gene postulated to exist at 7q.

Cells from some patients with CMML display a translocation between chromosomes 5 and 12. This fusion gene at the translocation junction has been cloned and analysed, and has been found to contain portions of both the *TEL* and *PDGF* genes (Figure 6.5). This is unusual since the *TEL* gene is a putative transcription factor and the *PDGF* gene is a cell surface receptor. The fusion gene product contains the amino terminal portion of the *TEL* gene, which includes a canonical helix–loop–helix domain, a protein structural motif believed to mediate multimerisation of nuclear transcription factors. In the fusion gene product, the helix–loop–helix domain of *TEL* is fused to a portion of the *PDGF* gene which contains both the transmembrane domain and the cytoplasmic signalling domain. Interestingly, the helix–loop–helix domain of TEL likely mediates dimerisation of the TEL–PDGF fusion protein. The functional consequences of the dimerisation mimic the ligand-mediated dimerisation of the native PDGF receptor. In the TEL–PDGF fusion protein, dimerisation leads to constitutive activation of the PDGF cytoplasmic kinase domain. As a result the PDGF-related intercellular signalling cascades are activated and neoplastic transformation results.

The discovery of excessive apoptosis in the bone marrow in MDS has led to speculation regarding genes involved in this process. High levels of c-*MYC* expression are correlated with an increased rate of apoptosis, and high levels of BCL-2 protein are correlated with a decreased rate of apoptosis. It is possible that the trisomy 8 cytogenetic abnormality leads to increased levels of c-MYC protein, with the functional consequence being increased levels of apoptosis. It is tempting to speculate that in the setting of higher rates of apoptosis, which would lead to peripheral blood cytopenias, there would initially be a compensatory increase in haematopoietic cytokine synthesis. The morphologic consequence of this would be a hypercellular bone marrow induced by cytokine stimulation with even higher rates of apoptosis induced by the high levels of c-MYC.

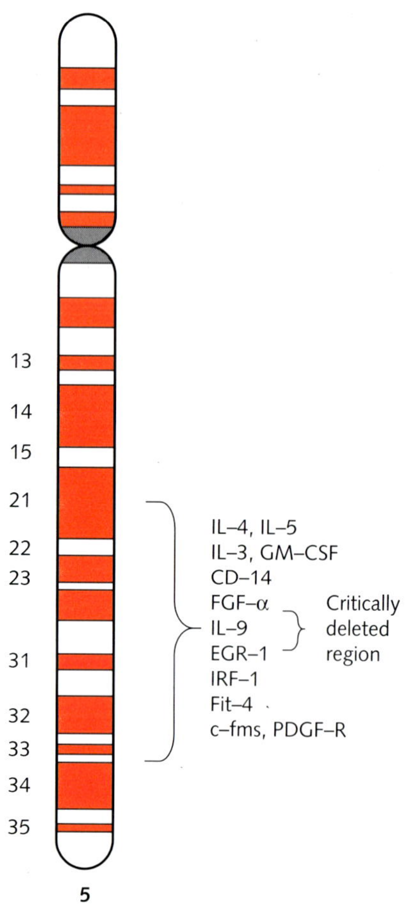

Fig. 6.4 Chromosome 5
Genes on critically deleted region located on long arm of chromosome 5. (Courtesy of D. Gary Gilliland, MD PhD.)

Molecular approaches to therapy

One obvious approach to molecular-based therapy of MDS involves the use of the haematopoietic cytokines. Granulocyte colony-stimulating factor, granulocyte-macrophage colony-stimulating factor and erythropoietin have all been investigated in patients with MDS. Although administration of myeloid growth factors leads to a higher white blood cell count, this effect has not been shown to confer major clinical benefit either in

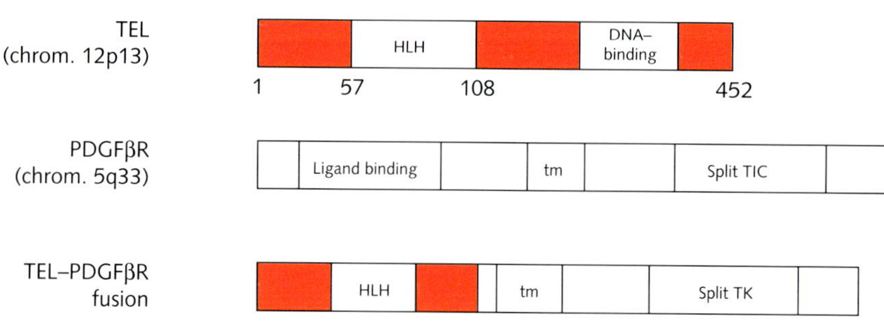

Fig. 6.5 The TEL/platelet-derived growth factor β receptor fusion in t(5;12) CMML
HLH, helix–loop–helix; tm, transmembrane domain; TK, tyrosine kinase. (From Carroll, M *et al.* (1996) *PNAS (USA)* 93, 14,845.)

terms of survival or reducing infections. Fortunately, early concerns that these growth factors might initiate leukaemic transformation have not been validated. Whether or not cytokines, such as thrombopoietin or interleukin-11, will be able to ameliorate the thrombocytopenia seen in MDS remains to be determined. Proximally acting growth factors such as interleukin-3 or interleukin-6 have not been particularly helpful in this regard.

There has been an attempt to employ recombinant human erythropoietin (EPO) to treat the MDS-associated anaemia. While EPO therapy is quite safe, only about 20%—usually those with inappropriately low endogenous EPO levels—will respond. However, individual cytokines *alone* may not be sufficient to stimulate the appropriate differentiation of haematopoietic stem cells. Therefore, cytokine combinations have been evaluated in patients with MDS. A recent study has suggested that the combination of granulocyte colony-stimulating factor and EPO may be superior to either cytokine alone for ameliorating anaemia. Of particular note, one study suggests that the combination of these two cytokines resulted in decreased rates of apoptosis in the bone marrow.

The discovery that the pathophysiology of MDS might be related to elevated levels of inhibitory or pro-apoptotic cytokines (e.g. IL-1β, TNF-α, TGF-β) has led to the concept of 'anti-cytokine' therapy. Specifically, the common lipid-based signalling pathway shared by these cytokines might represent a novel therapeutic target in MDS. Agents that affect this pathway include the methyl xanthine derivatives, lisophylline and pentoxifylline, as well as the fluoroquinolone antibiotic ciprofloxacin and the steroid dexamethasone. In theory, these agents may be effective in MDS by blocking the negative effects of the inhibitory and pro-apoptotic cytokines. Preliminary studies with a combination of these agents have reported a few clinical responses. Amifostine, a reducing agent licensed for use as a chemotherapy protectant, has been subjected to clinical trials in patients with MDS and some multilineage responses have been noted.

Observations that cells from patients with MDS fail to mature normally have led to trials of differentiating agents. Multiple agents have been observed to enhance differentiation of MDS or AML cells *in vitro*. These include low-dose cytarabine, 5-azacytidine, hexamethylene bisacetamide, interferons, butyrates, retinoids, derivatives of vitamin D and recently the protein kinase C agonist (Figure 6.6), bryostatin. Although intriguing *in vitro* results have been obtained, the clinical value of these agents remains to be determined.

It has been difficult to demonstrate the ability of specific available therapies to change the natural history of this disease. Preliminary results of a co-operative

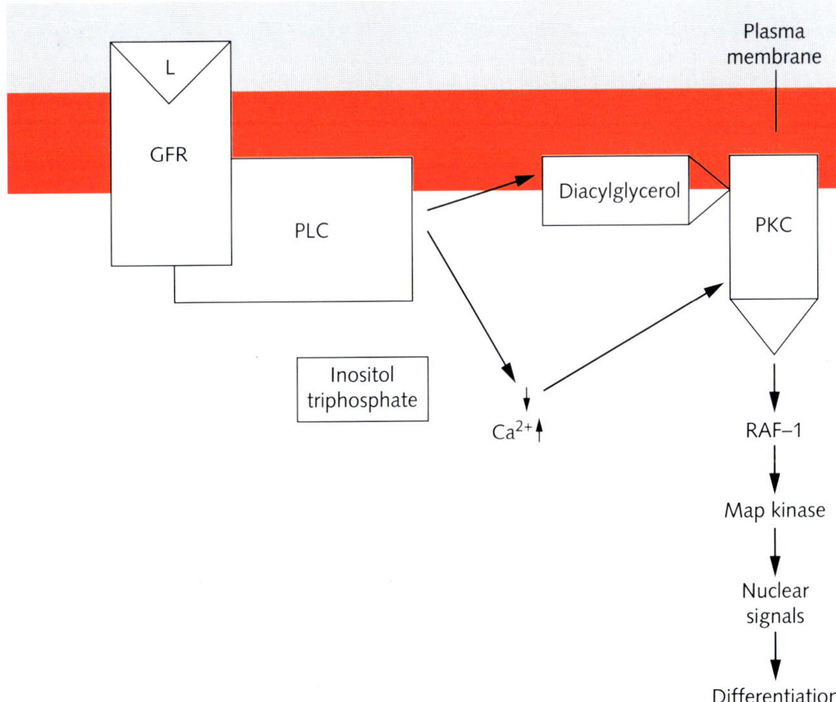

Fig. 6.6 Signal transduction via protein kinase C
GFR, growth factor receptor; L, ligand; PLC, phospholipase C; PKC, protein kinase C.

group trial in which patients with MDS were randomised either to receive the differentiating agent 5-azacytidine (mechanism is via DNA methylation), or undergo observation, were encouraging in that the treated group had a lower incidence of transformation to AML and a better quality of life. Allogeneic bone marrow transplantation is potentially curative in young patients (below age 60–65 years) with MDS. Not surprisingly, this approach is much more effective for those with low-risk disease. Recent work has suggested that those with MDS respond just as well as those with AML to antileukaemic (e.g. myelosuppressive) chemotherapy, with topotecan being a particularly interesting cytotoxic drug for this purpose. In other words, the likelihood of response to induction chemotherapy depends not on the number of bone marrow blasts but on other more biologically relevant factors (e.g. cytogenetics).

Conclusions

It is hoped that further understanding of the molecular basis for MDS will provide better tolerated and much more effective therapies than those now available. Such innovative future approaches could include gene therapy to correct the acquired defect in the disease, small molecule therapy to restore a disrupted transcriptional apparatus (e.g. the use of all-*trans*-retinoic acid for acute promyelocytic leukaemia) or prevent apoptosis, or strategies which could allow the immune system to recognise and destroy the altered MDS bone marrow progenitor cell. At the moment, the best recommendation for most patients with MDS is to be managed supportively with transfusions (a trial of EPO ± G-CSF warranted) or preferably to enrol on a clinical trial evaluating a new agent.

Further reading

Bennett JM, Catovsky D, Daniel MT *et al.* (1982) Proposals for the classification of the myelodysplastic syndromes. *British Journal of Haematology*, **51**, 189–199.

Estey E, Thall P, Beran M *et al.* (1997) Effect of diagnosis (refractory anemia with excess blasts, refractory anemia with excess blasts in transformation, or acute myeloid leukemia [AML]) on outcome of AML-type chemotherapy. *Blood*, **90**, 2969–2977.

Forman ST. (1996) Myelodysplastic syndrome. *Current Opinion in Hematology*, **3**, 297–302.

Gaenser A, Karthous M. (1997) Clinical uses of hematopoietic growth factors in the myelodysplastic syndromes. *Leukemia and Lymphoma*, **26**, 13–27.

Greenberg P, Cox C, Lebeau MM. (1997) International scoring system for evaluating prognosis in myelodysplastic syndromes. *Blood*, **89**, 2079–2088.

Karp JE. (1998) Molecular pathogenesis and targets for therapy in myelodysplastic syndrome (MDS) and MDS-related leukemias. *Current Opinion in Oncology*, **10**, 3–9.

Koeffler HP. (1996) Myelodysplastic syndromes. *Seminars in Hematology*, **33**, 87–94.

List AU. (1998) Hematopoietic stimulation by amifostine and sodium phenylbutyrate: what is the potential in MDS? *Leukemia Research*, **22**, suppl. 1, S7–S11.

Nevill TJ, Fung HC, Shepherd JD *et al.* (1998) Cytogenetic abnormalities in primary myelodysplastic syndrome are highly predictive of outcome after allogeneic bone marrow transplantation. *Blood*, **92**, 1910–1917.

Parker JE, Mufti GJ. (1998) Ineffective haemopoiesis and apoptosis in myelodysplastic syndromes. *British Journal of Haematology*, **101**, 220–230.

Stone RM. (1994) Myelodysplastic syndrome after autologous transplantation for lymphoma: the price of progress? *Blood*, **83**, 3437–3440.

van der Berghe H, Michaux L. (1997) 5q−, twenty-five years later: a synopsis. *Cancer Genetics and Cytogenetics*, **94**, 1–7.

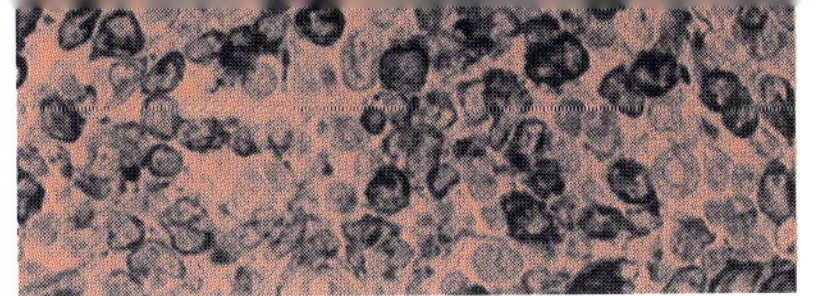

Chapter 7 Myeloproliferative disorders

Anthony J Bench, Brian J P Huntly, Elisabeth P Nacheva, Kim M Champion & Anthony R Green

Introduction and classification

The myeloproliferative disorders (MPDs) comprise polycythaemia vera (PV), essential thrombocythaemia (ET) and idiopathic myelofibrosis (IMF). They were first classed together as an overlapping spectrum of pre-leukaemic disorders along with chronic myeloid leukaemia (CML) by Dameshek in 1951. CML, with its pathognomonic chromosomal translocation, greater clinical homogeneity and increased leukaemic potential, is now considered a separate entity. The MPDs are believed to result from acquired genetic changes in haematopoietic stem cells which perturb stem cell behaviour and result in the overproduction of one or more cells of the myelo-erythroid series leading to a predisposition to acute leukaemia. These disorders are not mutually exclusive and considerable overlap is seen between distinct categories with progression from one disease to another a regular occurrence (Figure 7.1). The MPDs also have pre-leukaemic potential transforming to acute myeloid leukaemia (AML) in a number of patients.

The MPDs are relatively uncommon disorders. PV has an annual incidence of 5–10 cases per million population. Less is known about the incidence of ET. However, it is likely to be similar to, if not greater than, that for PV. Although little is known of the epidemiology of IMF, it is thought to have an incidence of 5 cases per million population annually but, since many patients are diagnosed coincidentally, and up to 25% are asymptomatic at the time of diagnosis, this figure is likely to represent an underestimate. The diagnosis of the MPDs is made according to strict diagnostic criteria (Table 7.1a–c), but there is still considerable emphasis on the exclusion of secondary causes since there is no *single* pathognomonic abnormality. Even with these strict criteria, it can be difficult to differentiate the MPDs, especially ET, from reactive causes. The identification of target genes in these disorders would produce much needed diagnostic tools for clinicians as well as providing important insights into the regulation of normal haematopoiesis.

X-linked clonality assays

Evidence that MPDs arise as a result of transformation of a haematopoietic stem cell has come from two main sources: analysis of karyotypic abnormalities and analysis of X-chromosome inactivation patterns to determine the clonality of different cell lineages. X-inactivation assays offer a means of assessing the clonality of a population of cells without any acquired cytogenetic or molecular markers. X inactivation occurs in females as a means of dosage compensation so that equal levels of expression of X-linked genes occur between males and females. Early in embryogenesis one X chromosome is inactivated at random in each cell—a process termed *Lyonisation*. The progeny of each cell inherits this inactivation pattern. As a consequence, the adult female is a *mosaic*—some cells carry an active maternal X chromosome, some an active paternal X chromosome.

A population of cells, such as a tumour, which is clonally derived from a single cell will therefore carry either an active maternal X chromosome or an active paternal X chromosome. By contrast, a polyclonal population contains some cells with an active maternal X chromosome and some with an active paternal X chromosome. Assessment of X-inactivation patterns requires an ability to distinguish paternal and maternal X chromosomes and so the various assays are all based on polymorphic X-linked genes. It is also necessary to determine which X chromosome is active. This can be achieved by monitoring expression of an X-linked gene at the protein or RNA

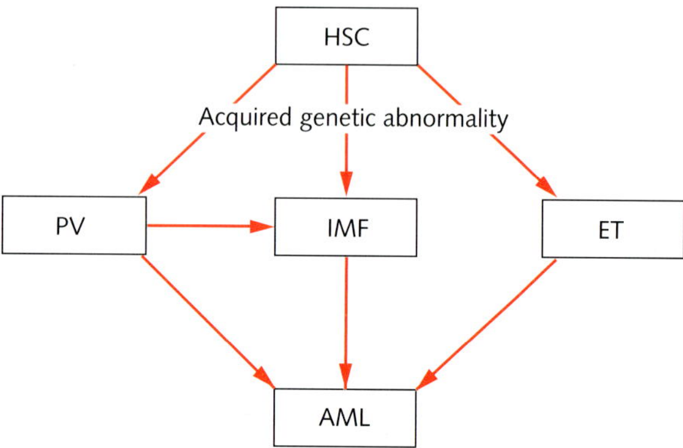

Fig. 7.1 Relationships of the myeloproliferative disorders and transformation to acute myeloid leukaemia
The percentage of patients who transform varies according to the initial disease, duration of disease and treatment. HSC, haematopoietic stem cell; PV, polycythaemia vera; IMF, idiopathic myelofibrosis; ET, essential thrombocythaemia; AML, acute myeloid leukaemia.

level. Alternatively, DNA methylation can be used as a surrogate marker for gene inactivity since, for many genes, methylation status correlates well with transcriptional activity. An example of a DNA-based technique, the human androgen receptor assay (HUMARA), is shown in Figure 7.2.

Initial studies on clonality used a rare polymorphism in the G6PD gene which results in two distinct protein products. In patients with PV, a single isoform was present in erythrocytes, granulocytes, platelets and bone marrow buffy coat implying that these cells were clonally derived. Both isoforms were expressed in lymphocytes and skin fibroblasts. The majority of erythroid and granulocyte progenitors were also clonally derived. Similar patterns were also observed for ET and IMF.

Subsequent studies using methylation of X-linked genes as a marker of gene inactivity have demonstrated an unbalanced pattern of methylation consistent with clonality in white blood cells or bone marrow cells from a high proportion of patients with ET, PV or IMF (*reviewed in* Hinshelwood *et al.*, 1997). However, in the

Table 7.1 Diagnostic criteria for myeloproliferative disorders.

(a) Proposed modified criteria for the diagnosis of polycythaemia vera
A1 Raised red cell mass (>25% above normal predicted value)
A2 Absence of cause of secondary polycythaemia
A3 Palpable splenomegaly
A4 Acquired cytogenetic abnormality

B1 Thrombocytosis (platelet count >400 × 10^9/l)
B2 Neutrophil leucocytosis (neutrophil count >10 × 10^9/l)
B3 Splenomegaly demonstrated on isotope/ultrasound scanning
B4 Characteristic BFU-E growth or reduced serum erythropoietin

A1 + A2 + A3 or A4 establishes PV. A1 + A2 + two of B establishes PV.

(b) Diagnostic criteria for essential thrombocythaemia
1 Platelet count >600 × 10^9/l
2 Packed cell volume (PCV) <0.51 for males or <0.48 for females or normal red cell mass in those with a high/normal PCV and splenomegaly
3 Stainable iron in marrow or normal serum ferritin or normal red cell mean corpuscular volume (MCV). If measurement suggests iron deficiency then PV cannot be excluded unless a trial of iron therapy fails to increase the red cell mass into the erythrocytotic range
4 No Philadelphia chromosome or *BCR-ABL* gene rearrangement
5 Collagen fibrosis of marrow either absent or less than one-third of biopsy area without marked splenomegaly and leucoerythroblastic reaction
6 No cytogenetic or morphological evidence for a myelodysplastic syndrome
7 No cause for reactive thrombocytosis

(c) Diagnostic criteria for idiopathic myelofibrosis
1 Bone marrow fibrosis
2 Extramedullary haematopoiesis
3 Splenomegaly
4 Leucoerythroblastic blood picture
5 Absence of another chronic myeloproliferative disorder
6 Absence of a condition associated with secondary bone marrow fibrosis

Information derived from Pearson 1998; Reilly 1997.

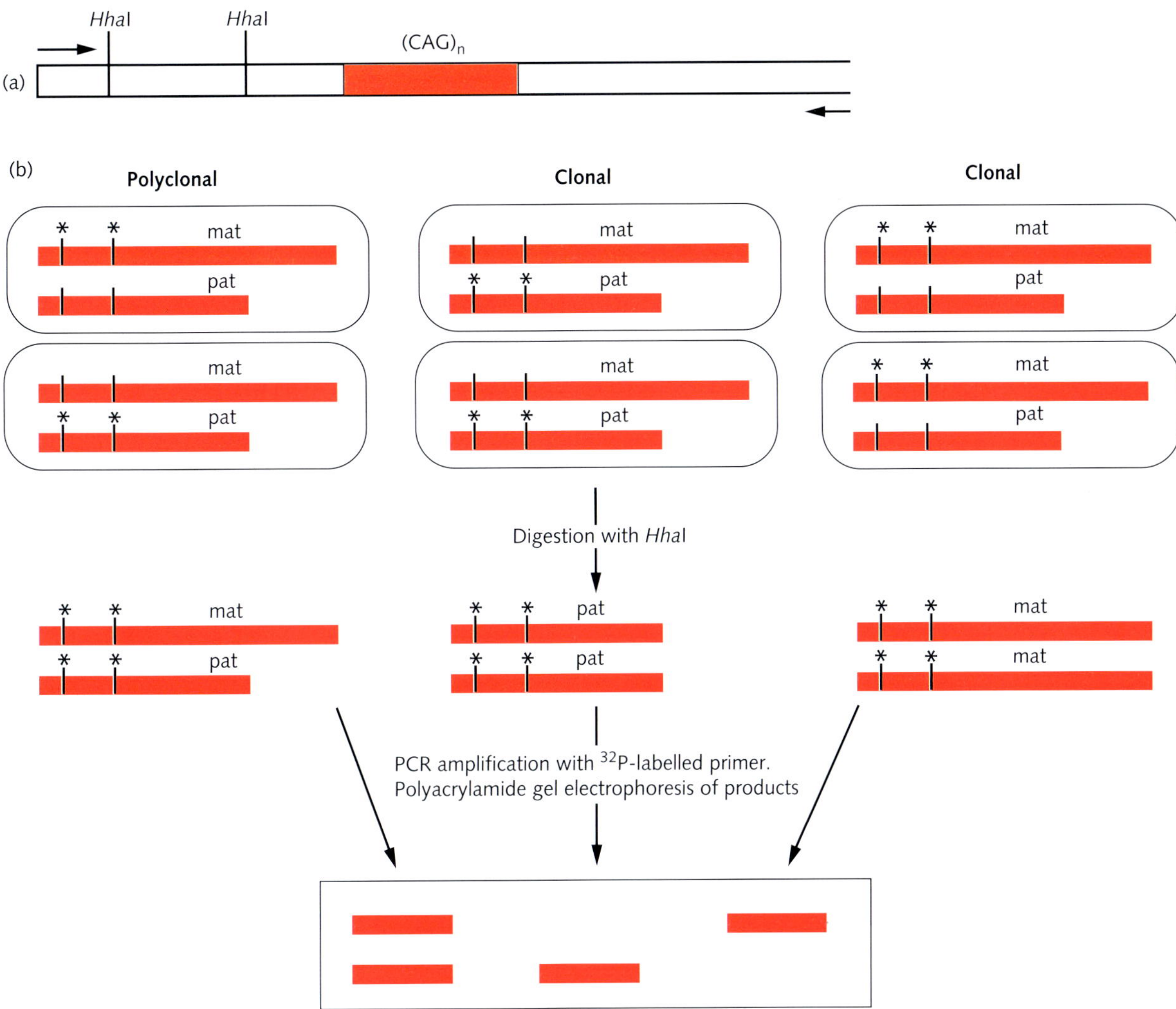

Fig. 7.2
(a) First exon of the human androgen receptor locus (HUMARA). The first exon contains two recognition sites for the methylation sensitive restriction enzyme, *Hha*I. Methylation of these sites correlates with X-chromosome inactivation. The sites lie very close to a highly polymorphic (CAG)n repeat. PCR primers can therefore be designed which flank both the *Hha*I site and the polymorphic (CAG)n repeat.

(b) Determination of clonality of a population of cells using the HUMARA. * = methylated restriction site. *Hha*I sites on the active X chromosome are unmethylated and are therefore digested with the enzyme, whereas methylated sites will not be cleaved. If the maternally and paternally derived alleles contain different numbers of the (CAG) repeat, their size can be distinguished following amplification by PCR and separation by polyacrylamide gel electrophoresis. (*Adapted from* Allen *et al.*, 1992.)

majority of early studies, no control was performed to exclude the possibility of skewed Lyonisation, a situation which can mimic true clonality. The most appropriate tissue to use for such a control is T-cells, and the demonstration of a polyclonal pattern in T-cells and a clonal pattern in granulocytes (or other appropriate lineage) in female patients has generally been considered as evidence for the presence of a clonal myeloid malignancy. Using these criteria, it was hoped that a test for clonality would be a useful diagnostic tool. Early reports demonstrated that the majority of patients who could be assessed by these criteria fell into this category (Figure 7.3).

Interestingly, a small number of well-characterised patients with PV and ET possess polyclonal T-cells and polyclonal granulocytes (Figure 7.3). These results suggest that, in some patients, only a small proportion of granulocytes are part of the neoplastic clone or that the granulocytic lineage is not involved at all. Alternatively, polyclonal haematopoiesis may still be present in some

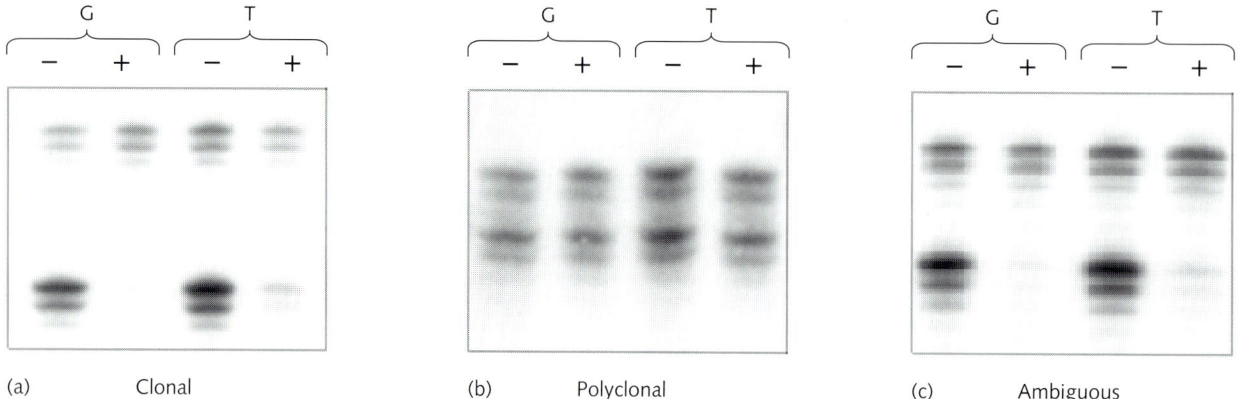

Fig. 7.3 HUMARA assay results
Examples of results obtained with three MPD patient samples are shown.
G, granulocytes; T, T-cells; + and − refer to presence and absence of predigestion with the methylation sensitive restriction enzyme, *Hha*I. (a) Clonal pattern observed in the majority of MPD patients. T-cells exhibit balanced X inactivation whereas granulocytes display a skewed pattern; (b) a small number of patients have polyclonal T-cells and polyclonal granulocytes; (c) result is ambiguous since both the granulocytes and T-cells give a skewed pattern. This is consistent with either excessive Lyonisation or with T-cells arising from the malignant clone.

patients fulfilling current criteria for an MPD. These results have been confirmed in patients with ET by analysis of polymorphisms at the level of mRNA and hence do not merely reflect alterations in the methylation status of these patients' granulocytes. The use of RNA-based methods has also shown that a small number of ET patients possess clonal platelets but polyclonal granulocytes and T-cells. These various observations have contributed to a growing realisation that heterogeneity exists within individual MPDs.

Although a minority of MPD patients possess polyclonal granulocytes, the finding of a clonal pattern in granulocytes with polyclonal T-cells was thought to be a potentially useful test for a positive diagnosis of MPD. Initial studies suggested that this pattern was rare in normal women. However, these control women were usually young and the MPDs are mainly observed in the elderly. When a large number of normal elderly women were studied, a significant number showed a clonal pattern in unfractionated blood cells. It has subsequently been found that a clonal pattern in granulocytes with polyclonal T-cells, identical to that found in MPD patients, is present in 25–50% of normal elderly women.

A number of mechanisms could account for this observation. Firstly, an acquired mutation could lead to clonal growth as is believed to be the case for MPD and myelodysplastic syndrome (MDS). However, it would seem unlikely that a significant number of otherwise normal women over the age of 60 years have a clonal haematological malignancy. Secondly, stem cell depletion may occur with increasing age. Transplantation studies have demonstrated that a small number of stem cells can lead to clonal dominance by what appears to be a stochastic process. However, old mice have an increased number of stem cells arguing against such a depletion mechanism. Thirdly, a possible mechanism is selection for allelic X-linked differences. Polymorphisms of X-linked loci may result in a small selective advantage for stem cells whose active X chromosome is of one particular parental type. The observation that elderly cats develop skewing towards one parental G6PD allele supports this concept and implies the presence of one or more X-linked genes which regulate stem cell kinetics.

Whatever the mechanism underlying these results, they have important clinical and practical implications. Firstly, determination of the clonality status using the HUMARA is clearly not a useful diagnostic tool in elderly women. It will be important to extend this analysis to younger women using RNA-based techniques. Secondly, in a number of patients, a clonal pattern may precede rather than follow neoplastic transformation. This has consequences for experimental strategies which entail identifying genetic changes in 'clonal' populations of cells. Thirdly, the data raise questions about the current dogma that clonal haematopoiesis in patients with MPD and MDS necessarily reflects transformation of a multipotent stem cell.

Chromosome abnormalities

Unlike the Philadelphia chromosome in CML, there is no

Table 7.2 Summary of karyotypic abnormalities identified by G-banding in PV and IMF in eight published series.

	Polycythaemia vera		Idiopathic myelofibrosis	
Abnormality	Number of occurrences of abnormality	% of all patients	Number of occurrences of abnormality	% of all patients
Deletion of 20q	36	8.6	26	9.6
Deletion of 13q	15	3.6	20	7.4
Trisomy 8	27	6.4	9	3.3
Trisomy 9	25	6.0	1	0.4
Duplication of 1q	14	3.3	8	3.0
Deletion of 7q or monosomy 7	5	1.2	4	1.5
Deletion of 5q or monosomy 5	17	4.1	1	0.4
Total number of patients with one or more abnormality	145	34.6	91	33.7
Total patients	**419**		**270**	

(Data taken from Diez-Martin *et al.*, 1991; Dupriez *et al.*, 1996; Reilly *et al.*, 1997; Swolin *et al.*, 1988; Berger *et al.*, 1984; Rege-Cambrin *et al.*, 1987; Demory *et al.*, 1998; Mertens *et al.*, 1991.)

pathognomonic chromosomal abnormality associated with the MPDs. However, a number of recurrent chromosomal abnormalities have been documented in the MPDs. Chromosomal abnormalities are seen in approximately one-third of patients with PV and IMF. The most frequent chromosomal abnormalities in these disorders, as detected by G-banding, are shown in Table 7.2. Detection of cytogenetic abnormalities is infrequent in ET patients.

In PV, there is some evidence that the survival of patients with a chromosomal abnormality is less than that of patients with a normal karyotype. Although the numbers of patients were small or not well matched, this suggests that an abnormal karyotype may be a poor prognostic indicator. For IMF, studies with large numbers of patients have demonstrated that an abnormal karyotype at diagnosis is associated with a poorer prognosis.

Some chromosomal changes such as deletions or monosomies of chromosomes 5 and 7 are almost invariably seen after exposure to myelosuppressive therapy and frequently as part of a complex karyotype. It is therefore unlikely that these chromosomes contain genes involved in the aetiology of the MPDs. By contrast, deletions of part of the long arm of chromosomes 20 (del 20q) and 13 (del 13q), trisomies of chromosomes 8 and 9 and duplication of part of the long arm of chromosome 1 have all been seen in untreated patients and are frequently present as sole abnormalities. They are likely, therefore, to mark the site of genes which play an early role in the pathogenesis of the MPDs.

Deletions

20q deletion

The importance of del(20q) is exemplified in a study of 3996 consecutive abnormal bone marrow samples performed by Dewald *et al.* (1993). Almost 3000 of these samples possessed a sole chromosomal abnormality and, of these, del(20q) was the second most common structural abnormality after t(9;22). In addition to the MPDs, 20q deletions are also seen in approximately 4% of patients with MDS and in 1–2% of patients with AML. However, 20q deletions are rarely seen in lymphoid malignancies. This pattern of disease association suggests that the deleted region of chromosome 20 marks the site of one or more genes, loss or inactivation of which perturbs the regulation of haematopoietic progenitors. The finding of 20q deletions at diagnosis and as a sole abnormality suggests that, in at least some cases, it plays an early role in disease pathogenesis.

There have been a number of studies concerning the prognostic significance of the 20q deletion in both MPD and MDS. As far as MPD is concerned, there is no significant difference in the survival rate of patients with and without a 20q deletion although only a small number of patients have been studied. For MDS, a 20q deletion is associated with a relatively good prognosis, if it is observed *without* any other karyotypic abnormalities.

Since both MPD and MDS are believed to result from transformation of a haematopoietic stem cell, it was of

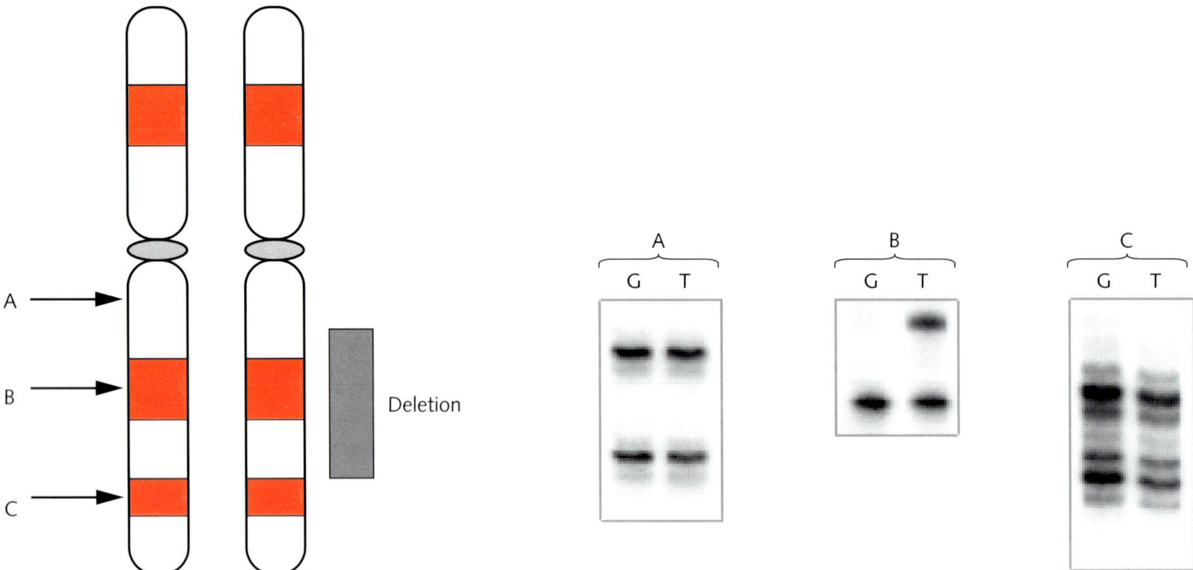

Fig. 7.4 Use of microsatellite PCR to map deletions
G, granulocytes; T, T-cells. Granulocytes contain the deletion whereas T-cells do not. Using markers A and C, two alleles are present in granulocytes and therefore these markers lie outside the deletion. Using marker B, two alleles are present in T-cells, but only one in granulocytes. Hence, marker B lies within the deletion. (*Reproduced from* Bench *et al.*, 1998b.)

interest to determine whether 20q deletions arise in a pluripotent progenitor or a later, committed progenitor. White *et al.* (1994) described a patient with MDS whose granulocytes and monocytes were clonal (as assessed by X-inactivation patterns) and clearly contained the deletion, whereas B-cells and T-cells were polyclonal and did not contain the deletion. However, EBV-transformed B-cell lines carrying the 20q deletion were derived from this patient. Similarly, in another patient, a 20q deletion was reported in EBV-transformed B-cell lines as well as in CFU-GM, CFU-GEMM and BFU-E. Clearly, the 20q deletion can arise in a very early progenitor with both lymphoid and myeloid potential.

In most patients with a 20q deletion, the deletion can readily be detected in peripheral blood neutrophils using microsatellite PCR (Figure 7.4). However, this is not always the case. Asimakopoulos *et al.* (1996) described an interesting subset of patients with a 20q deletion in the majority of bone marrow metaphases but with no deletion detectable in peripheral blood granulocytes by microsatellite PCR. This observation suggests that, in some patients, granulocytes carrying the deletion may be preferentially destroyed or retained within the bone marrow. Granulocytes from the female patients displayed a clonal pattern of X inactivation implying that either the 20q deletion was not the initiating event or the clonal X-inactivation pattern in granulocytes was age-related (*see above*) and not part of the pathogenesis of these disorders.

Deletions of chromosome 20q may be particularly associated with a subset of myeloid disorders characterised by megakaryocytic and erythroid dysplasia with only infrequent granulocytic dysplasia. However, no comparison was made with any control group of patients lacking a 20q deletion and so the significance of these findings is unclear.

Molecular analysis of the 20q deletion has been undertaken to identify the gene or genes involved (*reviewed in* Asimakopoulos & Green, 1996). Using FISH, microsatellite PCR (Figure 7.4) and quantitative Southern blotting, a common deleted region spanning 20q11–20q13 has been defined and is likely to contain one or more tumour suppressor genes. Loss of heterozygosity (LOH) of loci from 20q has also been demonstrated during transition from chronic phase to blast crisis of five of 17 CML patients. No fine mapping has yet been undertaken in CML blast crisis patients and so it is not yet clear whether the same target gene is affected.

Given that MPD and MDS are overlapping but clinically different diseases, it remains possible that different or additional genes are involved in the two disorders. Therefore, two overlapping common deleted regions have been defined. The MDS common deleted region spans a distance of 7–8 megabase pairs (Mb) whereas the

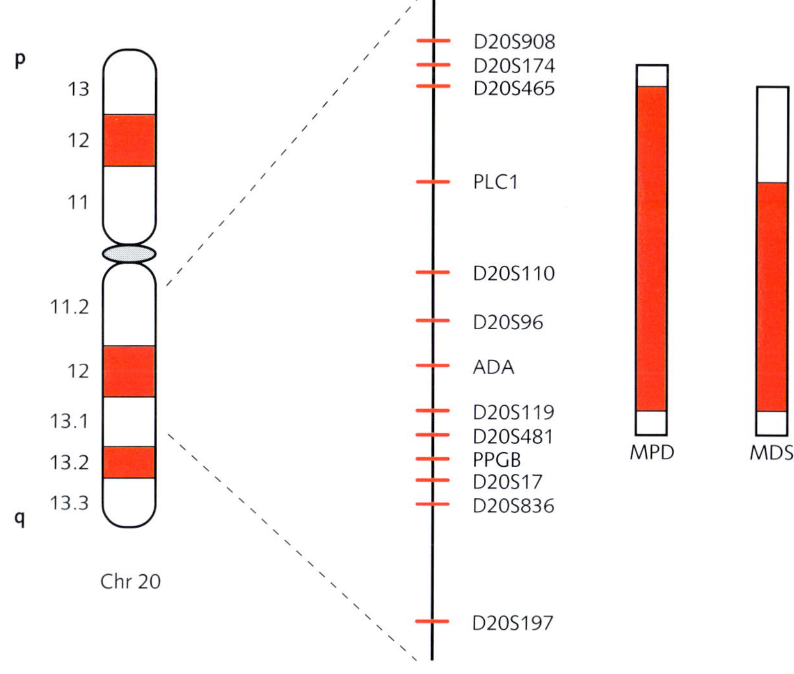

Fig. 7.5 Summary of common deleted regions on 20q for MPD and MDS
The MPD common deleted region is bordered by D20S174 and D20S481; the MDS common deleted region is bordered by D20S465 and D20S481. Open boxes represent the region within which the deletion breakpoints lie. *(Reproduced from* Bench *et al.*, 1998a.*)*

MPD common deleted region encompasses a slightly larger region of 8–9 Mb (Figure 7.5). Physical maps of this region have been constructed to facilitate gene identification. A total of 36 expressed sequences have been placed on the transcription map of this region, of which 12 represent known genes. These include genes encoding transcription factors (*MafB, MYBL2, TCF14*) and signal transduction components (*PLCG1, YWHAB*).

Loss and/or inactivation of candidate genes on 20q may be responsible for the pathogenesis of these disorders by a number of possible mechanisms (Figure 7.6). A simple 'two hit' model with a single target gene, reminiscent of Knudson's two hit hypothesis, might involve inactivation of one copy of the gene by a subtle genetic alteration such as a point mutation followed by loss of the second copy by deletion. Alternatively, the 'intact' copy may be transcriptionally silenced, for example by methylation as has been demonstrated for the *VHL*, *p16* and *p15* genes. In a 'one hit' model, loss of only a single copy of the gene may result in haploinsufficiency and be sufficient to contribute to disease pathogenesis. So far, we have assumed that 20q deletions result in loss of a single critical gene, but loss of two or more genes may be required (Figure 7.6). Again, inactivation of one or both copies of critical genes may be necessary to perturb progenitor cell behaviour. Perhaps inactivation of different combinations of genes is responsible for distinct myeloid disorders.

13q deletion

In contrast to 20q deletions, molecular analysis of chromosome 13q deletions in myeloid malignancies has only recently been initiated. La Starza *et al.* (1998) identified a common deleted region of 4 centiMorgans (cM) in MDS patients and of 14 cM in MPD patients. Furthermore, preliminary results from Gardiner *et al.* (1997) have defined a common deleted region of 1.5 Mb in IMF patients. Two lines of evidence have suggested that molecular alterations of chromosome 13q may be more common in MPD than cytogenetic observations suggest. Firstly, LOH at the RB1 locus has been observed in the bone marrow or peripheral blood from 13 of 30 MPD patients. Secondly, of five IMF patients without a visible 13q deletion analysed using FISH by Gardiner *et al.* (1997), two showed loss of loci on 13q. A case of IMF with a homozygous deletion of the RB gene was also identified implying that a two hit model of tumorigenesis applies for the 13q deletion. No mutations of the *RB1* gene have been found in MPD patients.

Deletion of chromosome 13q is the commonest structural chromosomal abnormality seen in chronic lymphocytic leukaemia (CLL). Deletions and unbalanced

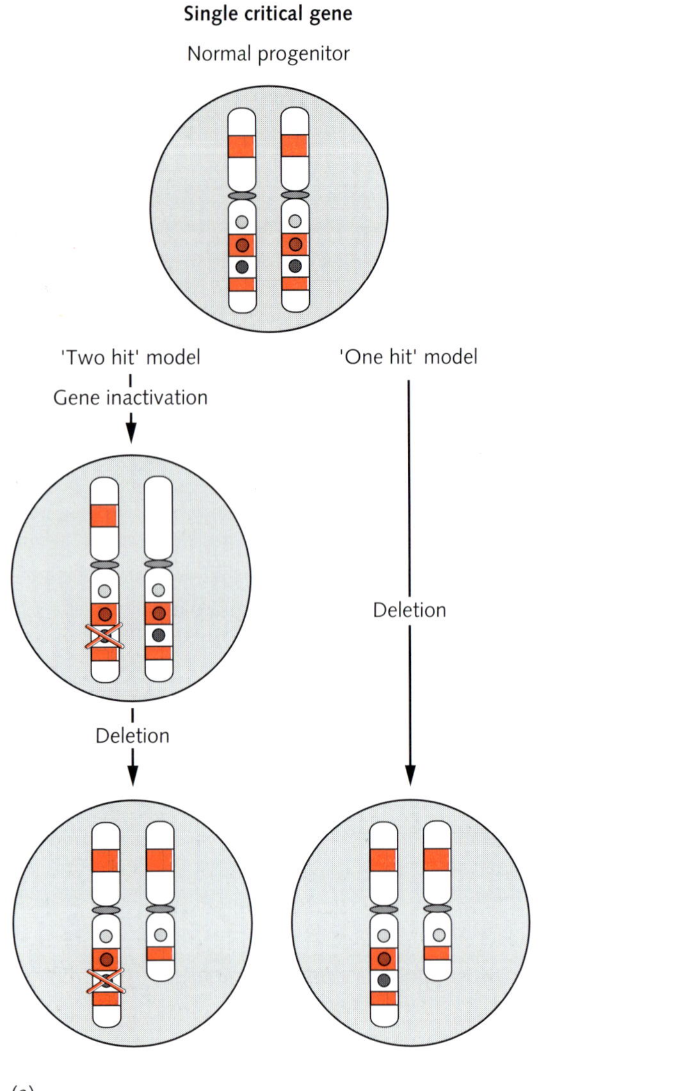

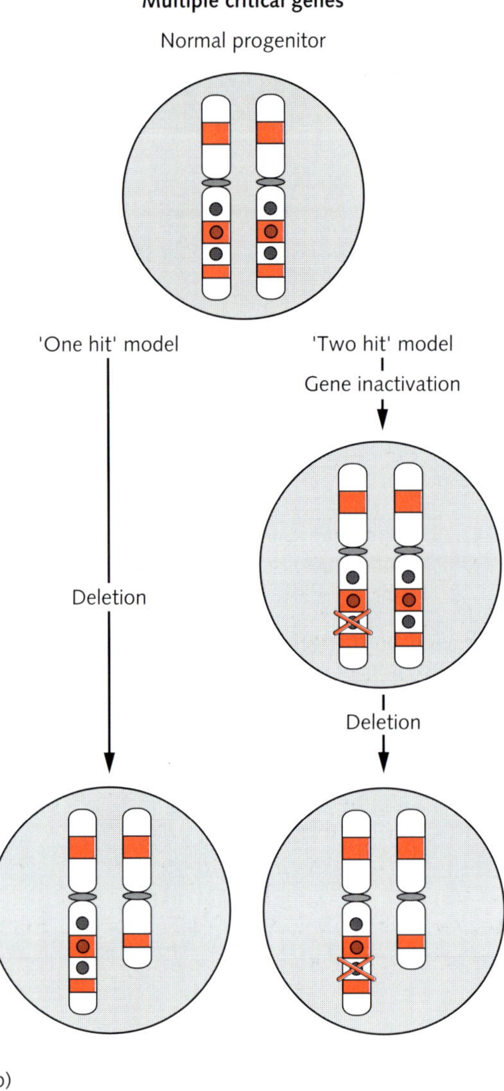

Fig. 7.6 Potential mechanism of the pathogenesis of 20q deletions
(a) If there is a single target gene on 20q (●), it may be necessary for both copies to be lost/inactivated ('two hit' model). Alternatively, loss of a single copy (haploinsufficiency) may be adequate to produce a phenotypic effect ('one hit' model). (b) If there is more than one target gene, the 'one hit' model would entail haploinsufficiency for two or more genes, perhaps scattered over a large distance of the chromosome. In contrast, the 'two hit' model would involve biallelic inactivation of at least one of the target genes. (*Adapted from* Asimakopoulos & Green, 1996.)

translocations involving 13q14 are seen in approximately 18% of all CLL cases. Several groups have identified very small common deleted regions (Figure 7.7) and a number of genes have been isolated, although no mutations found. The 13q MPD common deleted region partially overlaps some of these CLL common deleted regions (Figure 7.7). However, the very different biology of the MPDs and CLL argues against a single gene playing a role in both disorders. Isolation of a CLL tumour suppressor gene will provide the reagents to test this.

Gain of chromosomal material

Duplication of segments of 1q

Duplication of part of 1q has been demonstrated in a number of patients with MPD as well as other myeloid

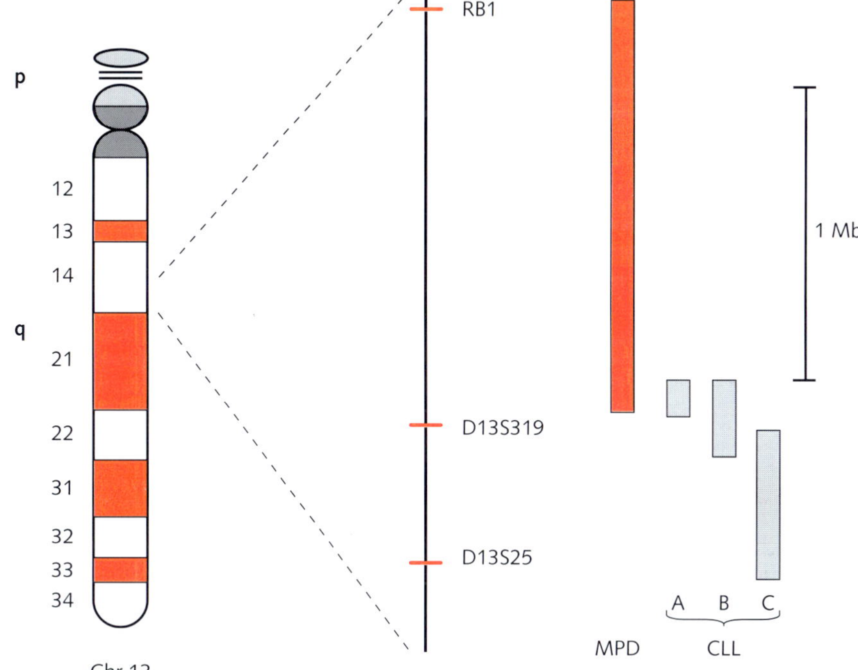

Fig. 7.7 Summary of common deleted regions on 13q for MPD and CLL
Three common deleted regions have been published for CLL. A (Corcoran *et al.*, 1998); B (Kalachikov *et al.*, 1997); C (Bouyge-Moreau *et al.*, 1997). The size of the MPD common deleted region (Gardiner *et al.*, 1997) is approximately 1.5 Mb. (*Adapted from* Bench *et al.*, 1998b.)

malignancies. It has been found at all stages of disease progression, including at diagnosis. Dupl(1q) was found in both erythroid and myeloid precursors of an MPD patient, confirming its origin within a multipotent progenitor. A common duplicated region spanning 1q23–q32 has been identified but, as yet, no molecular analysis has been undertaken.

Trisomy 8 and 9

An additional copy of both chromosome 8 and 9 is frequently observed in the same karyotypically abnormal clone. Trisomy 8 has been detected in 10–15% of patients with MDS and 5% of AML patients. The detection of trisomy 8 and 9 is particularly amenable to FISH-based techniques using centromeric probes and chromosome painting which are particularly useful for the analysis of samples in which metaphases are absent or of poor quality.

The use of such techniques has provided a number of interesting observations. Firstly, in some patients, it has been suggested that cells with trisomy 8 have a proliferative advantage over normal cells, at least in culture, since the frequency of trisomy 8 cells is greater in bone marrow metaphases than in interphase nuclei. Secondly, trisomy 8 has been detected in minor subclones of a small number of patients for whom conventional karyotyping showed no such aberration, indicating that trisomy 8 may be present in a greater proportion of patients than originally thought.

Combining FISH with immunophenotyping, it has been possible to follow the lineage involvement of trisomy 8. Price *et al.* (1992) demonstrated trisomy 8 in the majority of BFU-E and CFU-GM colonies from two patients with PV and trisomy 8. Furthermore, trisomy 8 was present in CD34+ cells and mature myeloid cells but not in lymphoid cells. In AML patients, trisomy 8 has been detected in multipotent progenitor cells as well as in a subpopulation of flow-sorted lymphoid and erythroid cells. Therefore, it seems likely that, in MPD and MDS, trisomy 8, like del(20q), arises in primitive progenitor cells with myeloid and lymphoid potential. The genetic consequence of chromosome 8 and 9 duplication is not clear as no molecular mapping has yet been undertaken.

Translocations

Consistent balanced translocations are uncommon in MPDs but may provide important insights into the pathogenetic mechanisms.

The 8p11 syndrome is a rare, atypical MPD with a balanced translocation involving chromosome 8p11. Patients commonly present with lymphadenopathy and general malaise. Bone marrow and peripheral blood show myeloid proliferation frequently with eosinophilia and there is a high incidence of T-cell non-Hodgkin's

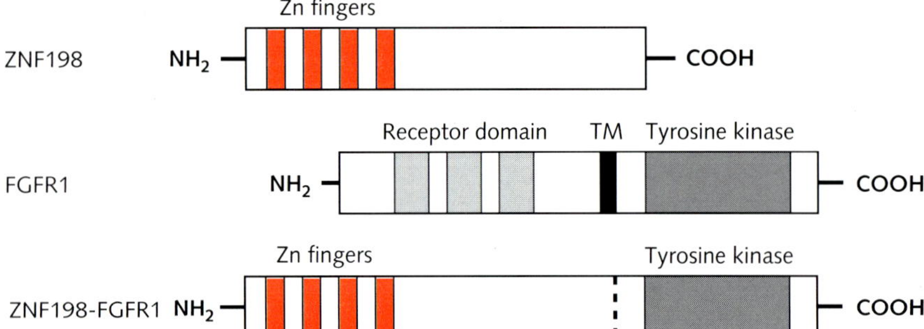

Fig. 7.8 Generation of ZNF198-FGFR1 fusion protein
TM, transmembrane domain. (*Adapted from* Bench *et al.*, 1998b.)

lymphoma. Almost invariably, the disease progresses to AML and has a poor prognosis. Cytogenetic examination has revealed a t(8;13)(p11;q12) translocation in the majority of cases although other translocation partners of 8p11 include 6q27 and 9q32–q34. This syndrome appears to result from transformation of a progenitor with both myeloid and lymphoid potential since cytogenetic analysis of lymph node and bone marrow from the same patient revealed the same chromosomal abnormality.

A candidate gene which mapped to chromosome 8p11 was the *FGFR1* gene which encodes fibroblast growth factor receptor 1, a member of the receptor tyrosine kinase family. Southern hybridisation revealed rearrangements of this gene in tumour DNA from patients with the t(8;13) translocation. The *FGFR1* gene, or a different gene very close to it, is also disrupted in patients with t(6;8) and t(8;9) translocations.

The fusion partner of *FGFR1* has been identified in patients with the t(8;13) translocation. This novel gene, termed *ZNF198* (also called *RAMP* or *FIM*), contains four putative novel zinc finger domains. The fusion protein, expressed in tumorigenic cells, is made up of the N-terminal portion containing the zinc finger domains of the ZNF198 protein fused with the tyrosine kinase domain of FGFR1 (Figure 7.8). Since this fusion protein lacks both the extracellular and the transmembrane domains of FGFR1 and does not have a nuclear localisation signal, it is presumably located in the cytoplasm.

Fusion proteins involving tyrosine kinases have been found in a number of other haematological malignancies. The first to be described was the *BCR-ABL* fusion gene generated by the t(9;22) translocation in CML. The BCR-ABL fusion protein contains the coiled-coil oligomerisation motif from BCR fused to the majority of the ABL protein containing a tyrosine kinase domain. The t(5;12) translocation in patients with chronic myelomonocytic leukaemia (CMML) results in the fusion of the helix–loop–helix domain of the ETS-like transcription factor, TEL, with the tyrosine kinase domain of the PDGFRβ protein. The *TEL* gene is also fused to the *ABL* gene in a small number of patients with AML or undifferentiated acute leukaemia. A number of common features are shared by all these fusion proteins as well as by ZNF198-FGFR1. Firstly, all contain oligomerisation domains from one protein linked to the tyrosine kinase domain (Figure 7.9). Secondly, all are potentially linked to the RAS signalling pathway.

These shared features suggest that the most likely mechanism of oncogenic activation by the ZNF198-FGFR1 fusion protein is ligand-independent dimerisation mediated by the zinc finger domains. Dimerisation would result in activation of the tyrosine kinase domain of the fusion protein with consequent phosphorylation of downstream targets. Indeed, the fusion protein has been shown to possess constitutive kinase activity. This would mimic constitutive activation of signalling pathways and may perturb proliferation and/or differentiation. By analogy, TEL-PDGFRβ self-association and transforming ability are dependent upon the TEL helix–loop–helix domain. Furthermore, this fusion protein associates with a number of signalling molecules known to be activated by PDGFRβ. However, a possible alternative mechanism is a dominant negative effect by heterodimerisation of the ZNF198-FGFR1 fusion protein with normal ZNF198 protein.

The partners of FGFR1 from chromosomes 6 and 9 have not been identified. Furthermore, additional genes on chromosome 13 may be involved in some t(8;13) patients with breakpoints distinct from the ZNF198 locus. Thus, a number of novel oncogenic fusion proteins involving FGFR1 remain to be identified.

Molecular genetic alterations

Clues about the molecular pathogenesis of the MPDs have also been obtained from the biology of the diseases. Prchal and Axelrad (1974) first demonstrated that erythropoietin (EPO)-independent BFU-E colonies could be grown from PV patients. Spontaneous BFU-E colonies

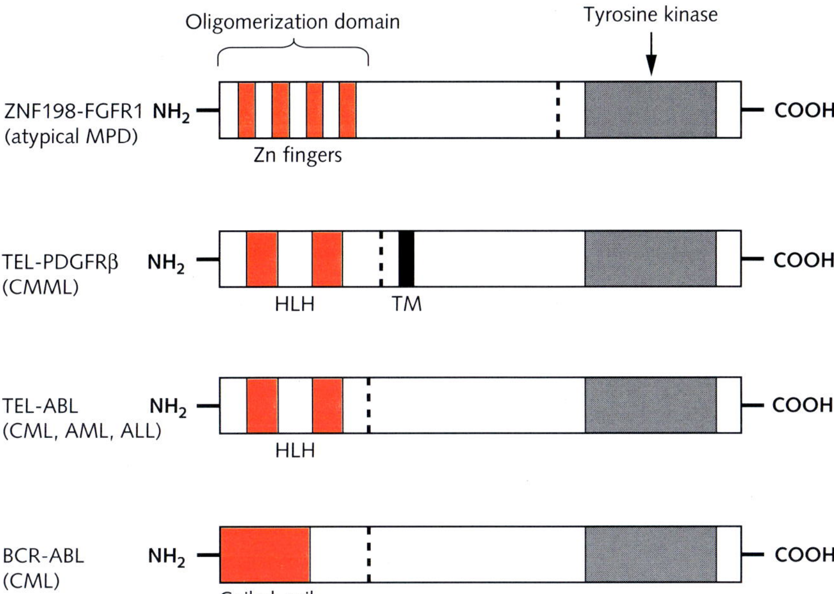

Fig. 7.9 Comparison of fusion proteins involving tyrosine kinase proteins in myeloid malignancies
Each fusion protein includes an oligomerisation domain plus a tyrosine kinase domain. HLH, helix–loop–helix domain; TM, transmembrane domain. (*Reproduced from* Bench *et al.*, 1998b.)

have been observed in the majority of PV patients as well as in a large number of ET patients. Similarly, spontaneous CFU-MEG colony formation occurs, without the addition of exogenous growth factors, in the majority of ET patients. Although it is now believed that progenitors are hypersensitive to a number of growth factors, these results have focused attention on the EPO and TPO signalling pathway (Figure 7.10).

Receptors and ligands

Mutations in the erythropoietin receptor gene, *EPOR*, have been found in some families with primary familial and congenital polycythaemia (PFCP). The majority of these mutations result in truncation of the polypeptide and loss of part of the cytoplasmic negative regulatory domain, although missense mutations in the same region have also been reported. Interestingly, not all families with PFCP have *EPOR* mutations, suggesting the existence of other target genes, in which mutations can give rise to polycythaemia. The finding of *EPOR* mutations in some cases of PFCP stimulated an intensive search for acquired mutations of the *EPOR* gene in PV. However, no acquired mutations in the *EPOR* gene have yet been identified in patients with PV or other MPDs.

Rare examples of familial thrombocythaemia exist. A mutation in the *TPO* gene has been detected in one such family. The consequence of this mutation is to increase the expression level of TPO. However, other families show no linkage to either the *TPO* or the *C-MPL* (TPO receptor) loci implying the existence of other genetic loci which contribute to familial thrombocythaemia. No acquired mutations in the TPO gene have been found in patients with acquired ET.

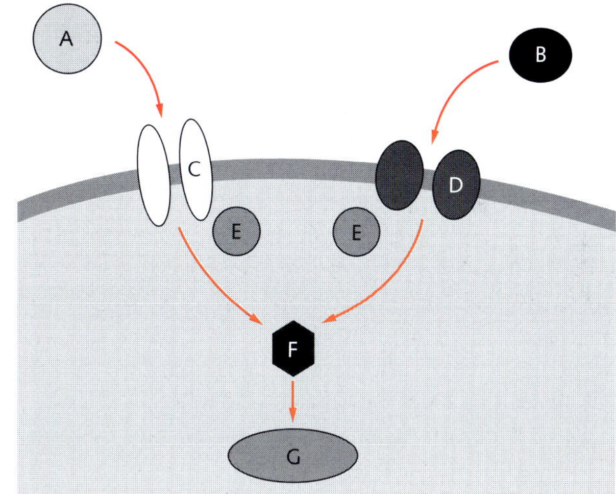

Fig. 7.10 Possible defects in signal transduction in MPD
Progenitor cells from patients are hypersensitive to a number of cytokines (A and B) such as EPO which act through specific receptor molecules (C and D). There may be a defect in a common receptor component (E), a common signalling intermediate (F) or a common effector molecule (G) such as a transcription factor. (*Reproduced from* Hinshelwood *et al.*, 1997.)

Reduced expression of *C-MPL*, at both the RNA and

protein level, has been reported in the platelets from 17 of 17 ET patients. By contrast, Moliterno *et al.* (1998) demonstrated reduced expression in 34 of 34 PV and 13 of 14 IMF patients but not in any of the four ET patients they analysed. Reasons for this discrepancy are not clear, but may involve differences in diagnostic criteria or may reflect pathogenetic heterogeneity. Indeed, it seems likely that what we currently call ET includes several distinct disorders.

Whether restricted to PV or not, the reduced level of the receptor for TPO remains an intriguing observation which could be diagnostically useful. It may reflect reduced RNA stability, possibly due to an acquired mutation. Alternatively, it may reflect reduced c-mpl transcription, due to either promoter or enhancer mutations (*cis*-acting) or to alterations in *trans*-acting factors. Although not exhaustively analysed, no acquired mutations have been found in the *C-MPL* gene of ET patients suggesting that reduced expression is a secondary consequence of alterations in *trans*-acting factors.

Signalling pathways

In retrospect, lack of receptor and ligand mutations may not be surprising. It is now recognised that PV progenitor cells are abnormally responsive to multiple growth factors. This suggests that the defect may be in a common signalling pathway (Figure 7.10). Protein phosphorylation plays a key role in several signalling pathways thought to drive cellular proliferation. Phosphatases that negatively regulate such pathways therefore represent candidate tumour suppressor proteins. The SHP-1 (HCP) phosphatase gene appeared a likely candidate for the genetic defect in PV for a number of reasons. Firstly, it interacts with a number of cytokine receptors including EPOR and negatively regulates EPO-induced signal transduction. Secondly, loss of the SHP-1 binding domain from EPOR results in congenital polycythaemia. Thirdly, mice with a SHP-1 mutation (*motheaten*) display hypersensitivity of progenitors to EPO. The SHP-1 gene was therefore characterised in a total of 17 PV and three ET patients but no mutations found. Furthermore, mRNA and protein levels were normal. In clonal granulocytes from nine PV patients, the methylation status of the promoter was identical to that of normal controls. These data, therefore, exclude SHP-1 as a target gene in PV.

Other oncogenes and tumour suppressor genes

Mutations in the p53 and *RAS* genes have been observed in a small proportion of patients with a MPD. However, the majority of such mutations were found in patients with a later or acute phase of the disease. Therefore, mutations of p53 and *RAS* genes are more frequently associated with disease progression and transformation to acute leukaemia rather than initiation of the MPD itself.

Future prospects

In addition to positional cloning strategies, several other approaches are being pursued to identify genetic defects which contribute towards the pathogenesis of MPD. One approach is to search for differentially expressed genes between progenitor cells from normal individuals and PV patients. This approach has a number of inherent problems. Firstly, progenitor cell populations are heterogeneous, so differences in gene expression may be secondary to shifts in the composition of the progenitor cell compartment. Secondly, genes which are affected by point mutations but whose expression level is unchanged will not be identified. However, even if the primary target is not identified, this approach may uncover consistent secondary changes and shed light on the altered behaviour of progenitor cells in PV.

A second approach is based on an expression cloning strategy. A plasmid expression library, constructed from purified CD34+ cells obtained from a PV patient, was transfected into normal CD34+ cells. The cells were then grown in semi-solid medium without EPO and the resultant EPO-independent colonies were isolated and plasmids recovered. Any recovered cDNAs would presumably be capable of inducing EPO-independent growth of erythroid progenitors and may play a role in the pathogenesis of PV.

Other approaches being undertaken involve genome-wide scans to identify changes at the DNA level. DNA from the granulocytes and T-cells of patients can be compared by Alu-PCR fingerprinting. This approach may identify novel fragments which are rearranged in the granulocytes of MPD patients. New molecular cytogenetic techniques now available offer the researcher the ability to analyse cytogenetic changes in much greater detail. In particular, colour karyotyping (M-FISH) permits the identification of cryptic translocations not previously detectable by G-banding and also reveals the chromosomal origin of genetic material present in marker chromosomes. Comparative genomic hybridisation is a complementary technique which detects quantitative changes (gain or loss of sequences) throughout the genome without the need to obtain metaphase chromosomes.

It is likely that one or more of the strategies described

will result in identification of target genes mutated in MPD. Identification of causal genes will be of considerable interest both to clinicians, who currently lack a specific and sensitive diagnostic test, and to scientists interested in fundamental issues of stem cell behaviour.

Acknowledgements

We thank Pam Stockham for secretarial assistance. Work in the authors' laboratory is supported by the Leukaemia Research Fund, the Medical Research Council and the Wellcome Trust.

Figure 7.5 is redrawn from Bench *et al.* (1998a), with permission of Academic Press.
Figure 7.10 is redrawn from Hinshelwood *et al.* (1997), *Blood Reviews*, **11**, 224–232, by permission of Churchill Livingstone.

Further reading

Classification

Dameshek W. (1951) Some speculations on the myeloproliferative syndromes. *Blood*, **6**, 372–375.

Pearson TC. (1998) Diagnosis and classification of erythrocytosis and thrombocytosis. In: Green AR, Pearson TC, eds. *Myeloproliferative Disorders*. London: Baillière Tindall (in press).

Reilly JT. (1997) Idiopathic myelofibrosis: pathogenesis, natural history and management. *Blood Reviews*, **11**, 233–242.

X-linked clonality assays

Adamson JW, Fialkow PJ, Murphy S, Prchal JF, Steinman L. (1976) Polycythemia vera; stem cell and probable clonal origin of the disease. *New England Journal of Medicine*, **295**, 913–916.

Allen RC, Zoghbi HY, Moseley AB, Rosenblatt HM, Belmont JW. (1992) Methylation of HpaII and HhaI sites near the polymorphic CAG repeat in the human androgen-receptor gene correlates with X chromosome inactivation. *American Journal of Human Genetics*, **51**, 1229–1239.

Asimakopoulos FA, Gilbert JGR, Aldred MA, Pearson TC, Green AR. (1996) Interstitial deletion constitutes the major mechanism for loss of heterozygosity on chromosome 20q in polycythemia vera. *Blood*, **88**, 2690–2698.

Busque L, Mio R, Mattioli J *et al.* (1996) Nonrandom X-inactivation patterns in normal females: Lyonization ratios vary with age. *Blood*, **88**, 59–65.

Champion KM, Gilbert JGR, Asimakopoulos FA, Hinshelwood S, Green AR. (1997) Clonal haemopoiesis in normal elderly women: implications for the myeloproliferative disorders and myelodysplastic syndromes. *British Journal of Haematology*, **97**, 920–926.

El-Kassar N, Hetet G, Briere J, Grandchamp B. (1997) Clonality analysis of hematopoiesis in essential thrombocythemia: advantages of studying T lymphocytes and platelets. *Blood*, **89**, 128–134.

Hinshelwood S, Bench AJ, Green AR. (1997) Pathogenesis of polycythaemia vera. *Blood Reviews*, **11**, 224–232.

Chromosome abnormalities

Berger R, Bernheim A, LeConiat M *et al.* (1984) Chromosome studies in polycythemia vera patients. *Cancer Genetics and Cytogenetics*, **12**, 217–223.

Demory JL, Dupriez B, Fenaux P *et al.* (1988) Cytogenetic studies and their prognostic significance in agnogenic myeloid metaplasia: a report on 47 cases. *Blood*, **72**, 855–859.

Diez-Martin JL, Graham DL, Petitt RM, Dewald GW. (1991) Chromosome studies in 104 patients with polycythemia vera. *Mayo Clinic Proceedings*, **66**, 287–299.

Dupriez B, Morel P, Demory JL *et al.* (1996) Prognostic factors in agnogenic myeloid metaplasia: a report on 195 cases with a new scoring system. *Blood*, **88**, 1013–1018.

Mertens F, Johansson B, Heim S, Kristoffersson U, Mitelman F. (1991) Karyotypic patterns in chronic myeloproliferative disorders: report on 74 cases and review of the literature. *Leukemia*, **5**, 214–220.

Rege-Cambrin G, Mecucci C, Tricot G *et al.* (1987) A chromosomal profile of polycythemia vera. *Cancer Genetics and Cytogenetics*, **25**, 233–245.

Reilly JT, Snowden JA, Spearing RL *et al.* (1997) Cytogenetic abnormalities and their prognostic significance in idiopathic myelofibrosis: a study of 106 cases. *British Journal of Haematology*, **98**, 96–102.

Swolin B, Weinfeld A, Westin J. (1988) A prospective long-term cytogenetic study in polycythemia vera in relation to treatment and clinical course. *Blood*, **72**, 386–395.

Chromosome deletions

Asimakopoulos FA, Green AR. (1996) Deletions of chromosome 20q and the pathogenesis of myeloproliferative disorders. *British Journal of Haematology*, **95**, 219–226.

Asimakopoulos FA, Holloway TL, Nacheva EP *et al.* (1996) Detection of chromosome 20q deletions in bone marrow metaphases but not peripheral blood granulocytes in patients with myeloproliferative disorders or myelodysplastic syndromes. *Blood*, **87**, 1561–1570.

Bench AJ, Aldred MA, Humphray SJ *et al.* (1998a) A detailed physical and transcriptional map of the region of chromosome 20 that is deleted in myeloproliferative disorders and refinement of the common deleted region. *Genomics*, **49**, 351–362.

Bench AJ, Nacheva EP, Champion KM, Green AR. (1998b) Molecular genetics and cytogenetics of myeloproliferative disorders. In: Green AR, Pearson TC, eds. *Myeloproliferative Disorders*. London: Baillière Tindall, *in press*.

Bouyge-Moreau I, Rondeau G, Avet-Loiseau H *et al.* (1997) Construction of a 780-kb PAC, BAC, and cosmid contig encompassing the minimal critical deletion involved in B cell chronic lymphocytic leukemia at 13q14.3. *Genomics*, **46**, 183–190.

Corcoran MM, Rasool O, Liu Y *et al.* (1998) Detailed molecular delineation of 13q14.3 loss in B-cell chronic lymphocytic leukemia. *Blood*, **91**, 1382–1390.

Dewald GW, Schad CR, Lilla VC, Jalal SM. (1993) Frequency and photographs of HGM11 chromosome anomalies in bone marrow samples from 3996 patients with malignant hematologic neoplasms. *Cancer Genetics and Cytogenetics*, **68**, 60–69.

Gardiner A, Corcoran M, Ibbotson R *et al.* (1997) An analysis of chromosome 13q14 deletions in myelofibrosis using FISH and Southern-based hybridisation. *Blood*, **90**, 292b.

Greenberg P, Cox C, LeBeau MM *et al.* (1997) International scoring system for evaluating prognosis in myelodysplastic syndromes. *Blood*, **89**, 2079–2088.

Hollings PE, Rosman I, Beard MEJ. (1994) A 20q deletion originating in a pluripotent stem cell. *Blood*, **83**, 305–306.

Kalachikov S, Migliazza A, Cayanis E *et al.* (1997) Cloning and gene mapping of the chromosome 13q14 region deleted in chronic lymphocytic leukemia. *Genomics*, **42**, 369–377.

Kurtin PJ, Dewald GW, Shields DJ, Hanson CA. (1996) Hematologic disorders associated with deletions of chromosome 20q. *American Journal of Clinical Pathology*, **106**, 680–688.

La Starza R, Wlodarska I, Aventin A *et al.* (1998) Molecular delineation of 13q deletion boundaries in 20 patients with myeloid malignancies. *Blood*, **91**, 231–237.

Liu Y, Corcoran M, Rasool O *et al.* (1997) Cloning of two candidate tumor suppressor genes within a 10 kb region on chromosome 13q14, frequently deleted in chronic lymphocytic leukemia. *Oncogene*, **15**, 2463–2473.

Mori N, Morosetti R, Lee S *et al.* (1997) Allelotype analysis in the evolution of chronic myelocytic leukemia. *Blood*, **90**, 2010–2014.

Pastore C, Nomdedeu J, Volpe G *et al.* (1995) Genetic analysis of chromosome 13 deletions in Bcr/Abl negative chronic myeloproliferative disorders. *Genes Chromosomes and Cancer*, **14**, 106–111.

White NJ, Nacheva E, Asimakopoulos FA *et al.* (1994) Deletion of chromosome 20q in myelodysplasia occurring in multipotent precursor of both myeloid cells and B cells. *Blood*, **83**, 2809–2816.

Gain of chromosomal material

Fugazza G, Bruzzone R, Dejana AM, Patrone F, Sessarego M. (1994) Trisomy 8 detection in Ph+ CML patients using conventional cytogenetic and interphase fluorescence *in situ* hybridization techniques. *Cancer Genetics and Cytogenetics*, **72**, 24–27.

Jenkins RB, Le Beau MM, Kraker WJ *et al.* (1992) Fluorescence *in situ* hybridization: A sensitive method for trisomy 8 detection in bone marrow specimens. *Blood*, **79**, 3307–3315.

Knuutila S, Ruutu T, Partanen S, Vuopio P. (1983) Chromosome 1q+ in erythroid and granulocyte-monocyte precursors in a patient with essential thrombocythemia. *Cancer Genetics and Cytogenetics*, **9**, 245–249.

Mehrotra B, George TI, Kavanau K *et al.* (1995) Cytogenetically aberrant cells in the stem cell compartment (CD34+lin−) in acute myeloid leukemia. *Blood*, **86**, 1139–1147.

Price CM, Kanfer EJ, Colman SM *et al.* (1992) Simultaneous genotypic and immunophenotypic analysis of interphase cells using dual-colour fluorescence: a demonstration of lineage involvement in polycythemia vera. *Blood*, **80**, 1033–1038.

Rowley JD. (1977) Mapping of human chromosomal regions related to neoplasia: Evidence from chromosomes 1 and 17. *Proceedings of the National Academy of Sciences (USA)*, **74**, 5729–5733.

Swolin B, Weinfeld A, Westin J. (1986) Trisomy 1q in polycythemia vera and its relation to disease transition. *American Journal of Hematology*, **22**, 155–167.

Translocations

Chaffanet M, Popovici C, Leroux D *et al.* (1998) t(6;8), t(8;9) and t(8;13) translocations associated with stem cell myeloproliferative disorders have close or identical breakpoints in chromosome region 8p11–12. *Oncogene*, **16**, 945–949.

Inhorn RC, Aster JC, Roach SA *et al.* (1995) A syndrome of lymphoblastic lymphoma, eosinophilia, and myeloid hyperplasia/malignancy associated with t(8;13) (p11;q11): Description of a distinctive clinicopathologic entity. *Blood*, **85**, 1881–1887.

Macdonald D, Aguiar RCT, Mason PJ, Goldman JM, Cross NCP. (1995) A new myeloproliferative disorder associated with chromosomal translocations involving 8p11: a review. *Leukemia*, **9**, 1628–1630.

Popovici C, Adélaïde J, Ollendorff V *et al.* (1998) Fibroblast growth factor receptor 1 is fused to FIM in stem-cell myeloproliferative disorder with t(8;13)(p12;q12). *Proceedings of the National Academy of Sciences (USA)*, **95**, 5712–5717.

Smedley D, Hamoudi R, Clark J *et al.* (1998) The t(8;13)(p11;q11–12) rearrangement associated with an atypical myeloproliferative disorder fuses the fibroblast growth factor receptor 1 gene to a novel gene RAMP. *Human Molecular Genetics*, **7**, 637–642.

Xiao S, Nalabolu SR, Aster JC *et al.* (1998) FGFR1 is fused with a novel zinc-finger gene, ZNF198, in the t(8;13) leukaemia/lymphoma syndrome. *Nature Genetics*, **18**, 84–87.

Molecular genetic alterations

Andersson P, Le Blanc K, Eriksson B-A, Samuelsson J. (1997) No evidence for an altered mRNA expression or protein level of haematopoietic cell phosphatase in CD34+ bone marrow progenitor cells or mature peripheral blood cells in polycythaemia vera. *European Journal of Haematology*, **59**, 310–317.

Asimakopoulos FA, Hinshelwood S, Gilbert JGR *et al.* (1997) The gene encoding hematopoietic cell phosphatase (SHP-1) is structurally and transcriptionally intact in polycythemia vera. *Oncogene*, **14**, 1215–1222.

Gregg XT, Prchal JT. (1997) Erythropoietin receptor mutations and human disease. *Seminars in Hematology*, **34**, 70–76.

Horikawa Y, Matsumura I, Hashimoto K *et al.* (1997) Markedly reduced expression of platelet c-mpl receptor in essential thrombocythemia. *Blood*, **90**, 4031–4038.

Moliterno AR, Hankins WD, Spivak JL. (1998) Impaired expression of the thrombopoietin receptor by platelets from patients with polycythemia vera. *New England Journal of Medicine*, **338**, 572–580.

Prchal JF, Axelrad AA. (1974) Bone marrow responses in polycythemia vera. *New England Journal of Medicine*, **290**, 1382.

Wiestner A, Schlemper RJ, van der Maas APC, Skoda RC. (1998) An activating splice donor mutation in the thrombopoietin gene causes hereditary thrombocythaemia. *Nature Genetics*, **18**, 49–52.

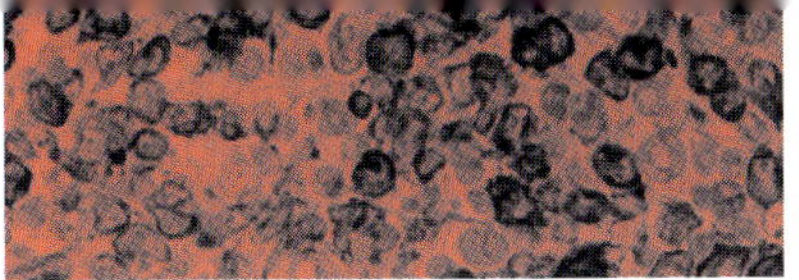

Chapter 8 Lymphoid neoplasms

Dennis Wright & David G Oscier

Introduction

For many years lymphoid neoplasms were defined on the basis of their clinical features and cytomorphology. The categorisation of these neoplasms was made more precise by the introduction of immunohistochemistry that permitted the determination of lineage, maturity and activation status of lymphoid cells. In recent years it has become apparent that many lymphoid neoplasms are characterised by non-random chromosomal abnormalities that may help to define these proliferations as entities. The practical use of these genetic abnormalities as defining features has been enhanced by the use of molecular techniques such as Southern hybridisation and polymerase chain reaction (PCR) that permit the identification of translocations and mutations in fresh, frozen or fixed archival material. The identification of the molecular genetic characteristics of some lymphoid neoplasms has not made the older diagnostic techniques of morphology and immunophenotyping redundant, but has rather been used to enhance and underpin these techniques. Knowledge of the molecular genetic abnormalities that characterise certain neoplasms has led to the development of antibodies to fusion proteins and oncogenes that can in turn be used to identify cells bearing the molecular genetic abnormalities.

During B- and T-cell ontogeny the antigen receptor genes (T-cell receptor and immunoglobulin genes) undergo recombination in the bone marrow. Within follicle centres the immunoglobulin genes of B-cells undergo mutation and selection in the process of antibody affinity maturation. Analysis of the antigen receptor genes using Southern hybridisation or PCR may be used to determine the clonality of a lymphoid proliferation. If sequencing the clonal product identifies a functional gene, a lineage (B- or T-cell) can be assigned to the proliferation. T-cell proliferations can be further categorised according to their antigen receptor usage as $\alpha\beta$ or $\gamma\delta$. Sequencing immunoglobulin variable (IgV) region gene products can be used to identify pre-germinal centre B-cells (unmutated IgV genes), post-germinal centre B-cells (mutated IgV genes) and follicle centre cell lymphomas (ongoing IgV gene mutations). Clustering of mutations in the third complementarity determining region (CDR3) of the IgV genes is suggestive of antigen drive.

The aim of this chapter is to show how an understanding of the molecular genetic characteristics of lymphoid neoplasms can be used in the diagnosis of these leukaemias and lymphomas.

The nature of chromosomal abnormalities in lymphoid neoplasms

Several of the common translocations that occur in malignant lymphomas involve the TCR or Ig genes. These presumably occur as recombination errors at the time of antigen receptor gene rearrangement. As a consequence of many such translocations, an oncogene is placed under the influence of the enhancer region of the antigen receptor gene. The abnormally regulated oncogene may result in uncontrolled cell proliferation or in a failure of cells to undergo apoptosis. Other translocations result in the production of fusion proteins such as the nucleophosmin (NPM)-anaplastic lymphoma kinase (ALK) chimera produced in anaplastic large cell lymphomas bearing the translocation t(2;5). In such tumours the abnormal distribution and kinetics of ALK presumably act as an oncogenic factor.

Translocations *in themselves* do not appear sufficient to induce malignancy in experimental animals, and they may be found in reactive lymphoid tissues from normal humans. Thus, in addition to the translocations that characterise a number of malignant lymphomas, it would appear that other events are necessary for malignancy to occur.

In addition to the primary genetic events that initiate the malignant phenotype, many lymphomas exhibit chromosomal instability, perhaps due to mutations in genes controlling DNA repair. These ongoing mutations may account for progression from low grade to high grade lymphoma, and for increasing pleomorphism in some high grade lymphomas. Mutations of the p53 gene appear to be particularly associated with progression of follicle centre cell lymphoma to large B-cell lymphoma.

Chronic lymphocytic leukaemia (CLL)

CLL is a clinically heterogeneous disorder. Most patients are elderly and are diagnosed on the basis of a routine blood count which shows a lymphocytosis. A minority present with lymphadenopathy and/or splenomegaly, infection, anaemia or constitutional symptoms. Progressive disease is usually accompanied by increasing hypogammaglobulinaemia and a tendency to autoimmune anaemia and thrombocytopenia. The reason why some patients pursue a benign stable course over many years while others have progressive disease is unclear.

The lymphocytes in the peripheral blood are typically small with scanty agranular cytoplasm and a round nucleus with coarsely clumped chromatin. In a minority of cases with atypical lymphocyte morphology, >10% of lymphocytes are larger and have a prominent nucleolus (*prolymphocytes*) (Plate 8.1, facing page 128). The lymph node in CLL is replaced by a diffuse infiltration of small lymphocytes with foci of larger cells with prominent nucleoli referred to as proliferation centres.

Immunophenotype (Table 8.1)

The majority of cases of CLL are of B-cell lineage and express the B-cell lineage markers CD19, CD20 and CD79a but have weak or absent expression of CD79b. Most cases express surface IgM either alone or with IgD. However, the expression is weak and may be below the level of detectability. The expression of CD23 helps to differentiate the immunophenotype of CLL from the other CD19/CD20/CD5 expressing lymphomas, e.g. mantle cell lymphoma (*see below*). Much more rarely CLL can be of T-cell lineage.

Molecular genetics

Cytogenetic analysis on peripheral blood using a B-cell mitogen such as TPA reveals clonal abnormalities in 50% of cases (Figure 8.1). The commonest abnormalities are deletions or translocations of chromosome 13q14 and trisomy 12.

Trisomy 12 is found in 10–15% of cases cytogenetically and in 20% of patients using interphase fluorescence *in situ* hybridisation (FISH) with a centromeric probe for chromosome 12. By using immunocytochemistry combined with FISH it has been shown that only a proportion of the malignant clone has trisomy 12 which is therefore a secondary genetic event. There is a strong correlation between the presence of trisomy 12, atypical lymphocyte morphology and progressive disease.

Deletions or translocations of chromosome 13 band q14 are found in 20% of patients cytogenetically and up to 60% of cases using interphase FISH. The translocations involve many different partner chromosomes,

Table 8.1 Lymphoid neoplasms: immunophenotypic and other markers.

	CLL	MCL	BL	FCC	MALToma	DLBCL	ALC
CD5	+	+	–	–	–	±	
CD10	–	–	+	±	–	±	
CD23	+	–	–	–	–	–	
CD19/20/22/79a	+	+	+	+	+	+	
SIg	±	+	+	+	+	±	
Light chain		λ > κ		κ > λ			
Other		Cyclin D1+	Ki67+				CD30+ ALK+

CLL, chronic lymphocytic leukaemia; MCL, mantle cell lymphoma; BL, Burkitt's lymphoma; FCC, follicle centre cell lymphoma; MALToma, extranodal marginal zone lymphoma; DLBCL, diffuse large B-cell lymphoma; ALC, anaplastic large cell lymphoma; SIg, surface immunoglobulin; + and –, positive and negative for cell marker; ±, weak expression.

resulting in the loss of genetic material rather than the activation of a proto-oncogene or the creation of a fusion gene (Figure 8.2). A commonly deleted region telomeric to the retinoblastoma gene has been identified. This region is particularly gene-rich, but the gene or genes which are important in the pathogenesis of CLL remain to be discovered.

Deletions of chromosome 11 band q23 are found in <5% of patients cytogenetically but in 20% of patients using interphase FISH. Chromosome 11q deletions are associated with bulky lymphadenopathy, progressive disease and a poor prognosis in patients under the age of 55 years. The deleted region contains the ATM gene (Ataxia Telangiectasia Mutation) which, on occasions, is associated with point mutations in the remaining allele. Mutations of the p53 gene occur in 10–15% of patients with CLL and are frequently accompanied by cytogenetic abnormalities of chromosome 17p leading to the homozygous loss of wild type p53. There is a strong association between p53 mutation and loss with advanced disease, drug resistance and poor prognosis.

Translocations involving the immunoglobulin heavy and light chain loci which are the hallmark of many B-cell neoplasms appear to be rare in CLL. Less than 5% of patients have a translocation between an immunoglobulin gene locus and the *BCL-2* gene. The *BCL-2* rearrangements are 5′ to those normally found in follicle centre cell lymphoma and preliminary data suggest that BCL-2 protein in these cases is expressed at a higher level than normally found in B CLL. The t(11;14) has been described in CLL, but there is controversy as to whether these cases represent the leukaemic phase of a mantle cell lymphoma. The t(14;19)(q32;q13) translocation occurs in 0.1% of cases. Lymphocyte morphology is frequently atypical and most patients have progressive disease. The breakpoint on chromosome 19 involves the *BCL-3* gene which encodes an I-kappa B-like transcription factor.

The consensus view has been that there is biased use of VH genes in CLL and that the VH genes retain the germline configuration. Our recent data on a large series of well-documented cases of CLL has confirmed

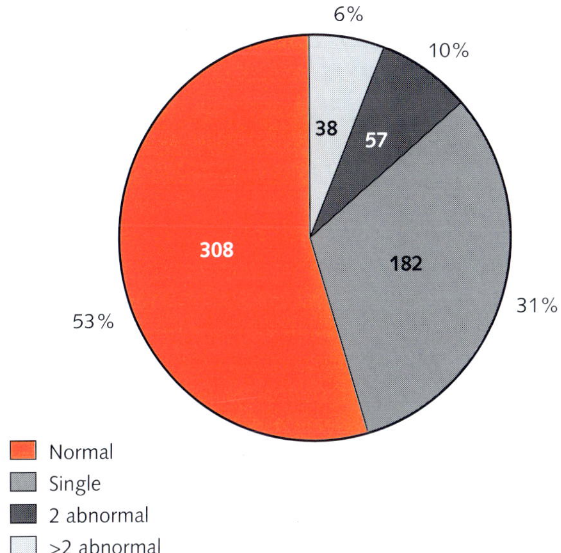

Fig. 8.1 Incidence of cytogenetic abnormalities in 585 patients with CLL investigated in Bournemouth
Whole blood was cultured with TPA as a mitogen.

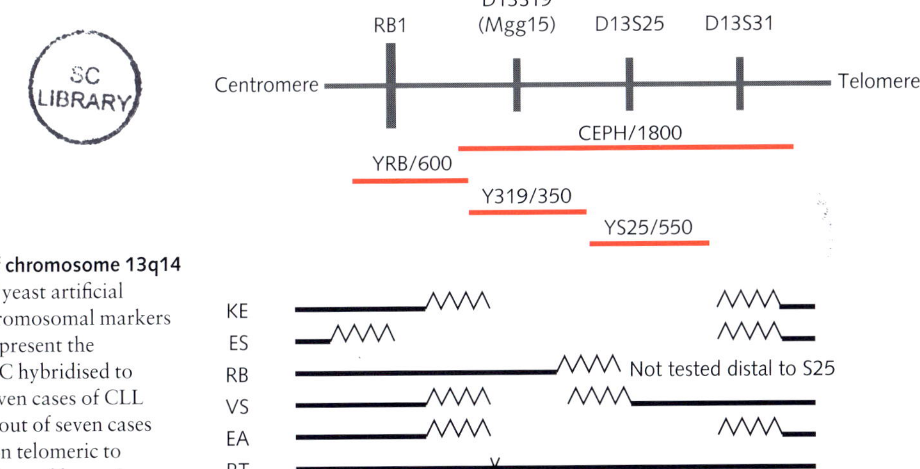

Fig. 8.2 Diagram showing part of chromosome 13q14
The relative position of a series of yeast artificial chromosomes (YACs) to other chromosomal markers is shown in red. The black lines represent the presence of a signal from each YAC hybridised to translocation metaphases from seven cases of CLL with 13q14 translocations. In six out of seven cases a signal was absent from the region telomeric to the retinoblastoma gene. Case 7 showed loss using cosmid probes.

overusage of an unmutated VI-69 gene and the presence of somatic mutation without clonal heterogeneity in 60% of cases. The patients showing somatic mutation were more likely to be Binet stage A with stable disease, to have typical lymphocyte morphology and to have abnormalities of chromosome 13q14. The absence of somatic mutation was associated with progressive disease, atypical morphology and trisomy 12. This suggests that CLL may exist in two forms deriving from cells that are either pre- or post-passage through the germinal centre.

No genetic abnormality which is present in all cases of CLL has been found. Familial CLL is rare but exhibits the phenomenon of anticipation since the age of onset in the younger generation is approximately 20 years less than in the older generation. This phenomenon is characteristic of the trinucleotide repeat expansion disorders, but is also consistent with the inheritance of a defective DNA repair gene which may predispose to the genetic abnormalities described above.

Mantle cell lymphoma

Mantle cell lymphoma has emerged as an entity having, for many years, been confused with lymphocytic lymphoma or a diffuse form of follicle centre cell lymphoma. The tumour shows a male predominance. It is often widespread at presentation with lymphadenopathy, splenomegaly and bone marrow infiltration. Extranodal tumour is common with involvement of Waldeyer's ring and the gastrointestinal tract where it may be manifest as lymphomatoid polyposis. The tumour usually runs an aggressive course with a median survival of three to five years.

The tumour cells are usually larger than those of lymphocytic lymphoma, and often have more angulated nuclei. In contrast to lymphocytic lymphoma, proliferation centres and paraimmunoblasts are not seen. The tumour cells appear initially to grow around pre-existing reactive follicles (mantle zone pattern) eventually invading and replacing the follicles. This pattern of evolution often leaves the tumour with an ill-defined nodular or follicular growth pattern. A more aggressive blastoid variant of the tumour occurs and may be difficult to distinguish morphologically from lymphoblastic lymphoma. An anaplastic variant of mantle cell lymphoma has also been described.

Immunophenotype

The tumour cells express the B-cell lineage markers CD19, CD20 and CD79a. They express strong surface immunoglobulin usually of IgM and IgD isotypes. λ light chain is found more frequently than κ light chain. In common with CLL the tumour cells express CD5 and CD43, but unlike CLL they are negative for CD23.

Molecular genetics

Mantle cell lymphoma is characterised by t(11;14)(q13;q32) which results in the juxtaposition of the immunoglobulin heavy chain promoter on chromosome 14 with the cyclin D1 gene on chromosome 11, and to overexpression of cyclin D1. Cyclin D1, together with a cyclin-dependent kinase (cdk4), phosphorylates retinoblastoma protein (pRB) which releases transcription factors (E2F) and histone deacetylase allowing the cell to proceed from G_1 to the S phase of the cell cycle (Figure 8.3). The overexpressed cyclin D1 can be detected in the nuclei of the tumour cells and provides a useful immunohistochemical marker for mantle cell lymphoma (Figure 8.4). In transgenic mice, overexpression of cyclin D1 is not in itself sufficient to cause lymphoma and it appears that the deletion of other genes is needed for tumour progression. Either homozygous or hemizygous deletion of the gene for p16/CDKN2, which suppresses the effects of CDK4/cyclin D1 on the phosphorylation of pRB, is frequent in mantle cell lymphoma, and correlates with the proliferative activity of the tumour.

Burkitt's lymphoma

Burkitt's lymphoma (BL) was originally described as a clinicopathological entity by Denis Burkitt, a surgeon working in East Africa. The tumour predominates in children with a peak age incidence of seven years. It is characterised by tumour involvement of the jaws, kidneys, liver, endocrine organs and gonads. The tumour is composed of sheets of uniform blast cells showing a high mitotic index and numerous apoptotic cells. The lymphoma cells are usually interspersed by foamy macrophages containing apoptotic bodies that give the tumour a characteristic 'starry sky' pattern. The tumour described by Denis Burkitt is designated as endemic BL (eBL).

Lymphomas with a similar cytomorphology are seen sporadically throughout the world (sporadic BL, sBL). These occur predominantly in children and young adults. They differ, however, in their clinico-anatomical features from eBL. The majority of patients have abdominal disease characteristically involving the ileocaecal region. Tumours of Waldeyer's ring are also common. Bone marrow involvement is uncommon in eBL, but

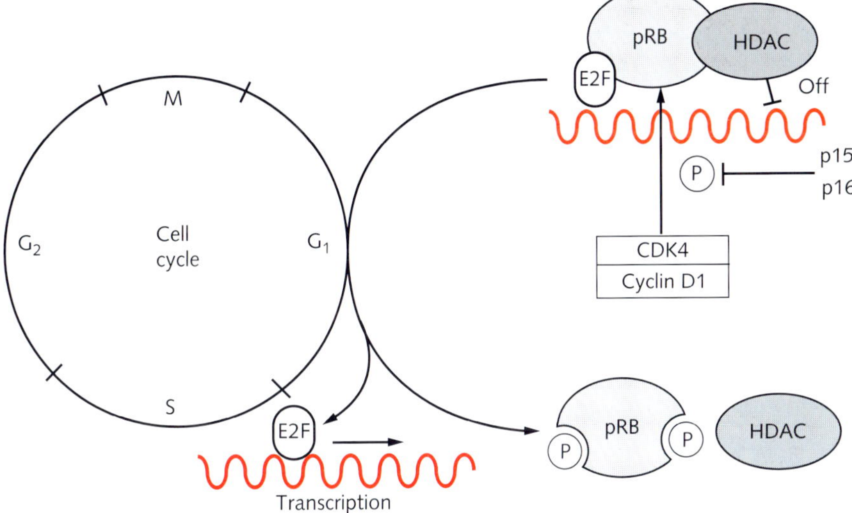

Fig. 8.3 Diagram showing the role of cyclin D1 in the G_1 to S phase transition
Retinoblastoma protein (pRB) binds to the transcription factors E2F and to histone deacetylase (HDAC). The histone deacetylase may convert the chromatin from a transcriptionally active (hyper-acetylated) to a transcriptionally repressed (hypo-acetylated) state. Cyclin D1 together with the cyclin-dependent kinase CDK4 phosphorylates pRB releasing E2F from the influence of HDAC allowing active transcription. The phosphorylation of pRB is inhibited by p15 and p16. P = phosphate groups.

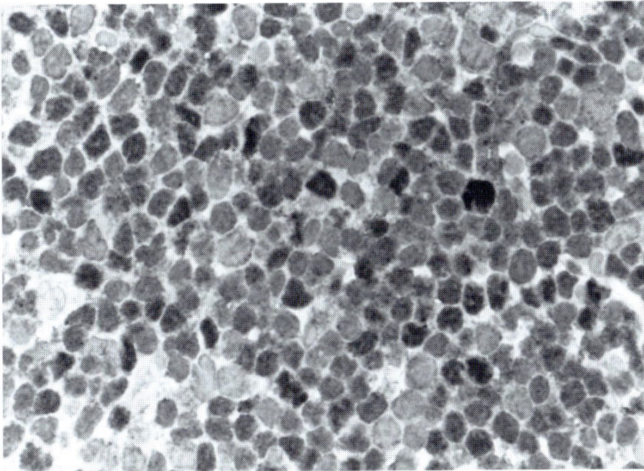

Fig. 8.4 Mantle cell lymphoma
Mantle cell lymphoma stained by the immunoperoxidase technique with an antibody to cyclin D1. There is positive staining of variable intensity of the tumour cell nuclei (immunoperoxidase).

occurs more frequently in sBL where it may be the predominant clinical feature. Such cases were designated as L3 in the French–American–British classification of lymphoblastic lymphomas.

A third subtype of BL is associated with AIDS. This lymphoma has a similar cytomorphology to other subtypes of BL and manifests most frequently as lymphadenopathy.

Immunophenotype

BL cells express CD19, CD20, CD21 and CD79a. They usually express surface IgM together with light chains. sBL secretes IgM which may appear as a serum monoclonal band, whereas eBL does not. A reciprocal relationship appears to exist between the expression of CD10 and CD23. Cell lines derived from eBL express more CD23 and less CD10 than those derived from sBL, which usually express CD10 but lack CD23.

Molecular genetics

All subtypes of BL are characterised by translocations between the *C-MYC* oncogene on chromosome 8q24 and one of the immunoglobulin genes. In 80% of cases this is the heavy chain locus on 14q32, the remainder involving either the κ light chain locus at 2p11/p12 or the λ light chain locus at 22q11. These translocations bring the *C-MYC* gene under the influence of the immunoglobulin gene regulatory regions. In a B-cell this leads to deregulation of C-MYC production. C-MYC protein forms a heterodimer with another cellular protein, MAX, and the ratio of these two proteins determines whether transcription expression or repression occurs. Deregulation of *C-MYC* expression following translocation leads to continuous cell growth without differentiation and probably accounts for the cytological uniformity of all types of BL. The continuous replication of BL cells can be measured using a proliferation marker such as Ki67 and provides a useful diagnostic aid since few lymphomas other than BL have a labelling index of 100% (Figure 8.5).

Although all subtypes of BL are characterised by translocations between the *C-MYC* oncogene and one of the immunoglobulin genes, the breakpoints on these genes are generally different (Figure 8.6); thus in sBL the breakpoints are usually immediately 5′ to the *C-MYC*

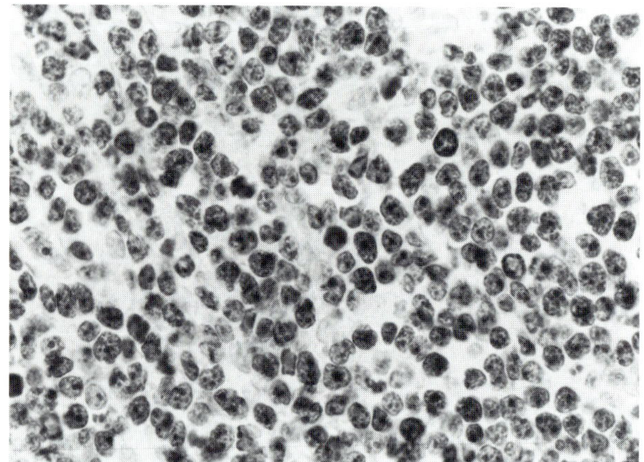

Fig. 8.5 Burkitt's lymphoma
Section of Burkitt's lymphoma stained with the antibody MIB1 which recognises a formalin resistance epitope of the Ki67 antigen (immunoperoxidase technique). The nuclei of all tumour cells show positive staining apart from those showing signs of apoptosis. Stromal cell nuclei are negative.

gene or within the first exon, whereas in eBL they are usually 100–300 kb 5′ to the gene. Similarly, on chromosome 14 the breakpoints in eBL usually cluster around JH, whereas in sBL and AIDS-BL they cluster in the switch region of the μ heavy chain gene. This may indicate that sBL and AIDS-BL arise later in B-cell ontogeny than eBL.

Experiments with transgenic mice suggest that t(8;14) and its variants are insufficient to cause lymphoma. Mutations of the C-*MYC* gene, of the p53 gene and of *BCL-6* have all been demonstrated in BL and may be of aetiological importance. Analysis of the mutation pattern in the variable region of immunoglobulin genes in eBL suggests that these are post-follicular centre cells (i.e. they have been exposed to the mutational influence of the germinal centre).

EBV has the ability to immortalise B-lymphocytes and was first identified in eBL. Latent EBV infection occurs in almost all cases of eBL. It is found in 15–20% of sBL in Europe and North America, but in up to 80% in South America and the Middle East. Latent EBV infection is found in 20–40% of AIDS-BL. These differences may be related to the different seroepidemiology of EBV in the different communities and possibly accounts for some of the clinicopathological differences between the subtypes of BL. Holoendemic falciparum malaria has been pro-

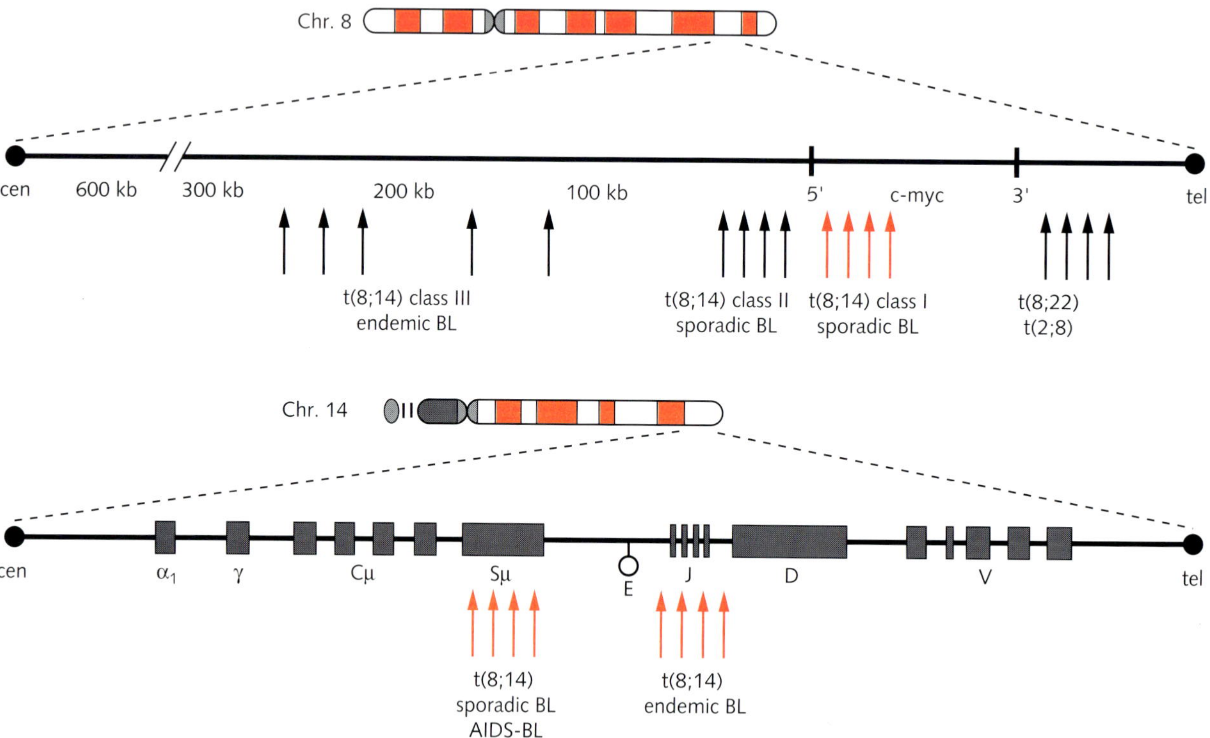

Fig. 8.6 Diagram of the breakpoints on chromosome 8 and chromosome 14 in the t(8;14) translocations found in eBL, sBL and AIDS-BL
The breakpoints on chromosome 8 in translocations involving chromosomes 2 and 22 are also shown. (Adapted with permission from Siebert *et al.* (1998).)

posed as a co-factor in the pathogenesis of eBL, and if proven would account for the geographical localisation of this tumour to the wet tropics.

Follicle centre cell lymphoma

Follicular lymphomas account for up to 40% of non-Hodgkin's lymphomas in North America and Western Europe, but are less prevalent elsewhere in the world. They usually present with lymphadenopathy and involvement of the spleen and bone marrow is frequent. The majority of patients present with stage III or IV disease. Follicle centre cell lymphomas usually have a follicular growth pattern that recapitulates many of the features of reactive germinal centres including the presence of follicular dendritic cells and CD4+ T-cells, as well as centroblasts and centrocytes in varying proportions. The differentiation between reactive and neoplastic follicles can be a major diagnostic problem.

Follicular lymphomas often follow an indolent course over many years. During this time they may show transformation to a more diffuse growth pattern with a greater proportion of blast cells.

Immunohistochemistry

Follicle centre cell lymphomas express CD19, CD20 and CD79a. They are CD5– and CD10+. The tumour cells usually express surface immunoglobulin, most frequently IgM and sometimes show cytoplasmic immunoglobulin.

Molecular genetics

Virtually all follicular lymphomas and a proportion of diffuse lymphomas are characterised by the t(14;18)(q32;q21) translocation which brings the *BCL-2* gene on chromosome 18 under the influence of the immunoglobulin heavy chain genes on chromosome 14, and leads to high levels of BCL-2 protein expression. BCL-2 protein is one of a family of proteins that controls apoptosis. Constitutive expression of BCL-2 in follicle centre cell lymphomas protects these cells from apoptosis.

In reactive germinal centre cells, the *BCL-2* gene is transcribed but not translated. The BCL-2-negative (BCL-2–) follicle centre cells are vulnerable to apoptosis when they undergo antibody affinity selection in the germinal centre. Only those cells capable of producing high affinity antibodies become plasma cells or memory B-cells, and switch on BCL-2 production. Staining for BCL-2 protein provides a useful means of distinguishing between reactive (BCL-2–) and neoplastic (BCL-2+) follicles (Figure 8.7). Staining for BCL-2 will not distinguish between follicle centre cell lymphomas and other low grade B-cell lymphomas, all of which express BCL-2 protein.

It is clear that t(14;18) alone is insufficient to cause neoplasia. Transgenic mice with constitutive expression of BCL-2 in all B-cells show follicular hyperplasia, but not lymphoma. It has also been shown that many normal individuals carry B-cells bearing t(14;18). Other events are necessary to transform cells bearing t(14;18) into

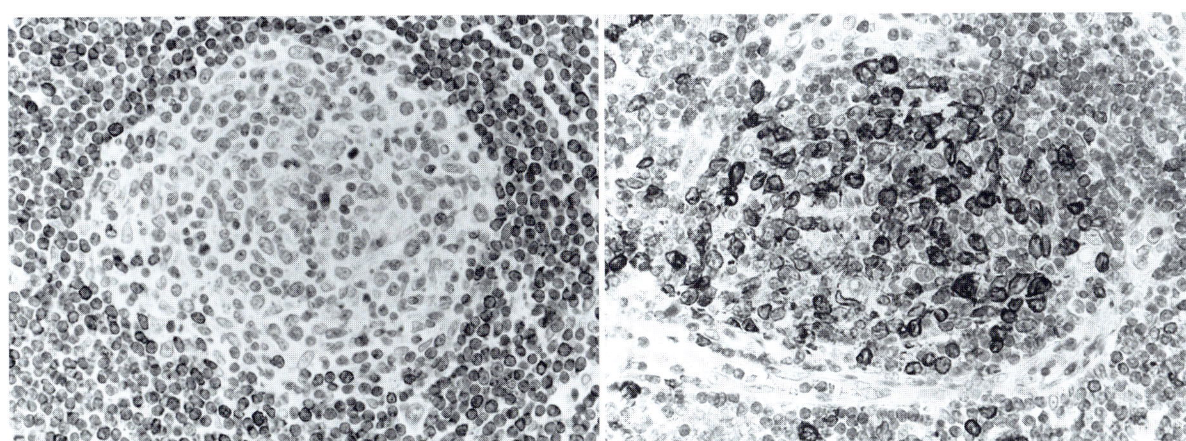

Fig. 8.7 (a) Reactive germinal centre stained for BCL-2
There is positive staining of the mantle cells and of scattered T-lymphocytes within the germinal centre. However, the germinal centre cells are unstained.
(b) Neoplastic follicle from a follicular lymphoma stained for BCL-2
Note very strong staining of neoplastic follicle centre cells (immunoperoxidase).

neoplastic cells. Further genetic events including p53 mutations are associated with the transformation of follicle centre cell lymphomas to high grade lymphomas.

Follicular lymphomas show a high level of mutations of the immunoglobulin genes with ongoing mutations in the CDRs suggestive of antigen drive, but it is not known whether antigenic drive is necessary for the continued proliferation in such cases. Approximately 5% of follicle centre cell lymphomas lack immunoglobulin expression in some cases due to mutations that have introduced stop codons. Such cases must presumably be independent of antigenic drive.

Extranodal marginal zone lymphomas

Extranodal marginal zone lymphomas (MALT lymphomas) are thought to arise from lymphocytes of the mucosal immune system. They occur most frequently in the stomach in the acquired lymphoid tissue associated with *Helicobacter pylori* induced gastritis. Other sites and predisposing causes are shown in Table 8.2. MALT lymphomas may remain localised for long periods of time, in contrast to all other low grade lymphomas. When they do disseminate, they may spread to other mucosal sites. Progression to high grade lymphoma may occur. If many blocks are examined from a high grade lymphoma of the stomach, it is often possible to identify areas of low grade lymphoma with the same immunoglobulin phenotype as the high grade tumour and it is assumed that this finding reflects transformation of a low grade to a high grade MALT lymphoma. It is often further assumed that high grade B-cell lymphomas occurring at extranodal sites have arisen by transformation from low grade lymphomas of MALT, and that the low grade tumour is no longer detectable, either because it has been overgrown by the high grade tumour, or because the tumour has not been adequately sampled.

MALT lymphomas have a good prognosis that may relate to their tendency to remain localised. Stage, rather than grade, appears to be the most important determinant of prognosis. A number of studies have shown that low grade MALT lymphomas of the stomach regress following eradication of *H. pylori*. The low grade lymphomas appear to require CD40 mediated signalling and Th2-type cytokines for growth and eradication of *H. pylori* presumably removes this T-cell dependent drive.

Table 8.2 Sites and predisposing causes of MALT lymphomas.

Site of MALT lymphoma	Predisposing causes of 2° MALT lymphoma tissue
Stomach	*Helicobacter pylori*
Liver	Hepatitis C
Skin	Lyme disease
Salivary gland	Autoimmune sialadenitis
Thyroid	Autoimmune thyroiditis
Lung	Sjögren's disease

Immunophenotype

Tumour cells express surface immunoglobulin, usually of the IgM class. They are negative for IgD. Cytoplasmic Ig is found in approximately 40% of cases, particularly those showing plasmacytic differentiation. Tumour cells express the B-cell associated antigens CD19, 20, 22, 79a. They are negative for CD5, CD10 and CD23.

Molecular genetics

Trisomy 3 has been reported to be the most common cytogenetic abnormality occurring in 50–85% of MALT lymphomas as detected by standard or interphase cytogenetics. A more recent report, however, found an incidence of 20% of trisomy 3 in low grade MALT lymphomas, a level similar to that found in other low grade B-cell lymphomas. The translocation t(11;18)(q21;q21) has been reported in approximately one-third of low grade MALT lymphomas. Currently, intense research is focused on the identification of the genes involved in these breakpoints. In the largest reported series of MALT lymphomas studied by conventional cytogenetics, t(11;18) was found in more than half of the low grade lymphomas with abnormal karyotypes, but in none of the high grade MALT lymphomas, including those with a mixed high and low grade component. The significance of this is uncertain and it may be that tumours with t(11;18) do not progress to high grade lymphomas. The high grade MALT lymphomas in this study did not show t(14;18) nor t(3;14), that characterised 10–35% of primary nodal large B-cell lymphomas. These tumours were, however, associated with t(8;14)(q24;q32) in three cases, and with chromosomal gains and losses in many cases.

Analysis of *V* genes in MALT lymphomas shows numerous point mutations relative to the germline genes and intraclonal sequence heterogeneity indicative of ongoing somatic hypermutation suggesting that low grade MALT lymphomas are under germinal centre influence.

Diffuse large B-cell lymphomas

Diffuse large B-cell lymphomas (DLBCL) account for

approximately 40% of all non-Hodgkin's lymphomas seen in Europe and North America. They present more frequently with localised disease than the usually widely disseminated low grade B-cell lymphomas, although a proportion of DLBCL are thought to be derived by transformation from follicle centre cell or other low grade B-cell lymphomas. Approximately 40% of DLBCL occur at extranodal sites.

Immunophenotype

The tumour cells usually express surface immunoglobulin and frequently show cytoplasmic immunoglobulin. They express the B-cell associated antigens CD19, CD20, CD22 and CD79a.

Molecular genetics

10–20% of DLBCL are found to have rearrangements of the *BCL-2* gene and this is often interpreted as evidence that these cases have transformed from pre-existing follicle centre cell lymphomas. The most frequent genetic abnormality in DLBCL involves the *BCL-6* gene on chromosome 3q27 which may be translocated with one of the immunoglobulin genes or with one of several other genes leading to promoter substitution. Whereas the expression of BCL-6 protein is found only during the germinal centre stage of B-cell differentiation, the products of most of the translocation partners are found also in post-germinal centre B-cells. Translocations involving *BCL-6* are found in 30–40% of DLBCL and in 5–10% of follicular lymphomas. More recently, it has been found that, independent of chromosomal rearrangements, somatic point mutations are detectable in the 5′ non-coding region of the *BCL-6* gene of 90% of DLBCL and 66.6% of AIDS-non-Hodgkin's lymphoma. Taken together, translocations and mutations of the *BCL-6* gene constitute the most common genetic abnormality found in human B-cell lymphomas.

The *BCL-6* gene codes for a zinc finger transcription factor that leads to transcriptional repression of promoters linked to its target sequence. It is expressed at high levels in lymphoid tissues being found within B-cells and CD4 T-cells within the germinal centres. It is not expressed in pre- or post-germinal centre B-cells. It is possible that deregulation of BCL-6 production does not allow terminal differentiation of B-cells, and thereby contributes to lymphomagenesis.

BCL-6 knock-out mice develop normally, but are unable to form lymphoid follicles, and have a defect in T-cell-dependent antibody responses. They also develop a Th2-mediated hyperimmune response with infiltration of multiple organs with eosinophils and IgE-bearing B-lymphocytes.

Anaplastic large cell lymphoma (ALCL)

This distinctive lymphoma was originally recognised because of its uniform strong expression of the CD30 antigen. Prior to this, many cases were categorised as histiocytic lymphomas. The tumour cells have blastic features with pleomorphic, often horseshoe-shaped nuclei. They have abundant cytoplasm and often grow in a cohesive pattern with a propensity to invade the sinuses of the lymph node. Involvement of the skin and other extranodal sites may occur. A distinction should be made between primary CD30+ ALCL of the skin, and systemic ALCL that involves the skin. The former appears to have a different molecular genetic basis and usually follows a very indolent course following local treatment alone. Rare cases of ALCL resemble Hodgkin's disease and in the REAL classification these have been placed in a provisional category of 'ALCL Hodgkin's like'. ALCL is one of the less common subtypes of AIDS-related non-Hodgkin's lymphomas.

Immunohistochemistry

The tumour cells may or may not express CD45. They show strong expression of CD30 on the cell membrane, and also usually in the Golgi region. Many cases express EMA in a similar fashion. Most cases are CD15–. There is variable expression of T-lineage markers giving tumours of T-cell or null-cell phenotype. Tumours of the B-cell phenotype with the morphology of ALCL are recognised, but in the REAL classification these have been included with the DLBCL. ALCL appears to be the only category of T-cell lymphoma that expresses the BCL-6 protein.

Molecular genetics

Approximately half the cases of ALCL show clonal rearrangements of the T-cell receptor genes, the remainder having germline T-cell receptor and immunoglobulin genes. The t(2;5)(p23;q35) translocation is a recurring cytogenetic abnormality in ALCL. The gene at 5q25 encodes the RNA binding phosphoprotein NPM, whereas the gene 2p23 encodes a receptor tyrosine kinase—ALK. The translocation results in the production of a fusion protein (NPM–ALK) (Figure 8.8) that leads to constitutive expression of ALK and deregulation of its mitogenic signal. Retrovirus transfer of NPM–ALK to mice leads to the development of

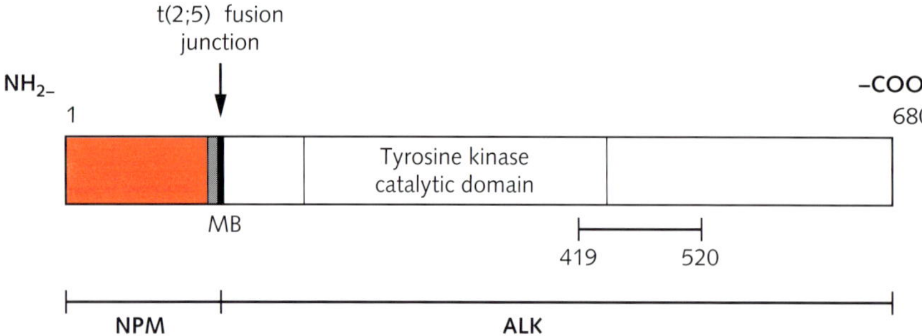

Fig. 8.8 Diagram of the t(2;5) translocation found in anaplastic large cell lymphoma
The translocation results in the production of an NPM–ALK fusion protein.

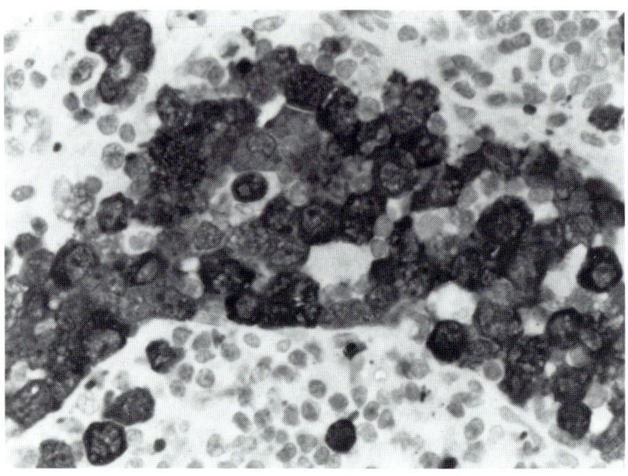

Fig. 8.9 Anaplastic large cell lymphoma
Anaplastic large cell lymphoma stained with an antibody to the NPM–ALK fusion protein (ALK-1). Note strong staining of both the cytoplasm and the nucleus. The sinusoidal distribution of the tumour cells is characteristic of ALCL (immunoperoxidase).

lymphomas within 4–6 months, suggesting a possible role for this activated fusion tyrosine kinase in oncogenesis. These lymphomas were phenotypically and genotypically of the B-cell lineage giving some support to those haematopathologists who recognise ALCL of the B-cell phenotype.

Antibodies have been raised to the NPM–ALK fusion protein and can be used to identify ALCL bearing t(2;5) (Figure 8.9). Approximately 50% of ALCL express this protein, the incidence being highest in children and young adults. Recognition of this protein can be of diagnostic importance. It may also be of prognostic significance since t(2;5)+ cases of ALCL have a good prognosis.

A rare subtype of large B-cell lymphoma expressing ALK has been reported. These tumours resemble ALCL in their abundant cytoplasm and sinusoidal growth pattern. They do not express CD30 but do express EMA and also show intracytoplasmic IgA. These tumours do not contain the t(2;5) translocation but express full length transcripts of the *ALK* gene. Most cases follow an aggressive clinical course.

Conclusions

In recent years the identification of non-random chromosomal abnormalities in many lymphoid neoplasms and the identification of the genes involved has given insight into the pathogenesis of these neoplasms. These molecular genetic abnormalities also aid in the identification and rational categorisation of lymphomas. It is possible that in the future they may provide targets for therapeutic intervention. There is a need to extend these molecular genetic studies to all lymphomas, particularly those of the T-cell phenotype where much confusion remains.

Further reading

Chronic lymphocytic leukaemia

Hamblin TJ, Oscier DG. (1997) Chronic lymphocytic leukaemia: The nature of the leukaemic cell. *Blood Reviews*, **11**, 119–128.

Horwitz M. (1997) The genetics of familial leukemia. *Leukemia*, **11**, 1347–1349.

Stankovic T, Weber P, Stewart G *et al.* (1999) Inactivation of ataxia telangiectasia mutated gene in B-cell chronic lymphocytic leukaemia. *Lancet*, **353**, 26–29.

Thompson A, Talley JA, Do HN *et al.* (1997) Aberrations of the B-cell receptor B29 (CD79b) gene in chronic lymphocytic leukemia. *Blood*, **90**, 1387–1394.

Mantle cell lymphoma

Banks P, Chan J, Cleary M *et al.* (1992) Mantle cell lymphoma: A proposal for unification of morphologic, immunologic and molecular data. *American Journal of Surgical Pathology*, **16**, 637–640.

Brehm A, Miska EA, McCance DJ *et al.* (1998) Retinoblastoma protein recruits histone deacetylase to repress transcription. *Nature*, **391**, 597–601.

Magnaghi-Javlin L, Groisman R, Naguibneva I *et al.* (1998)

Retinoblastoma protein represses transcription by recruiting a histone deacetylase. *Nature*, **391**, 601–605.

Rosenberg C, Wong E, Petty E *et al.* (1991) Overexpression of PRAD-1, a candidate BCL1 breakpoint region oncogene, in centrocytic lymphoma. *Proceedings of the National Academy of Sciences (USA)*, **88**, 9638–9642.

Burkitt's lymphoma

Adams JM, Harris AW, Pinkert CA *et al.* (1985) The c-myc oncogene driven by immunoglobulin enhancers induces lymphoid malignancy in transgenic mice. *Nature*, **318**, 533–538.

Cherney BW, Bhatia KG, Sgadari C *et al.* (1997) Role of the p53 tumor suppressor gene in the tumorigenicity of Burkitt's lymphoma cells. *Cancer Research*, **57**, 2508–2515.

Dalla-Favera R, Martinotti S, Gallo RC *et al.* (1983) Translocation and rearrangements of the c-myc oncogene locus in human undifferentiated B-cell lymphomas. *Science*, **219**, 963–967.

Hotchin N, Allday MJ, Crawford DH. (1990) Deregulated c-myc expression in Epstein–Barr virus-immortalized B-cells induces altered growth properties and surface phenotype but not tumorigenicity. *International Journal of Cancer*, **45**, 566–571.

Siebert R, Matthiesen P, Harder S *et al.* (1998) Application of interphase fluorescence *in situ* hybridization for the detection of the Burkitt translocation t(8;14) (q24;q32) in B-cell lymphomas. *Blood*, **91**, 984–990.

Follicle centre cell lymphoma

Bahler DW, Levy R. (1992) Clonal evolution of a follicular lymphoma: Evidence for antigen selection. *Proceedings of the National Academy of Sciences (USA)*, **89**, 6770–6774.

Bakhshi A, Jensen JP, Goldman P *et al.* (1985) Cloning the chromosomal breakpoints of t(14;18) human lymphomas: clustering around JH on chromosome 14 and near a transcriptional unit on 18. *Cell*, **41**, 889–906.

Cleary ML, Smith SD, Sklar J. (1986) Cloning and structural analysis of cDNA for bcl-2 and a hybrid bcl-2/immunoglobulin transcript resulting from the t(14;18) translocation. *Cell*, **47**, 19–28.

Korsmeyer SJ. (1992) Bcl-2 initiates a new category of oncogenes: Regulators of cell death. *Blood*, **80**, 879–886.

Limpens J, Stad R, Vos C *et al.* (1995) Lymphoma associated translocation t(14;18) in blood B-cells of normal individuals. *Blood*, **85**, 2528–2536.

LoCoco F, Gaidano G, Louie DC *et al.* (1993) P53 mutations are associated with histologic transformation of follicular lymphoma. *Blood*, **82**, 2289–2295.

McDonnell TJ, Deane N, Platt FM *et al.* (1989) Bcl-2-immunoglobulin transgenic mice demonstrate extended B-cell survival and follicular lymphoproliferation. *Cell*, **57**, 79–88.

Tsujimoto Y, Finger LR, Yunis J, Nowell PC, Croce CM. (1984) Cloning of the chromosome breakpoint of neoplastic B-cells with the t(14;18) chromosome translocation. *Science*, **226**, 1097–1099.

Zelenetz AD, Chen TT, Levy R. (1992) Clonal expansion in follicular lymphoma occurs subsequent to antigenic selection. *Journal of Experimental Medicine*, **176**, 1137–1148.

Extranodal MALT lymphomas

Auer IA, Gascoyne RD, Connors JM *et al.* (1997) t(11;18)(q21;q21) is the most common translocation in MALT lymphomas. *Annals of Oncology*, **8**, 979–985.

Chan JKC, Ng CS, Isaacson PG. (1990) Relationship between high-grade lymphoma and low-grade B-cell mucosa-associated lymphoid tissue lymphoma (MALToma) of the stomach. *American Journal of Pathology*, **136**, 1153–1164.

Greiner A, Knörr C, Qin Y *et al.* (1997) Low-grade B-cell lymphomas of mucosa-associated lymphoid tissue (MALT-type) require CD40-mediated signaling and TH2-type cytokines for *in vitro* growth and differentiation. *American Journal of Pathology*, **150**, 1583–1593.

Ott G, Kalla J, Steinhoff A *et al.* (1998) Trisomy 3 is not a common feature in malignant lymphomas of mucosa-associated lymphoid tissue type. *American Journal of Pathology*, **153**, 689–694.

Ott G, Katzenberger T, Greiner A *et al.* (1997) The t(11;18)(q21;q21) chromosome translocation is a frequent and specific aberration in low-grade but not high-grade malignant non-Hodgkin's lymphomas of the mucosa-associated lymphoid tissue (MALT) type. *Cancer Research*, **57**, 3944–3948.

Qin Y, Greiner A, Trunk MJ *et al.* (1995) Somatic hypermutation in low-grade mucosa-associated lymphoid tissue-type B-cell lymphoma. *Blood*, **86**, 3528–3534.

Wotherspoon AC, Finn TM, Isaacson PG. (1995) Trisomy 3 in low-grade B-cell lymphomas of mucosa-associated lymphoid tissue. *Blood*, **85**, 2000–2004.

Diffuse large B-cell lymphomas

Chen BW, Lida S, Louie DC, Dalla-Favera R, Chaganti RSK. (1998) Heterologous promoters fused to BCL6 by chromosomal translocations affecting band 3q27 cause its deregulated expression during B-cell differentiation. *Blood*, **91**, 603–607.

Gaidano G, Carbone A, Pastore C *et al.* (1997) Frequent mutations of the 5′ noncoding region of the BCL-6 gene in acquired immunodeficiency syndrome-related non-Hodgkin's lymphomas. *Blood*, **89**, 3755–3762.

Offit K, LoCoco F, Louie DC *et al.* (1994) Rearrangement of the bcl-6 gene as a prognostic marker in diffuse large cell lymphoma. *New England Journal of Medicine*, 331, 74–80.

Ye BH, Cattoretti G, Shen Q *et al.* (1997) The BCL-6 proto-oncogene controls germinal-centre formation and Th2-type inflammation. *Nature Genetics*, **16**, 161–170.

Anaplastic large cell lymphoma

Benharroch D, Meguerian-Bedoyan Z, Lamant L *et al.* (1998) ALK-positive lymphoma: A single disease with a broad spectrum of morphology. *Blood*, **91**, 2076–2084.

Delsol G, Lamant L, Mariamé B *et al.* (1997) A new subtype of large B-cell lymphoma expressing the ALK kinase and lacking the 2;5 translocation. *Blood*, **89**, 1483–1490.

Knefer MU, Look T, Pulford K *et al.* (1997) Retrovirus-mediated gene transfer of NPM–ALK causes lymphoid malignancy in mice. *Blood*, **90**, 2901–2910.

Pulford K, Lamant L, Morris SW *et al.* (1997) Detection of ALK and NPM–ALK proteins in normal and neoplastic cells with the monoclonal antibodies ALK-1. *Blood*, **89**, 1394–1404.

Wellmlum A, Otsuki T, Vogelbruch M *et al.* (1995) Analysis of the t(2;5)(p23;q35) translocation by reverse transcription-polymerase chain reaction in CD30+ anaplastic large-cell lymphomas, in other non-Hodgkin's lymphomas of T-cell phenotype, and in Hodgkin's disease. *Blood*, **86**, 2321–2328.

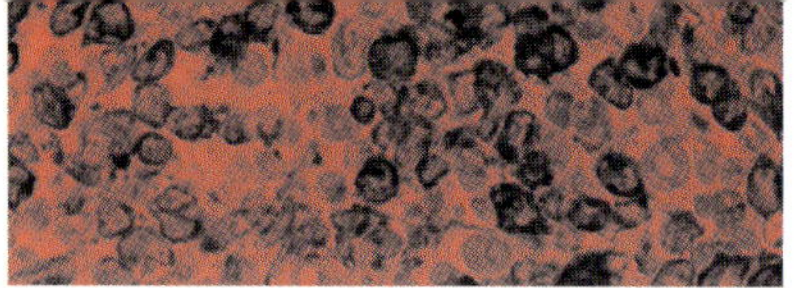

Chapter 9 The molecular biology of multiple myeloma

James R Berenson & Robert A Vescio

Introduction

Multiple myeloma is characterised by the accumulation of malignant plasma cells in the bone marrow compartment (Plate 9.1, facing page 128). These terminally differentiated B-lymphocytes all produce an identical immunoglobulin (Ig) known as a monoclonal protein, the laboratory hallmark of this malignancy. Although the predominant cell type in the bone marrow of these patients has the characteristics of a plasma cell, the low proliferative activity of these cells has raised the possibility that less mature B-lymphocytes represent the proliferating population which gives rise to the overabundant malignant plasma cell. Recent advances in molecular biological techniques have led to the determination of the stage of B-cell differentiation at which this disease begins. In addition, the finding of consistent chromosomal translocations involving the *Ig* gene locus has led to the identification of a number of potential oncogenes which may play a major role in the oncogenesis of this disease.

The tumour cells which reside within the bone marrow are supported by a non-malignant population of *stromal cells* which produce cytokines that enhance myeloma cell growth and prevent apoptosis. Moreover, the tumour cells themselves orchestrate the production of cytokines by these non-malignant bone marrow cells which can lead to a further increase in tumour cell burden. Recent demonstration of the human herpesvirus 8 (HHV-8) in some of these non-malignant cells provides an additional novel mechanism by which the bone marrow microenvironment may support this B-cell malignancy.

The malignant cell of origin

The low proliferative rate of the phenotypically identified malignant cell and inability of these cells to sustain tumour growth *in vivo* as demonstrated by kinetic and other studies imply that earlier precursor cells may be responsible for the proliferation of the malignant population. The presence of a circulating tumour component without obvious plasma cell morphology also suggests that less mature lymphocytes may be part of the clone, which could also explain the dissemination of the disease throughout the bone marrow. In addition, evidence for tumour cells at even earlier stages of haematopoietic differentiation came from studies showing the high rate of acute non-lymphoblastic leukaemia in these patients and the presence of non-lymphoid surface markers on malignant plasma cells. A variety of molecular biological techniques have subsequently been used to better define the cell types which are part of the malignant clone in this B-cell malignancy.

Immunogenotypes

Because of the monoclonal nature of the Ig synthesised by the malignant cells, the genes which lead to the production of this protein can be used as molecular markers capable of identifying surface markers on the malignant cells. In addition, specific characteristic changes in these genes occur at different stages of B-cell differentiation and thus allow determination of which cell types in this lineage are part of the tumour clone.

Each antibody-producing B-cell produces a single type of antibody. Early in normal B-cell development, rearrangement of four separate gene segments leads to the development of the heavy chain portion of a unique

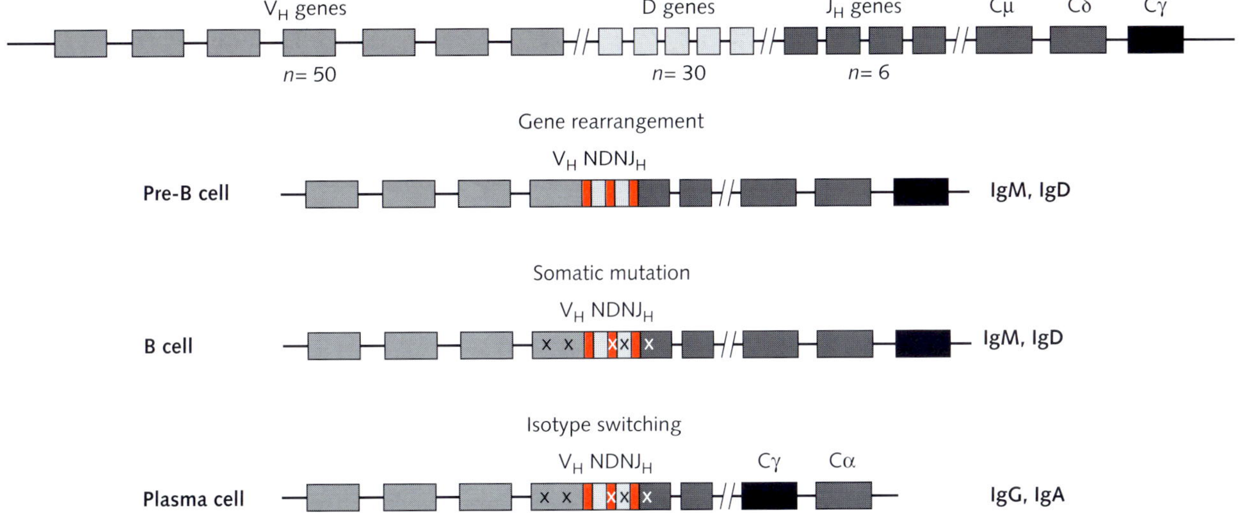

Fig. 9.1 Immunoglobulin gene rearrangement
Schematic diagram of the process of Ig gene rearrangement and Ig isotype switching which occurs during B-cell development. Exons are denoted by boxes, and introns by thin lines. The 'X's' represent mutations which occur within the Ig gene sequence during the process of somatic mutation.

functional antibody. These gene segments encode a constant region which determines the class of antibody (e.g. Cμ for IgM, Cγ for IgG, Cα for IgA). Three other gene segments encode the variable region of the heavy chain: *variable* (VH), *diversity* (D) and *joining* (JH). Since these latter three joined segments encode for the specific antigen recognition site of the final antibody, the recombination of genes which comprise this region must be unique to each antibody-producing cell. Thus, specific changes in these genes occur during the maturation of the antibody-producing B-cell. Most of a single functional heavy chain variable region is encoded by one of ~50 functional VH genes, whereas shorter stretches of amino acids are derived from one or more of ~30 D and one of six functional JH genes. In addition, increased antibody specificity is accomplished by the addition of non-germline nucleotides (N segments) at the VHD and DJH joints. Once a functional heavy chain rearrangement has occurred, the κ (and, if unsuccessful, the λ) light chain undergoes a similar rearrangement of V, J and C genes (Figure 9.1).

Additional specificity of the antibody is rendered by the mutation of nucleotides within the specific regions of the variable region which bind antigen directly, known as *complementarity determining regions* (CDRs), leading to enhanced avidity of the antibody for antigen. This process of somatic mutation occurs late in B-cell development in germinal centres. Following the secretion of a functional active antibody, this process ceases within this terminally differentiated B-cell (Figure 9.2).

In multiple myeloma, the properties of the Ig genes allow precise determination of the stage of B-cell development during which malignant transformation occurred (Table 9.1). Specifically, comparison of the myeloma VH gene sequence to the most homologous germline gene has shown marked somatic mutation (median 8%) of this gene segment. This frequency of somatic mutation is only found in the most differentiated B-cells after antigenic stimulation has occurred. In support of an antigenically driven process leading to these malignant clones, analysis of regions which bind antigen within these genes, the CDRs, demonstrates a marked predilection for somatic mutations compared to the other parts of the gene which are primarily responsible for maintaining the structural integrity of the molecule, the so-called *framework regions* (FRs). Moreover, in antigenically driven cells, mutations occurring within the CDRs should be more often associated with a change in the encoded amino acid compared to those changes occurring in the FRs. Indeed, the ratio of replacement to silent mutations is double in the CDRs compared to the FRs in multiple myeloma (Figure 9.3).

Importantly, analysis of multiple clones shows no clonal diversity in VH genes from myeloma patients, and determination of these sequences during the course of their disease shows no clonal evolution. These results differ from other B-cell tumours originating in germinal centres at earlier stages of B-cell differentiation. Analysis of CDR3 genes comprising of the D, JH and N segments

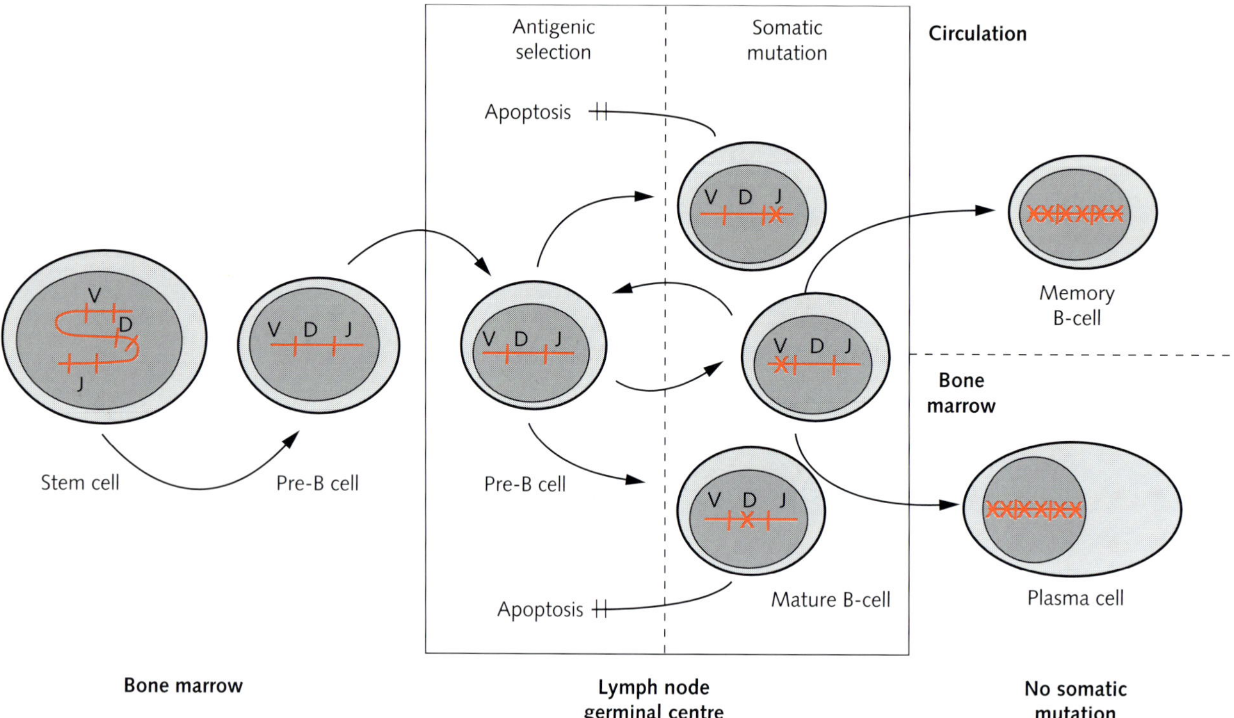

Fig. 9.2 Pre-B-cells which have undergone Ig gene rearrangement migrate to the lymph node where they are exposed to antigens If the B-cell surface antibody binds antigen, the cell undergoes replication whereby mutations within the Ig gene variable region occur by chance. If the resultant antibody is dysfunctional, the B-cell can no longer bind antigen and the cell undergoes apoptosis (programmed cell death). If, however, the mutation leads to improved antibody–antigen binding, the new B-cell preferentially binds to the lymph node antigens, survives and undergoes additional cycles of replication and somatic mutation. Once a B-cell has processed an antibody of high antigen affinity, the mature B-cell leaves the lymph node, undergoes class switching and differentiates into a plasma cell at which point no additional somatic mutation can occur.

Table 9.1 Characteristics of the VH genes in myeloma.

- High degree of somatic mutation
- Mutations occur in antigenically driven fashion
- No clonal diversity or evolution
- Lack of VH4.21 usage

further supports the high rate of somatic mutation with a high replacement to silent ratio. These segments also show a lack of clonal diversity.

Thus, these results suggest that the final oncogenic event in myeloma occurs very late in B-cell differentiation. Although some studies have suggested the existence of a pre-class switched (Cμ-containing) monoclonal cell in this disease, the frequency of these cells and their contribution to the malignant process have not been established. Using colony hybridisation techniques, our laboratory has not been able to demonstrate Cμ-containing clonal cells in myeloma.

Use of specific VH, D and JH genes

The approximately 50 functional VH genes have been divided into seven families based on sequence homology ranging in size from one (VH6) to 22 (VH3). In mature B-cells, VH gene family use is generally proportional to the number of functional genes. However, specific genes have been shown to be overused by immature B-cells including VH4.21. This same gene has also been frequently found in autoimmune diseases and several B-cell neoplasms. In fact, diffuse large cell lymphomas, which develop from relatively immature B-cells, use this VH gene in nearly two-thirds of cases.

In myeloma, although VH gene family usage closely parallels results found in normal B-cells, VH4.21 usage has been observed in only one case. Since this gene encodes antibodies capable of recognising self-antigens, the elimination of B-cells expressing this gene prior to plasma cell development would prevent production of possibly deleterious autoantibodies. Thus, this finding

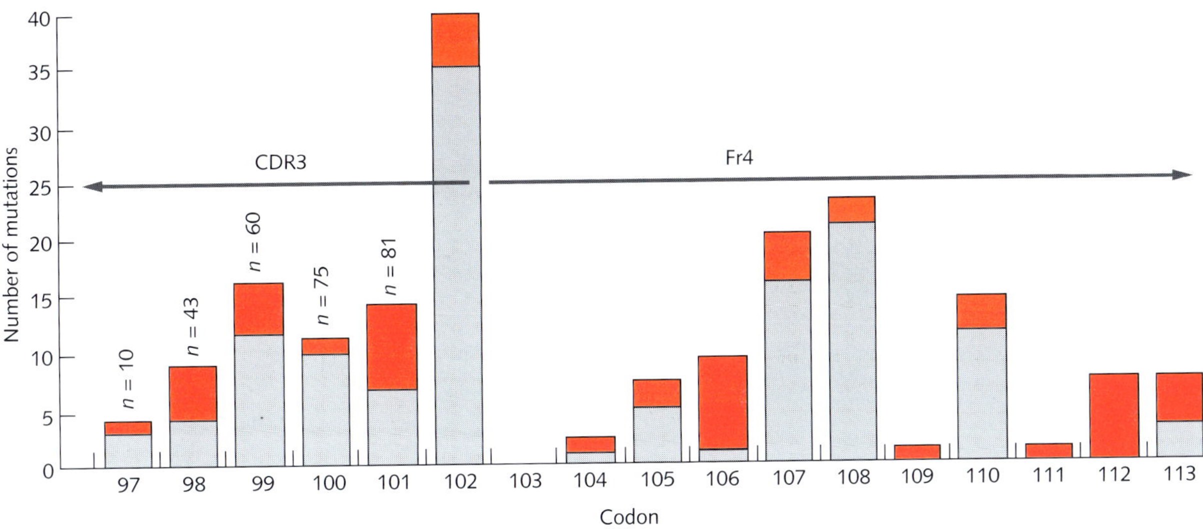

Fig. 9.3
Multiple myeloma Ig gene sequences were analysed from 83 patients and the JH region was compared to germline JH sequences to search for evidence of somatic mutation. Replacement mutations lead to a change in the antibody protein while silent mutations do not. The FR (framework region) of JH had relatively few replacement mutations, particularly in certain key codons, while numerous replacement mutations occurred in CDR3 which encodes for the antigen-binding portions of the antibody. (Key: red, silent mutations; grey, replacement mutations.)

also supports the view that the final transforming event occurs at the stage of terminal B-cell differentiation in myeloma. The CDR3 length in myeloma is comparable to normal B-cells, but fusion of multiple D genes is much more common than in normal B-cells. In myeloma CDR3s, N-region insertion is minimal compared to normal B-cells. Since studies of normal plasma cells have not been completed, it is unknown whether this increased frequency of D–D fusion and lack of N-region addition is specific to myeloma. Use of specific JH and D genes is quite comparable to usage in mature B-lymphocytes further supporting the late B-cell origin of myeloma.

Immunophenotype

Early studies using aneuploidy as a basis of malignant plasma cell determination suggested the existence of myeloid, megakaryocytic and T-cell markers on the malignant clone in myeloma. However, the use of these so-called 'lineage-specific markers' was problematic since it was learned that normal plasma cells could express these same antigens. The presence of a unique molecular marker, the Ig gene expressed by the malignant clone, has allowed a more precise determination of surface markers present on the malignant clone (Table 9.2).

Table 9.2 Surface phenotype of malignant cells.

Marker	Features
CD10	Subset
CD19 and CD20	Rarely expressed
CD28 and CD86	Occurs with progressive disease
CD34	Not expressed by malignant clone
CD38	High expression on most but not all malignant cells
CD56 (N-CAM)	Absent in MGUS and plasma cell leukaemia
CD95 (Fas antigen)	Mutations associated with lack of expression

MGUS, monoclonal gammopathy of indetermined significance; N-CAM, neural cell adhesion molecule.

CD34

CD34 is expressed on early haematopoietic precursors including the pluripotent stem cell. However, some B-cells also express this surface marker. Re-infusion of haematopoietic cells selected for CD34 can lead to rapid and sustained engraftment following myeloablative chemotherapy. Since we and others had previously demonstrated the presence of tumour cells in not only the bone marrow but also the blood of myeloma patients, it became of both biological and clinical importance to determine whether any malignant cells expressed this stem cell marker in myeloma patients. Initially, CD34+ cells were purified from a myeloma

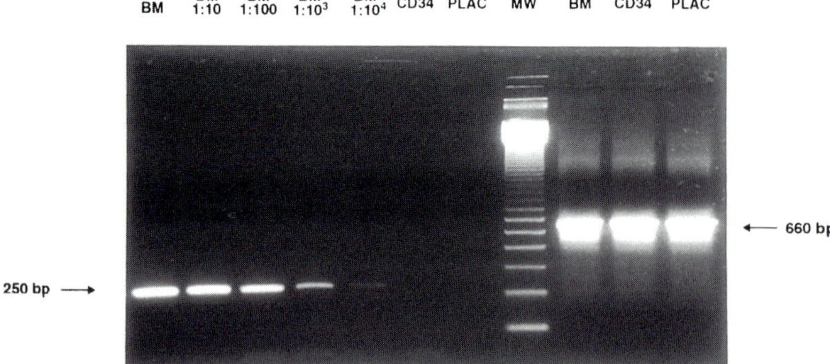

Fig. 9.4
Primers specific for the myeloma Ig gene sequence of patient WAD#12 were used to detect myeloma cell contamination of bone marrow (BM) successively diluted with placental DNA and an equivalent number of CD34+ cells purified from this same patient. The expected 250 bp product was detectable even in BM diluted 10,000-fold, but not in the CD34+ population of cells. Amplification of a 660 bp β-actin gene product served as a positive control.

patient's bone marrow using a combination of an immunoadsorption column and flow sorting. Using a sensitive polymerase chain reaction (PCR)-based assay with primers derived from the unique CDRs expressed by the patient's malignant clone, no tumour cells were detected in the CD34-expressing population (Figure 9.4) (*discussed in* Vescio *et al.*, 1994). Several other groups have confirmed this initial report, although other reports have suggested the existence of a CD34+ tumour cell in myeloma. However, CD34 selection with an immunoadsorption column (Ceprate, Cellpro Inc, Bothell, WA) on autologous peripheral stem cell autografts resulted in a reduction of autograft tumour burden by 2.7 to >4.5 logs as quantified using a PCR assay with patient-specific Ig gene primers. Results of a recently completed randomised phase III trial using the Ceprate® device confirmed this marked reduction in autograft tumour burden (3.3 logs) with the majority of autografts rendered 'tumour-free' to the sensitivity of the autograft (1 : 700,000). Despite this manipulation, engraftment was not different between the patients receiving CD34 selected compared to unselected autografts.

CD10

CD10, also known as the common acute lymphoblastic leukaemia antigen (CALLA), was originally described as a surface antigen present on the cells of some human acute lymphoblastic leukaemias. Subsequently, it has been shown that CD10 is expressed on a wide variety of haematopoietic cells including B-cells at early and late stages of differentiation. Studies of CD10 expression in myeloma have revealed that CD10-expressing myelomatous plasma cells are present in only a minority (average 25%; range, 10–60%) of cases, and that myeloma cells expressing this antigen comprised only a small fraction of the malignant population. However, these earlier studies were based on relatively insensitive immunohistochemical studies. Using PCR with patient-specific VH gene primers, our group has found a small CD10-bearing malignant population in all cases studied.

This malignant CD10-expressing population in myeloma may play an important role in the pathogenesis of this disease. Since CD10 is expressed on germinal centre B-cells with a high proliferative activity, this malignant subpopulation in myeloma may represent the part of the clone which leads to growth and disease progression. In support of this, some investigators have shown that the appearance of CD10-expressing tumour cells in the circulation occurs at the time of progression of myeloma.

CD19 and CD20

CD19 and CD20 are markers which become expressed during B-cell development, but are normally not present on terminally differentiated plasma cells. Although malignant bone marrow plasma cells also do not express these markers, controversy exists regarding their presence on the circulating malignant population. Most studies have suggested that these markers are rarely found on the circulating malignant cells in myeloma patients. In fact, a recent study suggests not only that these circulating CD20-expressing cells are polyclonal, but also that there is an inverse relationship between their numbers and prognosis in myeloma.

CD28 and CD28 ligand (CD86)

Although CD28 was originally identified as an antigen present on T-lymphocytes and responsible for T-cell activation, its presence has also been found on both malignant and non-malignant plasma cells. Its presence on the malignant plasma cells of myeloma patients is associated with disease progression and treatment failure. Interestingly, when CD28 is present on the malignant cells, it is accompanied by the presence of its ligand, CD86. By contrast, there is an inverse correlation between CD28 and the expression of the neural cell adhesion molecule marker CD56.

CD38

Previous studies have demonstrated the high expression of CD38 on normal and malignant plasma cells. Although this antigen is not expressed on the pluripotent stem cell, it is expressed weakly on early lineage-committed cells. If CD38 is expressed on all malignant cells, it may be possible to select for CD38-negative cells in autografts and render these products tumour-free. However, most studies of CD38 expression in myeloma have relied only on insensitive immunohistochemical techniques, which would be incapable of identifying an infrequent CD38-negative tumour population in myeloma patients. Using flow sorting with anti-CD38 antibodies on peripheral blood mononuclear cells from myeloma patients, we identified a CD38-negative tumour cell population with a PCR-based assay in all myeloma patients. However, the frequency of these circulating CD38 cells was markedly less than the CD38-expressing tumour cells in all cases. Thus, although tumour cells lacking CD38 exist in myeloma, they represent a relatively minor component of the malignant population. Since CD38 is not expressed on B-cells prior to the plasma cell stage, however, these CD38-negative malignant cells may represent less mature malignant cells with a more proliferative capability.

CD56 (N-CAM)

The neural cell adhesion molecule (N-CAM), CD56, is a member of the Ig superfamily, and as the name implies was originally detected on a wide variety of neural cells. However, it has also been recently identified on haematopoietic cells, especially on natural killer cells, and more recently on malignant plasma cells in the majority of myeloma patients, but not on the monoclonal plasma cells from patients with monoclonal gammopathy of undetermined significance (MGUS). Patients with plasma cell leukaemia are also often missing this adhesion molecule and most autonomously growing cell lines also do not show this surface marker. These studies may suggest that this adhesion molecule helps keep the plasma cell in the bone marrow microenvironment. On the other hand, with autonomous growth, i.e. development of plasma cell leukaemia, its presence is no longer required and allows cells to traverse to the bloodstream. More recent studies suggest serum levels of N-CAM predict outcome in these patients with higher levels associated with a poor clinical outcome. Moreover, it has been shown that low levels (<20 U/ml) can distinguish patients with MGUS from those patients with myeloma.

Chromosomal and genetic abnormalities

Although earlier studies suggested chromosomal abnormalities rarely existed in the malignant cells of these patients, more recent sophisticated techniques using fluorescence *in situ* hybridisation (FISH) and comparative genomic hybridisation have shown that anomalies exist in the malignant cells of most if not all myeloma patients (Table 9.3). Similar to the translocations common in other B-cell malignancies, these abnormalities often involve the Ig heavy chain gene locus on the long arm of chromosome 14 and a limited number of different non-Ig-containing partner chromosomes. However, the site of translocation within the Ig heavy chain gene loci is different from the region (JH) found in other B-cell malignancies involving the switch regions which are involved in heavy chain class switching from Cμ to another heavy chain class (Figure 9.5). The non-Ig partner chromosomes often involve 11q, 4p, 6p and 16q. Recent studies have demonstrated previously identified and potentially new oncogenes near these non-Ig breakpoints. Interestingly, the identified genes include cyclin D, oncogenic fibroblastic growth factors and other newly identified genes (11q), the fibroblastic growth factor receptor 3 (4p), the basic zipper C-MAF transcription factor (4p) and the interferon regulatory factor 4 (6p). At this point, it is impossible to invoke a common mechanism by which these different genes may lead to malignant plasma cell development.

Other frequent chromosomal abnormalities involve

Table 9.3 Common chromosomal abnormalities in myeloma.

Translocations (listed in order of frequency)	
14q32 *with*	11q13 (*cyclin D, other new fibroblastic growth factors*)
	4p16 (*fibroblastic growth factor receptor 3*)
	6p25 (*interferon regulatory factor 4*)
	16q23 (*C-MAF* transcription factor)
	8q24 (*C-MYC*)
	18q21 (*BCL-2*)
1q *with*	5, 8, 12, 14, 15, 16, 17, 19q, 21, 22
Losses	6q, 13q
Gains	3, 5, 7, 9q, 11q, 12q, 15q, 17q, 18, 19, 21, 22q

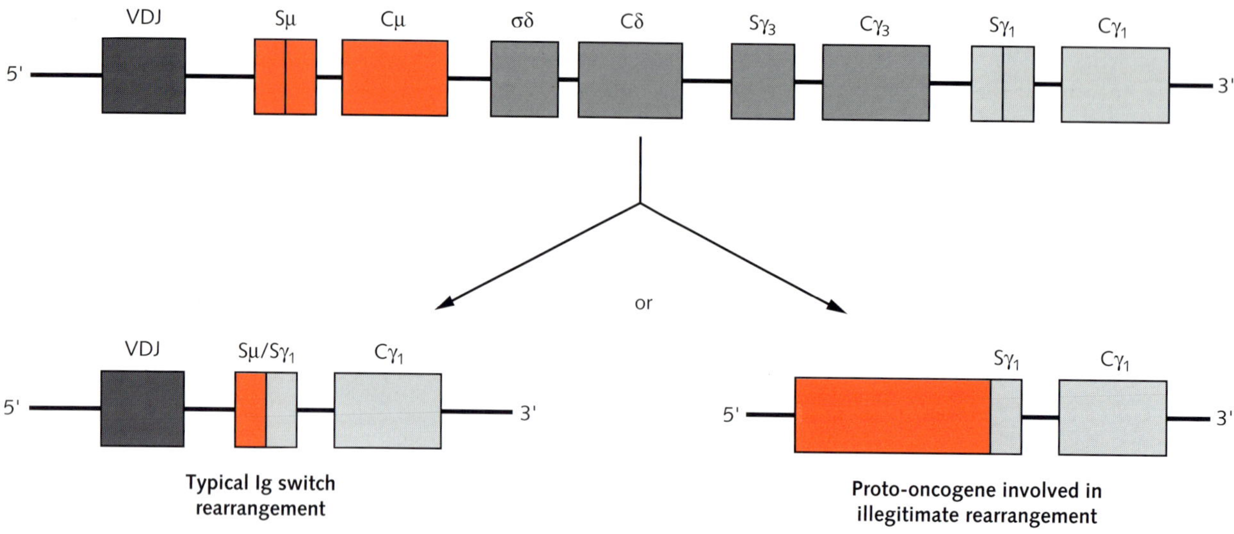

Fig. 9.5 Illegitimate Ig gene rearrangement
Proposed mechanism of illegitimate Ig gene rearrangement resulting in the translocation of an oncogene to the switch region of one of the constant region genes. This process would lead to the overproduction of the translocated oncogene due to the high transcription rate of the Ig gene sequences.

Table 9.4 Common oncogenic changes in myeloma.

Ras mutations	*—advanced disease*
N-*Ras*	
K-*Ras*	—associated with poor outcome
Rb loss	
p53 loss	—advanced disease and plasma cell leukaemia
Cyclin D overexpression (associated with 11q13 anomalies)	
Cylin D kinase inhibitor abnormalities loss of p15, p16 and p18 genes methylation of p15 and p16—advanced disease	

loss of chromosome 13 and a recently described jumping translocation of 1q. The presence of these anomalies, or 11q translocations, is associated with a poor outcome in myeloma. On the other hand, trisomies of 6, 9 and 17 have been associated with prolonged survival.

Interestingly, cytogenetic changes have also been observed in patients with MGUS suggesting that additional events are required to develop the malignant disorder in myeloma patients.

Other oncogenic changes have been observed in myeloma patients (Table 9.4). Ras mutations occur in a minority of patients and are associated with more aggressive disease and a poor clinical outcome. In addition, abnormalities of both the p53 and Rb genes have also been observed more frequently in patients with plasma cell leukaemia or more aggressive disease. Although cyclin D may be overexpressed in patients containing 11q anomalies, another mechanism leading to progression through the cell cycle involves loss of function of the cyclin D kinase inhibitors. Uncommonly, loss of some of these genes (p15, p16 and p18) may occur in myeloma patients. However, methylation of these genes occurs commonly in the malignant plasma cells, and also leads to loss of their expression. This phenomenon is often observed in patients with more advanced disease.

The Fas antigen, CD95, is a 45 kDa transmembrane protein which can induce apoptosis when bound to Fas ligand. Point mutations of the antigen have been described in patients with congenital autoimmune disease and *LPR* mice characterised by a lupus-like syndrome. Recently, similar mutations have been described in myeloma patients and are associated with lack of expression of this apoptosis-inducing molecule. However, the role of these mutations and the lack of Fas antigenic expression in the development or maintenance of myeloma remains unclear.

The role of the HHV-8-infected stroma in myeloma

Stromal cells in myeloma

In myeloma, the role of the bone marrow microenvironment has been shown to be of increasing importance in supporting the malignant plasma cell. Specifically, non-malignant stromal cells in the bone marrow from myeloma patients have been shown to promote the growth and prevent apoptosis of malignant plasma cells. The cytokine interleukin-6 (IL-6) is produced in large quantities by these cells, and has been demonstrated to enhance growth and prevent apoptosis of the tumour cells. The production of this cytokine by stromal cells from myeloma patients has been shown to be enhanced by the adherence of malignant plasma cells. Thus, there is a close 'symbiotic' relationship between bone marrow stromal cells and tumour cells which results in an increase in tumour burden in myeloma patients. Many years ago, Hamburger and Salmon suggested the existence of a specific factor only present in bone marrow macrophages from myeloma patients which was required for supporting the malignant clone.

HHV-8 in other diseases

In a case of Kaposi's sarcoma (KS), a new member of the herpesvirus family was discovered. In addition to being frequently found in KS associated with or without HIV infection, this virus, Kaposi's sarcoma-associated herpesvirus (KSHV), also known as HHV-8, has been identified in two other B-cell disorders, primary effusion lymphoma and multicentric Castleman's disease. Interestingly, this virus contains an IL-6 homologue and all three of these diseases also share IL-6 as a growth factor. In these cases, the virus has been localised to the malignant cells, although some controversy still exists in KS. Recently, HHV-8 has been found in cells bearing macrophage and dendritic cell markers cultured from the blood of KS patients. In one study, viral DNA has also been identified in peripheral blood B-cells from nearly half of KS patients. Moreover, although latent virus was present in the KS tumour itself, viral forms characteristic of HHV-8 replication were present in the peripheral blood of these patients. Thus, although HHV-8 has been associated with the malignant population, some studies support infection of non-malignant cells and suggest these cell types may disseminate the virus.

HHV-8 in myeloma bone marrow and peripheral blood (Table 9.5)

This new virus was also found to encode an IL-6 homologue which was capable of stimulating growth and preventing apoptosis of a murine myeloma cell line. Recently, it has been shown that this viral homologue can also stimulate growth of a human myeloma cell line. Previously our laboratory has demonstrated the presence of HHV-8 in the adherent non-malignant cell population from long-term cultures of bone marrow from myeloma patients (Plate 9.2). Moreover, approximately 25% of patients with MGUS also showed virus in these bone marrow-derived dendritic cells. Further characterisation of the virally infected stromal population showed characteristics of a dendritic cell phenotype.

Because the infected cells were initially found only in long-term cultures derived from fresh bone marrow aspirates obtained from these patients, further studies were performed on fresh bone marrow biopsies using both PCR and *in situ* hybridisation techniques with viral-specific primers and probes, respectively. In most cases, viral presence could be demonstrated using these techniques in myeloma bone marrow biopsy samples, whereas biopsies from patients with lymphomas, other cancers infiltrating the bone marrow and normal subjects did not contain HHV-8. The few myeloma patients in whom HHV-8 was not detected were either studied at diagnosis with earlier stage disease or in remission following chemotherapy. In patients with KS, the presence of circulating HHV-8 has been observed. Although whole peripheral blood mononuclear cells (PBMCs) from myeloma patients demonstrate amplified PCR product using viral-specific primers in a small minority of cases, enrichment of PBMCs for markers (CD68 or CD83) present on the virally infected bone marrow stromal cells allows detection of virus in most of the 137 cases analysed (70%). In addition, recent studies suggest a relationship between viral load and extent of KS in HIV-infected individuals. Similarly, although HHV-8 can be detected in most myeloma patients' blood following enrichment for dendritic cells at diagnosis, its absence is associated with a lower tumour burden at diagnosis. Moreover, myeloma patients in relapse are more likely to show amplified PCR product with HHV-8 primers than patients in remission.

Transmission of HHV-8 among family members and sexual partners of myeloma patients

HHV-8 has previously been demonstrated to be present in sexual and other body secretions. Recent studies suggest a close relationship between the presence of serology to HHV-8 and the number of sexual partners in homosexual men, and seroconversion is associated with the development of KS. Because of these findings, we sought to determine the transmissibility of HHV-8 among family members and sexual partners of myeloma patients. Although approximately 80% of myeloma patients demonstrate HHV-8 in PBMCs enriched for dendritic cells, only 2% of the family members or sexual partners show viral presence in the enriched PBMCs. This suggests either the absence of HHV-8 in this group at risk for viral exposure, or that the level is below the level of sensitivity of the PCR-based assay.

Sequencing of HHV-8 open reading frames (ORFs) in myeloma patients

Although we have consistently found HHV-8 in myeloma bone marrow biopsies and peripheral blood using primer pairs from many different HHV-8 ORFs (*T1.1. MIPs, ORF26, ORF65, ORF74, V-IRF, V-BCL-2, cyclin D*), other investigators have had difficulty identifying HHV-8 in bone marrow and peripheral blood samples from myeloma patients. Using the KS330233 primers derived from ORF26, three different tissue sources (long-term cultures of adherent bone marrow stromal cells, PBMCs enriched for dendritic cells and bone marrow core biopsies) were sequenced. Although interpatient differences exist in this ORF, these three tissues showed identical ORF26 sequences in the same patient except for a single base pair substitution in only one sample. In addition, compared to those sequences derived from both HHV-8-infected lymphomas and KS tissues, ORF26 derived from myeloma patients showed specific consistent changes.

A similar analysis of ORF65 also showed interpatient differences as well as a consistent deletion in all myeloma patients. Since this ORF is responsible for a major part of the serological response to HHV-8, deletion of a base pair, likely resulting in changes in the resulting protein product, may help explain the lack or low level of serological response to this virus observed in myeloma patients.

HHV-8 gene expression in myeloma bone marrow

Representational differential analysis (RDA) was performed using bone marrow dendritic cells from myeloma patients compared to normal subjects, and showed the presence of the vIRF homologue from HHV-8. Reverse transcriptase (RT)-PCR on RNA derived from fresh bone marrow biopsies from myeloma patients and normal subjects confirmed the presence of vIRF transcripts only in the myeloma patients. Transfection of this viral gene in murine fibroblasts leads to a transformed phenotype, and injection into nude mice produces stromal tumours. Moreover, vIRF transfection of these cells inhibits the normal induction of the *p21* cyclin D kinase inhibitor, a growth inhibitor, by interferon β, and results in a growth advantage for vIRF-transfected cells. The expression of this same gene in myeloma bone marrow dendritic cells may allow this virally infected population to 'outgrow' uninfected stromal cells.

Additional studies to determine expression of HHV-8-specific genes have also shown the presence of the viral homologue of IL-8R in fresh myeloma bone marrow samples. This viral gene also produces a transformed phenotype in transfected murine fibroblasts, and introduction into nude mice leads to stromal cell tumours. It has also been shown that this viral gene induces angiogenesis by induction of vascular endothelial growth factor (VEGF). Studies of myeloma bone marrow show marked staining with CD31, a vascular endothelial cell marker, consistent with the induction of VEGF in these HHV-8-infected samples. Recent studies also suggest an important role for this factor in regulating normal dendritic development.

By contrast, despite the expression of viral IL-6 transcripts in the adherent cells from long-term cultures from myeloma bone marrow, these transcripts are identified in only a small minority of patients' fresh bone marrow biopsies. Recent studies also show the relative lack of potency of the viral homologue compared to the human IL-6. Thus, other viral factors are likely involved in supporting the virally infected stromal cell as well as the malignant plasma cell (Figure 9.6).

Conclusions

Recent advances in molecular biology have clarified that the final malignant event must have occurred in a post-class switch terminally differentiated B-cell in multiple myeloma. The identification of a common chromosomal abnormality involving the Ig heavy chain switch region has allowed identification of potentially new genetic targets for therapy in this disease. Although recent studies suggest a potential role of HHV-8 in the pathogenesis of multiple myeloma (Table 9.5), further work is required to clearly establish this connection. The establishment of this link could lead to major changes in how clinicians approach this fatal malignancy.

Table 9.5 Characteristics of HHV-8 in myeloma patients.

- Infects non-malignant bone marrow dendritic cell
- Circulates in blood of most patients
- Presence in blood associated with poor outcome
- Viral sequence is unique to myeloma patients
- High RNA expression of vIL-8R and vIRF homologues
- Found in only one-quarter of MGUS patients
- Not found in other family members of myeloma patients

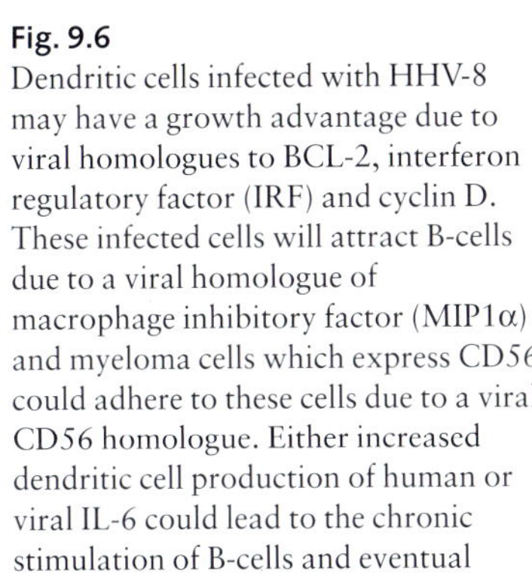

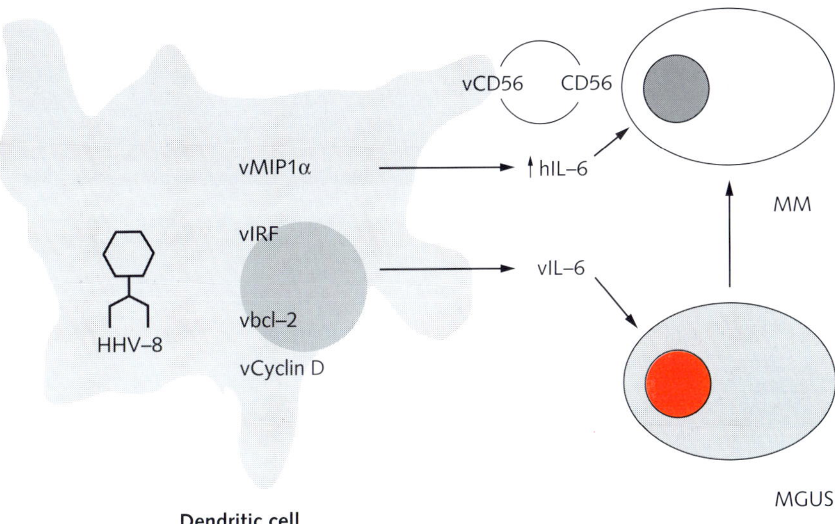

Fig. 9.6
Dendritic cells infected with HHV-8 may have a growth advantage due to viral homologues to BCL-2, interferon regulatory factor (IRF) and cyclin D. These infected cells will attract B-cells due to a viral homologue of macrophage inhibitory factor (MIP1α) and myeloma cells which express CD56 could adhere to these cells due to a viral CD56 homologue. Either increased dendritic cell production of human or viral IL-6 could lead to the chronic stimulation of B-cells and eventual MGUS or myeloma development.

Further reading

Biology and molecular genetics of myeloma

Bakkus MHC, Heirman C, Van Riet B, Van Camp B, Thielemans K. (1992) Evidence that multiple myeloma Ig heavy chain VDJ genes contain somatic mutations but show no intraclonal variation. *Blood*, **80**, 2326–2335.

Billadeau D, Ahmann G, Greipp P, Van Ness B. (1993) The bone marrow of multiple myeloma patients contains B-cell populations at different stages of differentiation that are clonally related to the malignant plasma cell. *Journal of Experimental Medicine*, **178**, 1023–1031.

Corradini P, Boccadoro M, Voena C, Pileri A. (1993) Evidence for a bone marrow B-cell transcribing malignant plasma cell VDJ joined to Cμ sequence in immunoglobulin (IgG)- and IgA-secreting multiple myelomas. *Journal of Experimental Medicine*, **178**, 1091–1096.

Rettig MB, Vescio RA, Cao J *et al.* (1996) VH gene usage in multiple myeloma: complete absence of the VH4.21 (VH4–34) gene. *Blood*, **87**, 2846–2852.

Vescio RA, Cao J, Hong CH *et al.* (1995) Myeloma Ig heavy chain V region sequences reveal prior antigenic selection and marked somatic mutation but no intraclonal diversity. *Journal of Immunology*, **155**, 2487–2497.

Immunophenotypic markers

Cao J, Vescio RA, Rettig MB *et al.* (1995) A CD-10 positive subset of malignant cells is identified in multiple myeloma using PCR with patient-specific primers. *Leukemia*, **9**, 1948–1953.

Ong F, Kaiser U, Seelen PJ *et al.* (1996) Serum neural cell adhesion molecule differentiates multiple myeloma from paraproteinemias due to other causes. *Blood*, **87**, 712–716.

Pilarski LM, Jensen GS. (1992) Monoclonal circulating B-cells in multiple myeloma: a continuously differentiating, possibly invasive, population as defined by expression of CD45 isoforms and adhesion molecules. *Hematology/Oncology Clinics of North America*, **2**, 297–322.

Ruiz-Arguelles GJ, Katzmann JA, Greipp PR *et al.* (1984) Multiple myeloma: circulating lymphocytes that express plasma cell antigens. *Blood*, **64**, 352–356.

Schiller G, Vescio R, Freytes C *et al.* (1995) Transplantation of CD34+ peripheral blood progenitor cells after high-dose chemotherapy for patients with advanced multiple myeloma. *Blood*, **86**, 390.

Sonneveld P, Durie BGM, Lokhorst HM, Frutiger Y, Schoester M, Vela EE. (1993) Analysis of multi-drug resistance (MDR-1) glycoprotein and CD56 expression to separate monoclonal gammopathy from multiple myeloma. *British Journal of Haematology*, **83**, 63–67.

Szczepek AJ, Bergsagel PL, Axelsson L *et al.* (1997) CD34+ cells in the blood of patients with multiple myeloma express CD19 and IgH mRNA and have patient-specific IgH VDJ gene rearrangements. *Blood*, **89**, 1824–1833.

Vescio RA, Hong CH, Cao J *et al.* (1994) The hematopoietic stem cell antigen, CD34, is not expressed on the malignant cells in multiple myeloma. *Blood*, **84**, 3283–3290.

Vescio R, Schiller G, Stewart AK *et al.* (1999) Multicenter phase III trial to evaluate CD34+ selected vs. unselected autologous peripheral blood progenitor cell transplantation in multiple myeloma. *Blood*, **93**, 1858–1868.

Chromosomal and cytogenetic abnormalities

Bergsagel PL, Chesi M, Nardini E *et al.* (1996) Promiscuous translocations into immunoglobulin heavy chain switch regions in multiple myeloma. *Proceedings of the National Academy of Sciences (USA)*, **93**, 13931–13936.

Chesi M, Bergsagel PL, Shonukan OO *et al.* (1998) Frequent dysregulation of the *c-maf* proto-oncogene at 16q23 by translocation to an Ig locus in multiple myeloma. *Blood*, **91**, 4457–4463.

Chesi M, Nardini E, Brents LA *et al.* (1997) Frequent translocation t(4;14) (p16.3;q32.3) in multiple myeloma is associated with increased expression and activating mutations of fibroblastic growth factor receptor 3. *Nature Genetics*, **16**, 260–264.

Cigudosa JC, Rao PH, Calasanz MJ *et al.* (1998) Characterization of nonrandom chromosomal gains and losses in multiple myeloma by comparative genomic hybridization. *Blood*, **91**, 3007–3010.

Corradini P, Inghirami G, Astolfi M *et al.* (1994) Inactivation of tumor suppressor genes, p53 and Rb1, in plasma cell dyscrasias. *Leukemia*, **8**, 758–767.

Ida S, Rao PH, Butler M *et al.* (1997) Deregulation of MUM1/IRF4 by chromosomal translocation in multiple myeloma. *Nature Genetics*, **17**, 226–230.

Landowski TH, Qu N, Buyuksal I, Painter JS, Dalton WS. (1997) Mutations in the fas antigen in patients with multiple myeloma. *Blood*, **90**, 4266–4270.

Liu P, Leong T, Quam L *et al.* (1996) Activating mutations of N- and K-ras in multiple myeloma show different clinical associations: Analysis of the Eastern Cooperative Oncology Group Phase III trial. *Blood*, **88**, 2699–2706.

Sawyer JR, Tricot G, Mattox S, Jaganath S, Barlogie B. (1998) Jumping translocations of chromosome 1q in multiple myeloma: Evidence for a mechanism involving decondensation of pericentromeric heterochromatin. *Blood*, **91**, 1732–1741.

Tasaka T, Asou H, Munker R *et al.* (1998) Methylation of the p16 gene in multiple myeloma. *British Journal of Haematology*, **101**, 558–564.

Tricot G, Barlogie B, Jaganath S *et al.* (1995) Poor prognosis in multiple myeloma is associated only with partial or complete deletions of chromosome 13 or abnormalities involving 11q and not other karyotype abnormalities. *Blood*, **86**, 4250–4256.

Zandecki M. (1996) Multiple myeloma: Almost all patients are cytogenetically abnormal. *British Journal of Haematology*, **94**, 217–227.

HHV-8

Bais C, Santomasso B, Coso O *et al.* (1998) G-protein-coupled receptor of Kaposi's sarcoma-associated herpesvirus is a viral oncogene and angiogenesis activator. *Nature*, **391**, 86–89.

Burger R, Neipel F, Fleckenstein B *et al.* (1998) Human herpesvirus type 8 interleukin-6 homologue is functionally active on human myeloma cells. *Blood*, **91**, 1858–1863.

Mackenzie J, Sheldon J, Morgan G *et al.* (1997) HHV-8 and multiple myeloma in the UK. *Lancet*, **350**, 1144–1145.

Marcelin A-G, Dupin N, Bouscary D *et al.* (1997) HHV-8 and multiple myeloma in France. *Lancet*, **350**, 1144.

Oyama A, Ran S, Nadaf S. (1998) Vascular endothelial growth factor affects dendritic cell maturation through the inhibition of nuclear factor activation in hematopoietic progenitor cells. *Journal of Immunology*, **160**, 1224–1232.

Rettig M, Ma H, Vescio R *et al.* (1997) Kaposi's sarcoma-associated herpesvirus infection of bone marrow dendritic cells from myeloma patients. *Science*, **276**, 1851–1854.

Said J, Rettig M, Heppner K *et al.* (1997) Localization of Kaposi's sarcoma-associated herpesvirus in bone marrow biopsy samples from patients with multiple myeloma. *Blood*, **90**, 4278–4282.

Uchiyama H, Barut B, Mohrbacher A, Chauhan D, Anderson K. (1993) Adhesion of human myeloma-derived cell lines to bone marrow stromal cells stimulates interleukin-6 secretion. *Blood*, **82**, 3712–3720.

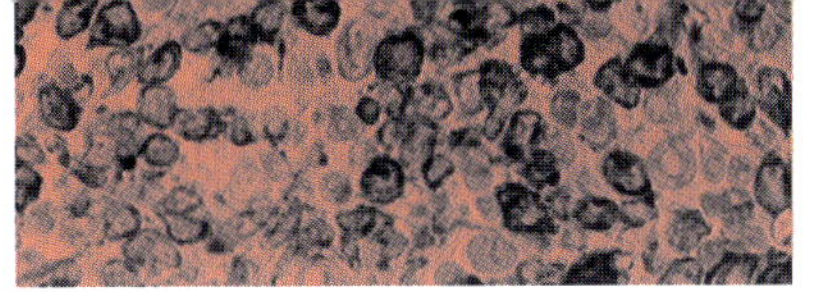

Chapter 10 Haemoglobinopathies due to structural mutations

Ronald L Nagel

Introduction

This chapter discusses those haemoglobinopathies that are caused by mutations in the exon (i.e. coding) portion of the α or β globin genes. Alterations of globin gene expression (*thalassaemias*) are reviewed in *Chapter 1*. We will limit ourselves only to the most frequent mutations that must be considered in the differential diagnosis of the common haemoglobinopathies.

Normal haemoglobin structure and function

The adult major haemoglobin molecule, Hb A, is a tetramer formed by four polypeptide chains: two α chains and two β chains. Each of these chains is attached to a prosthetic group (haem) formed by protoporphyrin IX in a complex with a single iron molecule (Figure 10.1).

The haem is semi-buried in the globin, surrounded by a hydrophobic niche that favours the maintenance of the ferrous state of the iron. The haem pocket is large enough for oxygen to penetrate, but large ligands (molecules capable of binding to the iron), such as carbon monoxide (CO) or the family of isocyanates, have progressive difficulty in finding the iron.

Oxygen transport to tissues, the ultimate purpose of haemoglobin, is dependent on blood flow which in turn is affected by cardiac output and by microcirculatory size and distribution, the haemoglobin concentration and O_2 extraction by the tissues, which in turn is dependent on the shape of the oxygen binding curve of the red cells and on tissue pO_2. The shape of the oxygen equilibrium curve for haemoglobin is sigmoidal. This shape is determined by the extent of co-operativity. The initial portion of the curve has a very low slope, reflecting a low affinity for oxygen by haemoglobin at the beginning of the loading process. In other words, when haemoglobin is totally deoxygenated it has a rather poor avidity for oxygen (Figure 10.2). As the loading proceeds, and as the molecule binds more oxygen molecules, the slope of the reaction begins to change rapidly and becomes steep indicating that the affinity for oxygen has markedly increased. After two molecules of oxygen have bound to two haems of deoxyhaemoglobin tetramers, the protein changes its avidity for oxygen. This property helps haemoglobin tetramers to become promptly fully oxygenated. Hence, in red cells that are exposed to sufficient oxygen to oxygenate only half of the haems available, most molecules will either not be oxygenated at all, or entirely oxygenated, with a very small compartment of partially oxygenated molecules.

At the molecular level, co-operativity is accounted for by the fact that haemoglobin can exist stably in only two different conformations, one for the oxygenated molecule (R state), and another for the deoxygenated molecule (T state), without intermediate conformations. The molecule of haemoglobin will bind two or three molecules of oxygen at low affinity (T state). While this concept has been challenged recently, postulated intermediate stable states have not been generally recognised.

The haem triggering mechanism for conformational change has been resolved. The iron in deoxyhaemoglobin is slightly out of the plane of the haem (domed configuration) because the pyrrole rings are also slightly pyramidal. When the ligand binds the sixth co-

Haemoglobin tetramer

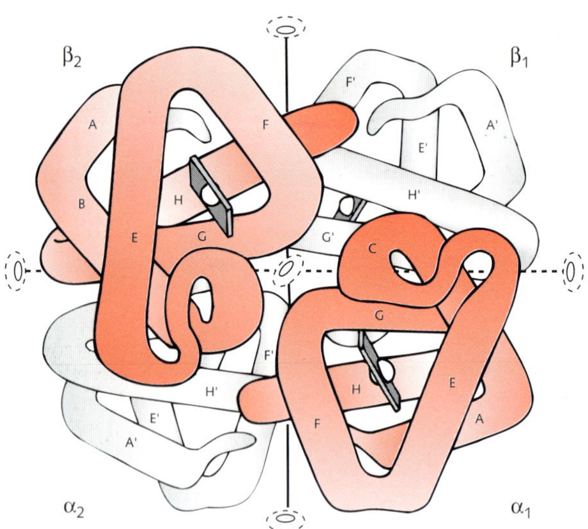

(a) Front view

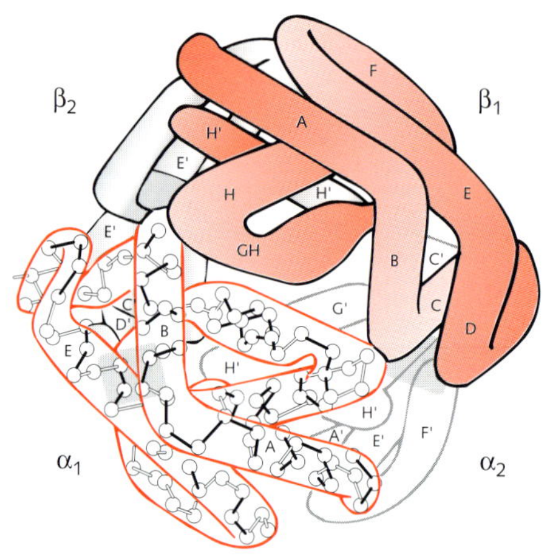

(b) Side view

Fig. 10.1 Haemoglobin molecule

Front view: depicts haemoglobin tetramer and the three axes of symmetry. The vertical line (marked by a solid ellipse) tracks the true twofold axis of symmetry (if you look down this axis you will see first the central cavity constituted by the β chains). The dashed ellipses and dashed lines mark the two pseudoaxes of symmetry, since the symmetry is only approximate. Only the 21 carbons are shown, with none of the side chains. Bold face numbers depict the residues in direct contact between the α_1 and β_2. In deep red the $\alpha_1\beta_2$ dimer, which never dissociates and interacts with the light colour $\alpha_1\beta_2$ dimer to change the conformation from T → R. Alterations in this area can produce high or low affinity haemoglobins. The side view of the tetramer depicts the stable dimer, the one that does not move or dissociate.

Horse methaemoglobin

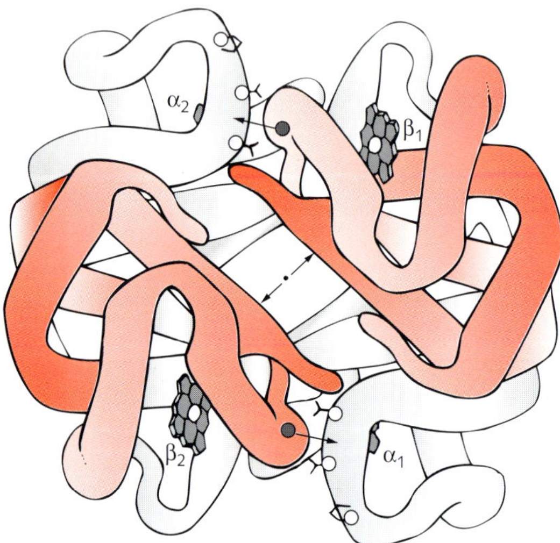

Horse deoxyhaemoglobin

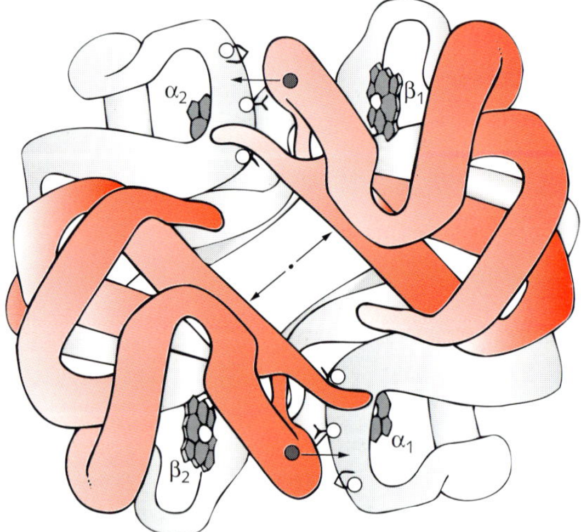

Fig. 10.2 The allosteric transition of haemoglobin: R → T

Left: Deoxygenated (T, tense) conformation of haemoglobin: notice that the centre cavity (space between the two β chains, in red) is larger than in the oxygenated tetramer (right). This space in the molecule is occupied by 2,3-diphosphoglycerate (2,3-DPG), when the tetramer is in the red cell. The allosteric effector, 2,3-DPG, is in a little over equimolar concentration with the tetramer. The T form has *low* affinity for oxygen. *Right:* Oxygenated (R, relaxed) conformational state of haemoglobin: the central cavity has been reduced in size by the movement of the β chains (red) towards each other. This tetramer cannot bind 2,3-DPG. The R form has *high* affinity for oxygen. The change in conformation forms and breaks bonds between the αβ dimers (red and white chains on each side of the central cavity).

ordinating position of the iron, significant steric stresses are introduced, and to relieve this strain the distal histidine moves 8° to become perpendicular to the haem, significantly decreasing the doming of the iron (the angle between iron and the haem falls to 4°). There is also the displacement of FG5 in the same direction of the histidine F8. The configuration around the haem has now changed to the oxygenated (R state), and a chain of events takes place involving the critical interactions that change the conformation of the haemoglobin tetramer.

Haemoglobin binds CO_2 while it is delivering O_2 and releases CO_2 when it is binding O_2, helping to dissipate the increase in concentration of CO_2 in the tissues and conveniently delivering this metabolic end product to the alveoli of the lungs. It accomplishes this particular task with ease because carbon dioxide is an inhibitor of haemoglobin oxygen-carrying capacity by decreasing the oxygen affinity of the molecule.

Haemoglobin binds hydrogen ions efficiently in a low pH environment and releases them when it encounters high pH (the *Bohr effect*). The Bohr effect describes the changes in oxygen affinity secondary to pH changes within a certain range—the lower the pH the lower the affinity or higher the p50. This means that an increased concentration of protons favours a low affinity state in haemoglobin. In other words, deoxyhaemoglobin binds more protons than the oxy conformer.

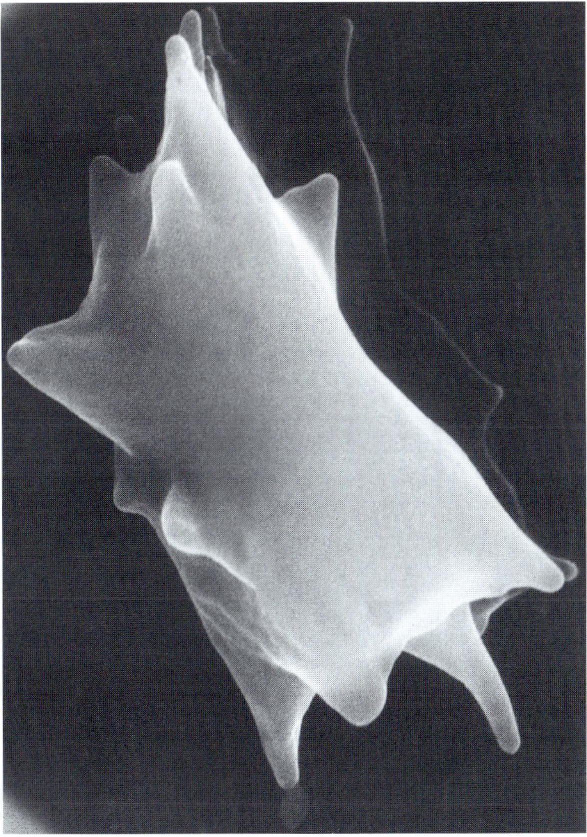

Fig. 10.3 Sickled cell
This is a Hb S homozygous (SS) red cell that has been deoxygenated. Notice the digitations stemming in all directions. These digitations are the product of the presence of fascicles of fibres, which are the polymerised form of deoxyHb S.

Sickle cell anaemia

Genetics

The genetic basis of sickle cell anaemia is central to the history of medical genetics. The disease was first described by Herrick (1910), a cardiologist, who observed 'sickle'-shaped red cells (Figure 10.3) in the blood of a medical student from Grenada, who suffered from chronic haemolytic anaemia. James V. Neel was the first to suggest that sickle cell anaemia was a homozygous state and sickle trait (the asymptomatic carrier state) was a heterozygous state of a not yet defined genetic character. Linus Pauling proposed that the sickling represented an abnormality of the haemoglobin molecule, based on the observation of the medical student that sickle cells, induced by deoxygenation, were birefringent. Birefringence indicated to Pauling that some type of molecular alignment or orientation existed inside these red cells, and since haemoglobin predominates overwhelmingly, it had to be this particular protein which was involved in the pathology. Electrophoretic studies confirmed this interpretation and the concept of *molecular disease* was born.

The biochemical definition of Hb S was achieved by Vernon Ingram, who developed a technique capable of probing the primary sequence of a protein, and revealed that sickle haemoglobin differed from normal haemoglobin by a single peptide, which was later found to have a single amino acid change in position 6 of the β chain in which a glutamic acid was substituted by a valine. At the gene level the change was A → T in the middle nucleotide of codon 6 of the β chain.

The globin genes were among the first to be located in the human genome with the β and β-like globin genes mapping to chromosome 11. Using 11 polymorphic sites located in the β gene cluster, it has been established that the β^S gene is associated with *three* distinctly different chromosomal haplotypes in Africa, identifiable by their specific array of DNA polymorphic sites (haplotypes), each one *exclusively* present in *three* separate geographical areas in Africa (Figure 10.4). Finally, a rather small

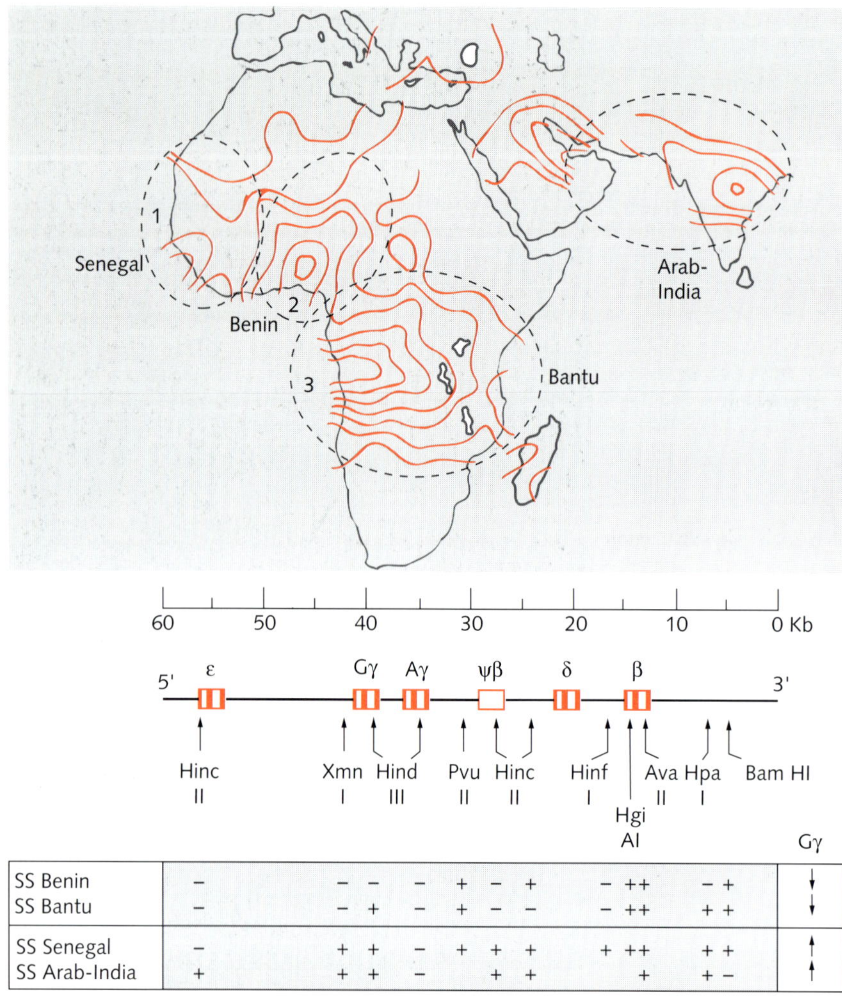

	Hinc II	Xmn I	Hind III	Hind III	Pvu II	Hinc II	Hinc II	Hinf I	Hgi AI / Ava II	Hpa I	Bam HI	Gγ
SS Benin	−	−	−	−	+	−	+	−	++	−	+	↓
SS Bantu	−	−	+	−	+	−	−	−	++	+	+	↓
SS Senegal	−	+	+	−	+	+	+	+	++	+	+	↑
SS Arab-India	+	+	+	−		+	+		+	+	−	↑

Fig. 10.4 β gene cluster haplotypes linked to β^S in Africa and Middle East/Pakistan/India
In the top of the figure the corresponding geographical distribution of the haplotypes described below is shown. A haplotype is a particular array of polymorphic sites (that is, sites variable among invividuals), defined here by the capacity of endonuclease enzymes to recognise the short sequence and cut the DNA.

ethnic group in southern Cameroon, the Eton people, have their own haplotype linked to the sickle gene.

The sickle gene has arisen around the world on at least five separate occasions, but the present-day gene frequencies demonstrate that the heterozygote is favoured, compensating the lower fitness of the homozygous state (balanced polymorphism). The selective pressure involved is the protective effect of Hb S in sickle carriers against *Plasmodium falciparum* malaria.

The multicentric origin of the sickle gene in the world expanded when a different haplotype was found to be associated with this gene in the eastern oasis of Saudi Arabia and among the 'tribals' of India. This Indo-European sickle mutation has been proposed to have originated in the Harappa of the Indus Valley, and then was distributed, probably during the Sassanian Empire, to the present sites (eastern Saudi Arabia, Bahrain, Kuwait and Oman).

The sickle gene has also spread through gene flow; for example, the Benin haplotype linked β^S has found its way to North Africa, Sicily, Greece, Turkey, most of the Arab world and the Americas, through the vagaries of wars of conquest (Sudanese troops in Sicily during the Arab conquest, for example) or the horrors of the Atlantic slave trade.

Clinical features

Sickle cell anaemia refers to the homozygous state for the β^S gene, in which the majority of the haemoglobin in the red cells is sickle haemoglobin (Hb S). This induces sickling (marked changes in red cell shape by intercellular Hb S polymers) when the oxygen tension is reduced, increases in red cell viscosity, decreased pliability and, by consequence, lowering of the sickle cell rheological competence, and haemolysis.

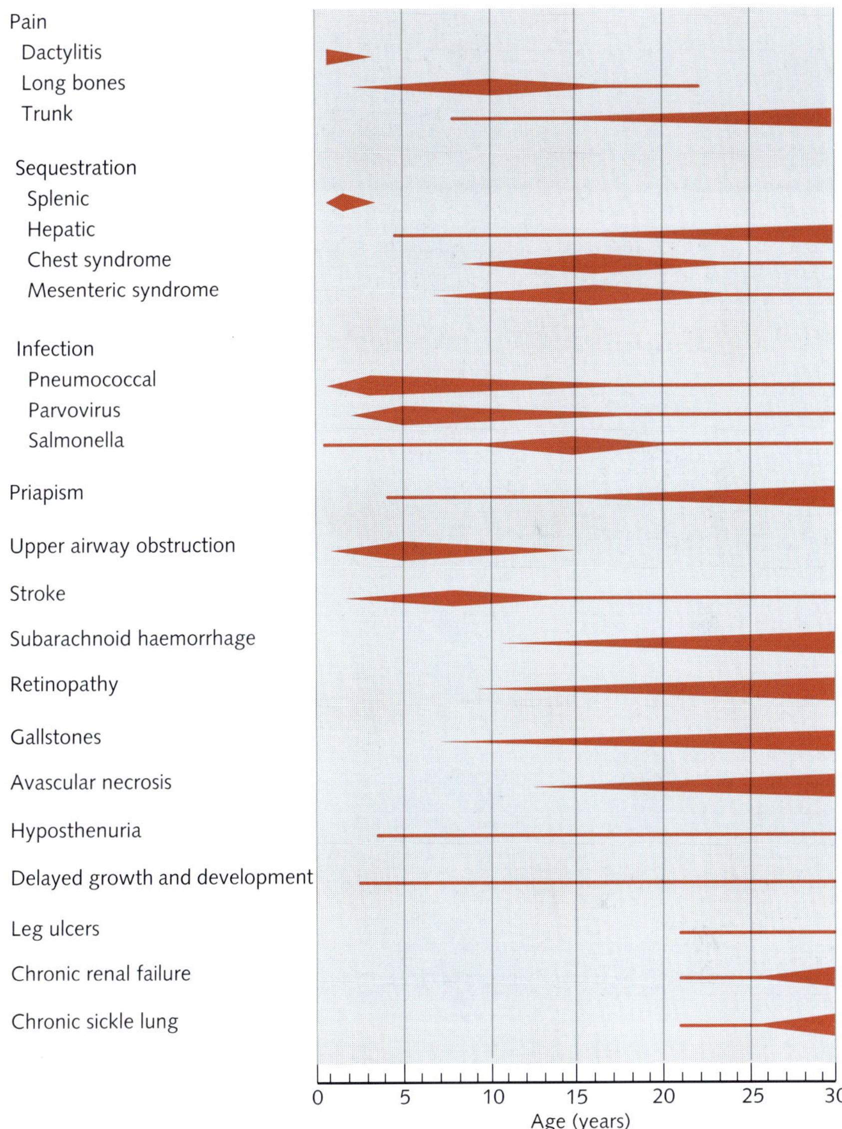

Fig. 10.5 Age dependency of complications in sickle cell anemia (From Davies S.C. & Oni L. (1997) Management of patients with sickle cell disease. *BMJ* **315**, 656–60. With Permission.)

In addition, there is a myriad of pleiotropic effects such as increased adherence of sickle cells to endothelium, induction of red cell dehydration and irreversibly sickled cell (ISC) status, autosplenectomy and urine concentration defects (Figure 10.5).

The primary events as well as the pleiotropic events are, in addition, affected by modifier or epistatic genes, which tend to be polymorphic, that is, different among individuals. The strong effect of all of these factors explains the great interpatient differences in the intensity of the phenotype: some patients are severely affected whilst others have only mild disease, and the majority span these two extremes.

Anaemia is present in all cases, with an average Hb of 8.4 g/dl, reticulocytosis varying between 5 and 20%, dense cell fraction between 5 and 40%, increased white cells ($10–20 \times 10^9$/l) and platelets in the upper limit of normal. Most of these features are modulated by the level of fetal haemoglobin (Hb F) in the sickle cells and the distribution function of the levels among red cells, since Hb F is heterogeneously expressed in reticulocytes and mature red cells. They are also modulated by the co-presence of α thalassaemia (–α/αα and particularly –α/–α), a feature quite common among sickle cell anaemia patients (between 20 and 50% of cases, according to age). Gender is also a factor, for example in females sickle cell anaemia is associated with higher Hb F concentrations, particularly when associated with the Senegal haplotype.

The kidneys are particularly affected in this disease: there is an increase in glomerular filtration rate early in life, as well as urinary concentration defect, papillary necrosis with haematuria, renal insufficiency and nephrotic syndrome (Plate 10.1, facing page 128). The lungs are the site of the acute chest syndrome that can be caused by infection (viral, bacterial and atypical organisms) as well as fat embolism. The latter gives the most severe cases and has the highest mortality. This life-threatening complication may be arrested by exchange transfusion. Neurological complications also occur, for example, in children, classical infarcts occur involving the major vessels, as well as small vessel infarcts. Some of these infarcts, particularly in the frontal lobe, have been associated with behavioural changes. The bones of patients with sickle cell anaemia show a fivefold increase in red marrow and may suffer aseptic osteonecrosis, particularly at the site of terminal circulation (head of the femur and humerus) and also in the calcaneus. Peripheral retinopathy characterised by new vessel formation and choroidal infarcts is well recognised in patients with sickle cell disease. Patients with homozygous Hb SS, and some heterozygotes, may suffer hyphaema secondary to eye trauma, since sickled cells cannot exit through the Schlemm canals (vitreous is very deoxygenated). The spleen is partially ineffectual during the first decade of life and essentially disappears (autosplenectomy), except in the co-presence of $-\alpha/-\alpha$ thalassaemia.

The liver can harbour bilirubin stones in the gall bladder as well as the common duct, but fortunately the patients have infrequent cholecystitis. They may also suffer hepatic crises, characterised by increase in serum bilirubin, abnormal liver functional tests, pain and fall in haemoglobin. Thick bile, due to suspended bilirubinate crystals, can be a factor, as well as sequestration of red cells, a hypermacrophage erythrophagia (Kupffer cells).

The heart may be affected by cardiomyositis leading to cardiac insufficiency and, in a small number of patients, small vessel obstruction. The lack of more vaso-occlusion in the heart may be the consequence of the very high perfusion pressure of coronary vessels as well as the 'squeezing' effect of the ventricular contraction. Finally, the ankles are the site for leg ulcers in sickle cell anaemia, and these may be painful and reduce quality of life.

In sickle cell anaemia, pregnancy poses a significant risk to the mother and newborn (lower birth weight). Previous protocols of exchange transfusion during pregnancy have been replaced by putting the patient into 'high risk track' obstetric care, involving frequent follow-ups, with good results and fewer complications.

The most devastating complication of sickle cell anaemia is painful crisis. This involves pain in extremities, joints, lower back, abdomen, cranium and parotid glands. The pain may be insidious or rapidly progressive, and may begin in one site and extend over time to others. It involves infarction of the circulation in marrow, bone or muscle, or a combination of the above. Further studies have demonstrated that the decrease in dense sickle cells is actually preceded by a decrease in light density sickle cells. The latter event might record light density sickle cell adhesion while the subsequent decrease in dense cells reflects their trapping in vessels bedecked by adherent cells. Fever is usually present even in the absence of intercurrent infection. Precipitating factors include dehydration, fever, infection, emotional stress, interference with the vascular circulation of limbs, intense exercise, use of cocaine, etc.

Pathophysiology: there are four major contributors to the pathophysiology of sickle cell anaemia

Polymerisation of Hb S

This chemical reaction, underlying sickling, is a nucleus-mediated reaction. That is, a nucleus of about 10 haemoglobin tetramers has to form first, before the polymerisation can start its characteristic exponential course, to form sickle fibres. The formation of a nucleus is a hit-and-miss affair, and it takes time to form the right structure. Hence, the reaction has a delay time, after deoxygenation, that is shortened by an increase in intracellular Hb concentration (over the normal 33 g/dl), by lowering the pH and by increasing the temperature. This explains why red cell dehydration and infections are serious in sickle cell anaemia patients. The final products of polymerisation are double-stranded fibres which lead to red cell deformity with protuberances (Figure 10.6).

Adhesion of sickle red cells to the endothelium

Young sickle red cells have a propensity to adhere to small post-capillary venules. This has been demonstrated both in the mesenteric circulation (*ex vivo*) as well as *in vivo* in the cremaster muscle of sickle transgenic mice. Evidence exists that obstruction of the microcirculation occurs primarily in the venule side, preceded by adhesion of young sickle red cells, and completed by the trapping of dense cells and ISCs in areas bedecked by adhered red cells.

The mechanism of adhesion is not completely understood, and is probably multifactorial, but von Willebrand factor and the vibronectin receptor ($\alpha_v\beta_3$) appear

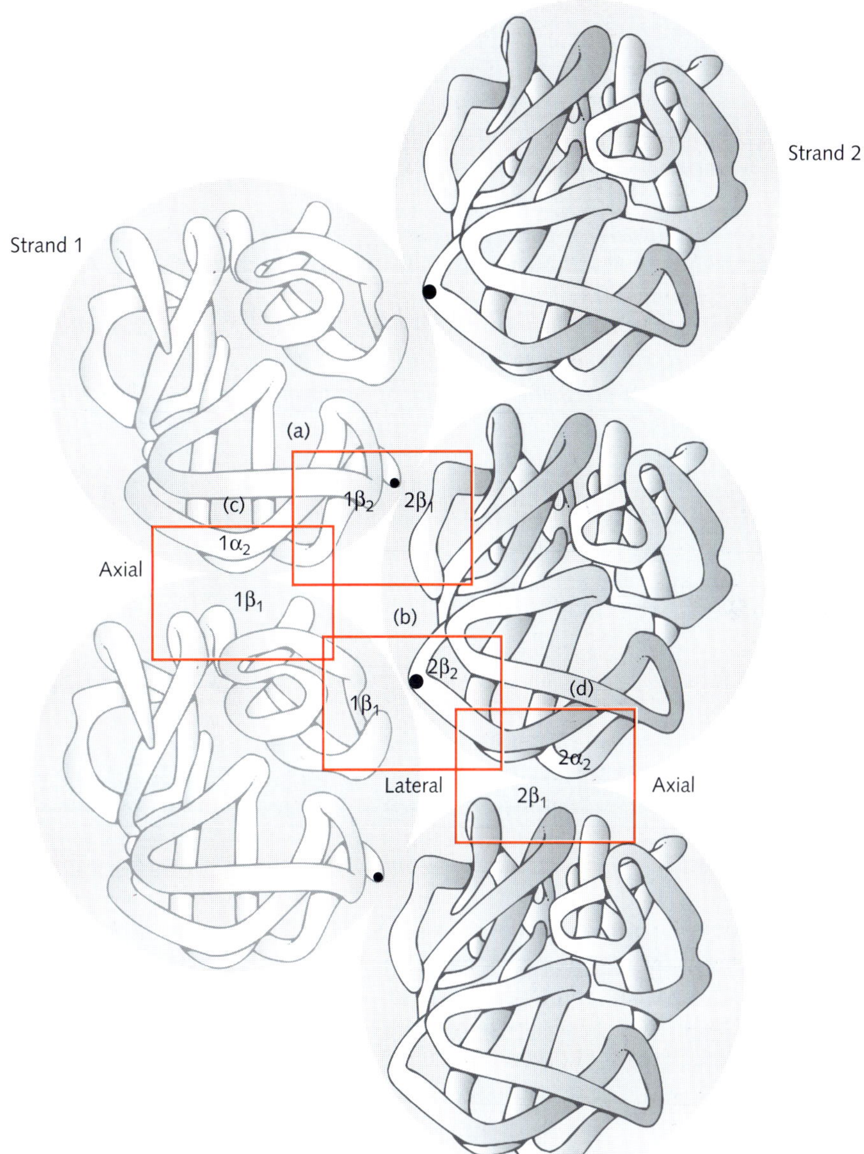

Fig. 10.6 Polymer Hb S structure
This is the assembly unit of the Hb S polymer: the Werner–Love double strand. This double strand is part of the Hb S crystal, but in the crystal it propagates in all directions to form a lattice. The sickle fibre wraps around to form a helical fibre. The squares depict the four different areas of contact that form the double strand.

to be excellent candidates, since antibodies against either of the members of the pair inhibit adhesion in living circulatory preparations. Other proposed mechanisms have not been fully validated in microcirculatory preparations nor have they been demonstrated to be operative in small venules.

Red cell dehydration

Some young sickle red cells undergo a fast process of dehydration after they enter the circulation. There are, in effect, intermediate dense cells and very dense cells. It is possible that different mechanisms are involved in each of these types. It is clear that Ca^{2+}-dependent K^+ efflux and probably deoxy-induced K^+ efflux are responsible for the latter, and that K:Cl co-transport overexpression, due to the relative youth of the red cells, is responsible for the former. K:Cl is no longer active in normal adult red cells, while reticulocytes retain a modicum of this system. Finally, cycles of oxy-deoxygenation seem to be required for dense cell formation. Patients with sickle cell anaemia who have high Hb F levels and co-existent α thalassaemia have fewer dense cells. Dense cells and ISCs both have very short lives (probably less than 5 days) and have markedly right shifted oxygen equilibrium curves.

Anaemia

Anaemia is not a simple product of haemolysis in sickle cell anaemia as demonstrated by the marrow expansion of only five times normal, compared to ten times normal seen in thalassaemia major. One reason for this is the right shift of the oxygen equilibrium curve described above: this type of O_2 binding curve results in increased oxygen delivery to the tissues. This explains why erythropoietin increases only below 9 g of Hb. In addition, the response to erythropoietin is blunted, that is inappropriately low for the anaemia, below the threshold of 9 g of haemoglobin. The reason for this is not understood, but the fact that age increases the deficiency of erythropoietin suggests that 'silent' renal damage might be involved in a reduction of erythropoietin response. Another contributor to the anaemia (a reduction of erythropoietin response) is the increase of 2,3-DPG found in sickle red cells.

The haemolysis is also complex: actually there are three red cell populations in sickle cell anaemia, the very dense red cells that live only 4–5 days, the F cells (these are sickle cells containing Hb F) that live close to normal life spans and the rest of the cells that fall in between. Co-existence of α thalassaemia and high Hb F reduces haemolysis considerably.

Interestingly, the level of Hb F also defines the properties of progenitors as well as the circulating haemopoietic cytokines. Low Hb F sickle cell anaemia patients have an increased number of circulating BFU-e, which are in active cycle. In addition, these patients have constitutively circulating GM-CSF and Steel factor, unlike normal individuals and high Hb F sicklers. In contrast, the low Hb F patients have IL-3 circulating in addition to a haemopoietic inhibitory factor, TNFα.

Sickle cell anaemia patients are susceptible to an acute anaemia superimposed on their chronic anaemia, due to infection with parvovirus B19, which can produce a life-threatening drop in haemoglobin which is generally self-limited (7–15 days). This results from its ability to infect BFU-E through the blood group P system that serves as receptor. Treatment is by transfusion of red cells in most cases.

Treatment

Hydroxyurea has been demonstrated to reduce the incidence of painful crises and acute chest syndrome by 50% in adult sickle cell (Hb SS) patients; in addition, hydroxyurea reduces their transfusion requirements. It has become apparent that the rise in Hb F alone does not explain the benefits of hydroxyurea fully, and it is felt that this drug must have other effects, for example reduction of sickle cell adhesion. Predictors of good results with hydroxyurea are high white cell count and the absence of the Bantu haplotype.

Bone marrow transplantation has been carried out in many patients with sickle cell anaemia with reasonably good results, including the regeneration of the spleen in some cases. Mortality is between 5 and 20% depending on the protocol used. Selection of patients because of history of CNS involvement in children initially produced strokes during convalescence, but adjustment of the protocol has reduced this risk. This procedure is generally restricted to the severely ill patient because of the mortality of graft rejection occurring in up to 20%.

Preventive measures have been very successful in this disease, particularly in the reduction of infant mortality. These include prophylactic penicillin, pneumoccocal vaccine and teaching patients about splenic sequestration.

The judicious use of exchange transfusion in acute chest syndrome, splenic sequestration, aplastic crises and liver crises has saved countless lives.

Treatment of painful crises remains a challenge. The best approach is a rapid assessment, preferably by quantitative instruments, of the intensity, quality and distribution of pain, the presence of co-morbidities and the state of dehydration. Rapid, aggressive, individually tailored analgesia treatment, with the additional use of NSAIDs has proven to be the best route. All of this is almost impossible in an Emergency Room; hence a Day Hospital dedicated to sickle cell anaemia is probably the best alternative service model.

Sickle/β thalassaemia

This syndrome is observed in locations in which both Hb S and β thalassaemia are frequent, such as Africa, Sicily, Greece, Turkey, the Arab countries and the regions of America with African and southern Mediterranean admixture.

The genotype may be S/β^+ thalassaemia, in which the red cells contain between 20–40% Hb A with the remainder comprising Hb S and Hb F; or S/β^0 thalassaemia in which the red cells contain only Hb S and Hb F. The latter genotype can only be diagnosed by pedigree or genetic analysis.

The clinical picture of S/β^0 thalassaemia is very similar to sickle cell anaemia but it is milder. Anaemia may be milder than Hb SS, and in some cases the mean cell

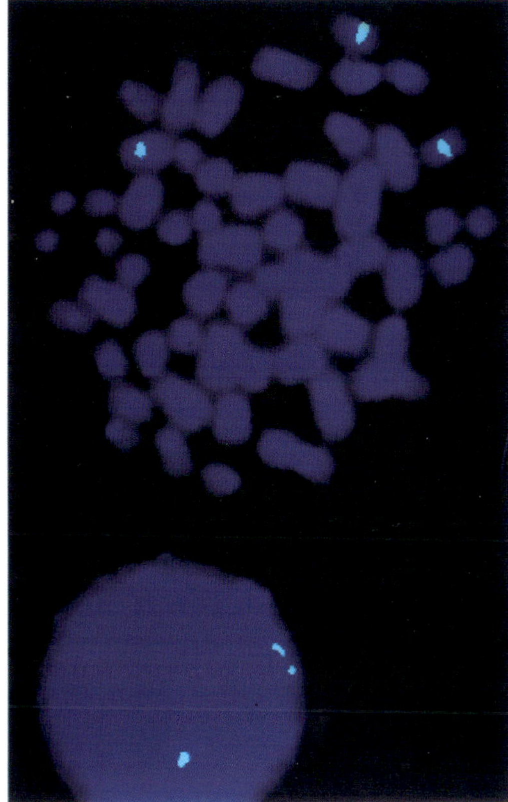

Plate 2.1 Detection of numerical abnormalities
Digoxigenin labelled α satellite probe for chromosome X (Oncor®) showing hybridisation to a metaphase and interphase cell from a patient with ALL. This patient has a hyperdiploid karyotype with several additional chromosomes including an extra copy of chromosome X as seen by FISH.

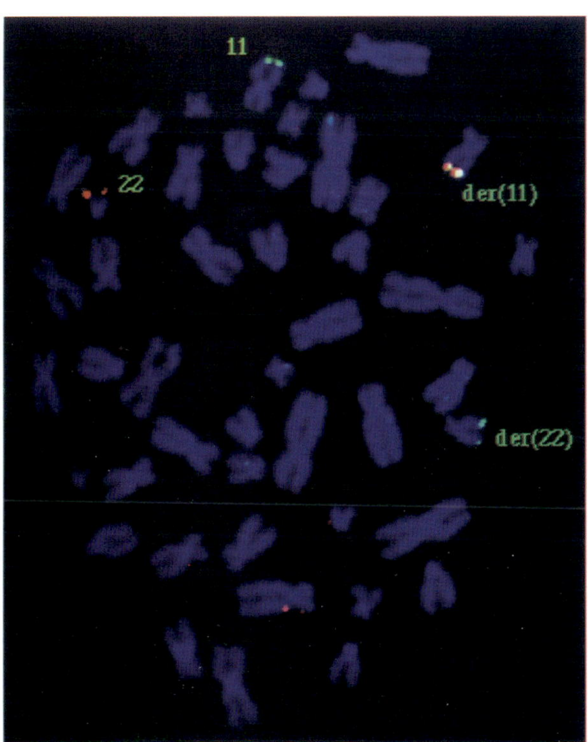

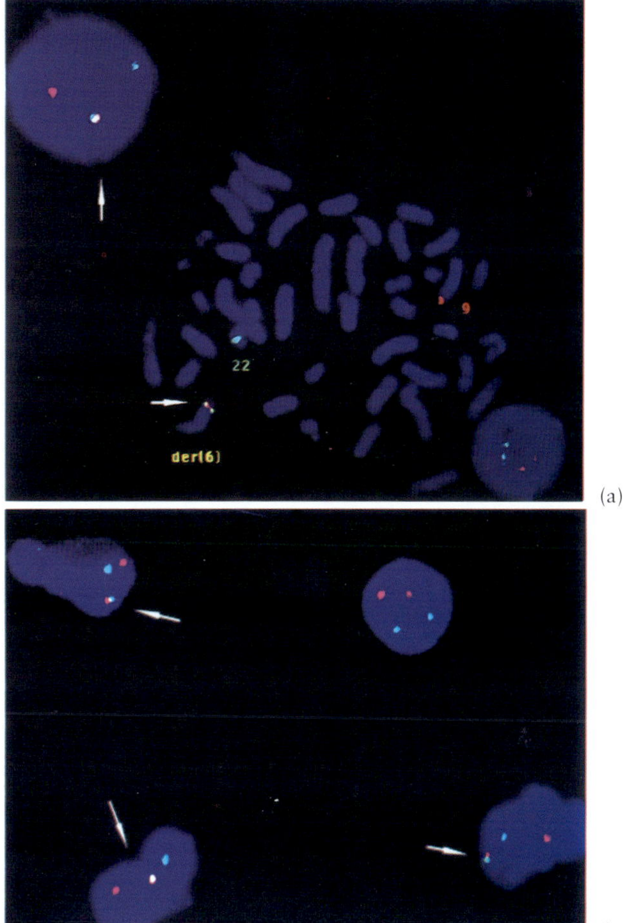

Plate 2.3 Unique sequence probes
(a) *BCR–ABL* fusion. Probes for the chimeric gene fusion resulting from the t(9;22), Philadelphia translocation, seen in chronic myeloid leukaemia. The *BCR* probe on chromosome 22 directly labelled with spectrum green, and the *ABL* probe on chromosome 9 directly labelled with spectrum orange (Vysis®) were applied to cells from a patient with a variant Philadelphia translocation. One interphase cell and the metaphase cell show the juxtaposition of one copy of *BCR* and *ABL* (arrowed), indicative of the chimeric gene fusion, on an abnormal chromosome 6. The other interphase cell is normal showing four discrete probe signals. (b) *PML–RARA* fusion. Probes for the chimeric gene fusion resulting from the t(15;17) specifically associated with acute promyelocytic leukaemia. The *PML* probe is directly labelled with spectrum orange and the *RARA* probe is directly labelled with spectrum green. Three interphase cells from this patient with APML show juxtaposition of one copy of *PML* and *RARA* (arrowed) whilst the fourth cell represents a normal cell.

Plate 2.2 (left) YAC probe spanning 11q23 (MLL) breakpoint region
The YAC 13HH4 labelled with biotin and visualised using avidin-FITC hybridised to a patient metaphase containing a t(11;22)(q23;q13). A digoxigenin labelled probe mapping to 22q13 was also applied to the slide and visualised with antidigoxigenin-rhodamine. The YAC probe is split by the t(11;22) and consequently hybridises to both the der(11) and the der(22) as well as the normal 11. The probe for 22q13 is translocated to the der(11) and co-localises with the proximal end of the YAC.

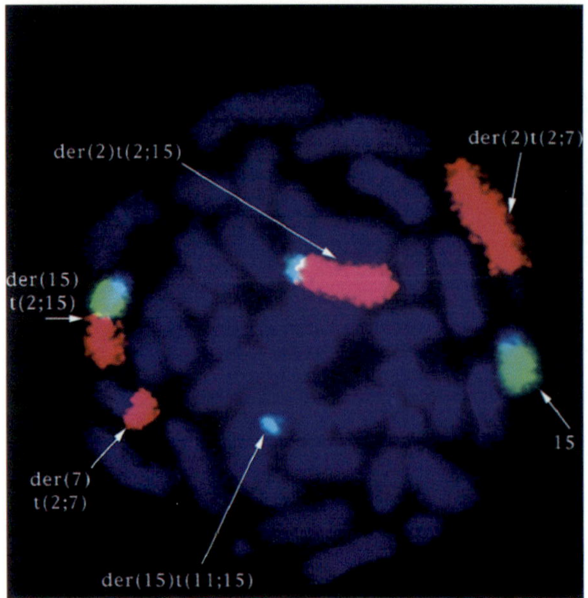

Plate 2.4 Whole chromosome paints
Whole chromosome paint for chromosomes 2 (Texas Red) and chromosome 15 (FITC) applied to a metaphase from a patient with a complex karyotype. FISH analysis allowed better characterisation of the chromosome abnormalities which included a der(2)t(2;15), der(15)t(2;15), der(7)t(2;7), der(2)t(2;7) and der(15)t(11;15).

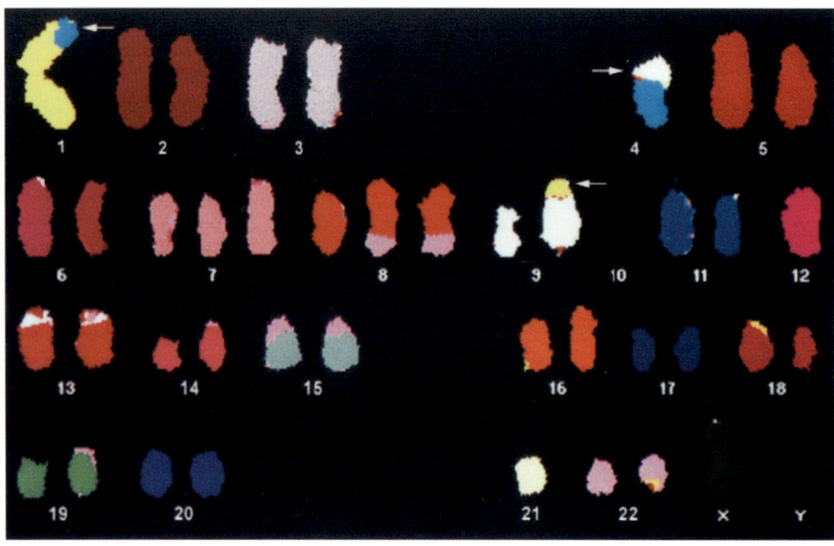

Plate 2.5 M-FISH
Whole chromosome paints for each of the 24 chromosomes labelled with differing combinations of fluorochromes (applied spectral imaging) and hybridised to a patient metaphase with a complex karyotype. The patient has ALL L3 (Burkitt's type) with the Burkitt's translocation t(8;22) plus an additional copy of the der(8). M-FISH also showed the presence of a three-way translocation affecting one copy of each of chromosomes 1, 4 and 9.

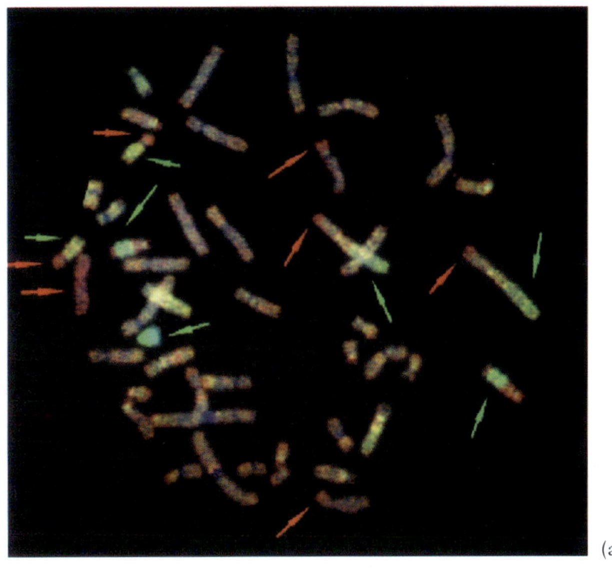

(a)

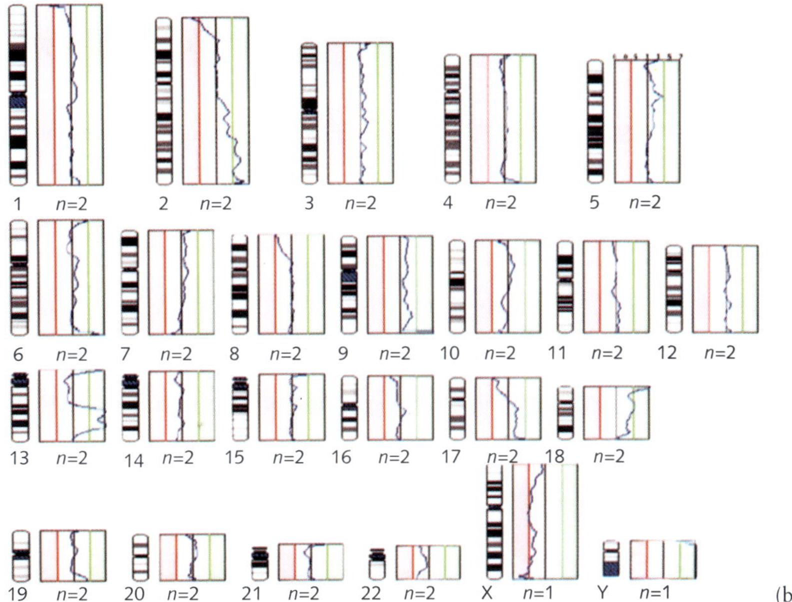

(b)

Plate 2.6 Comparative genomic hybridisation
(a) Tumour DNA (test) from a patient with follicular lymphoma was directly labelled with spectrum green. Normal DNA (reference) was directly labelled with spectrum red and then equal quantities of test and reference DNA were combined and applied to normal metaphases. The green arrows represent regions which were amplified in the tumour, and the red arrows represent regions of deletion in the tumour. (b) The CGH computer profile measures the green : red fluorescence intensities along each chromosome. Regions of amplification in the tumour include 2q, 13q, 17q, 18q and Y. Regions which are deleted include 2p, 8p, 17p and X.

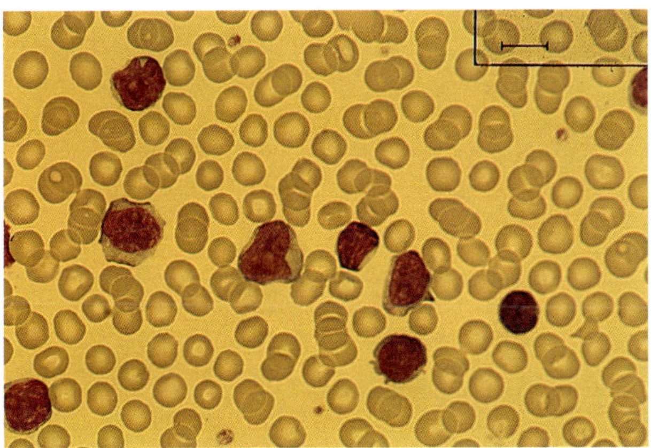

Plate 8.1
Blood film showing a mixture of small lymphocytes and prolymphocytes from a patient with atypical CLL (×100).

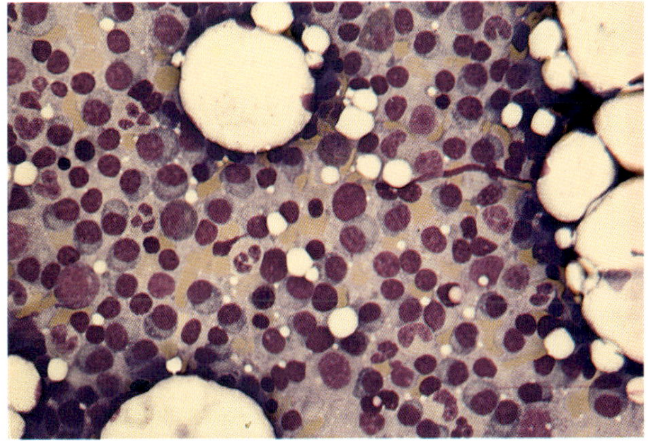

Plate 9.1 Multiple myeloma
Bone marrow aspirate obtained from a patient with multiple myeloma. The plasma cells are characterised by the eccentric nucleus and the perinuclear halo, or clearing, due to the Golgi apparatus.

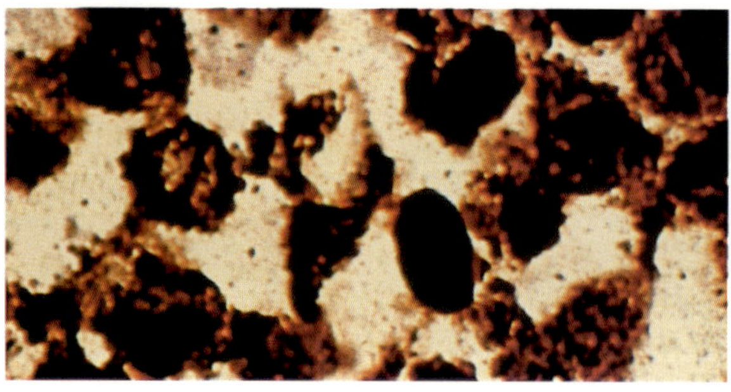

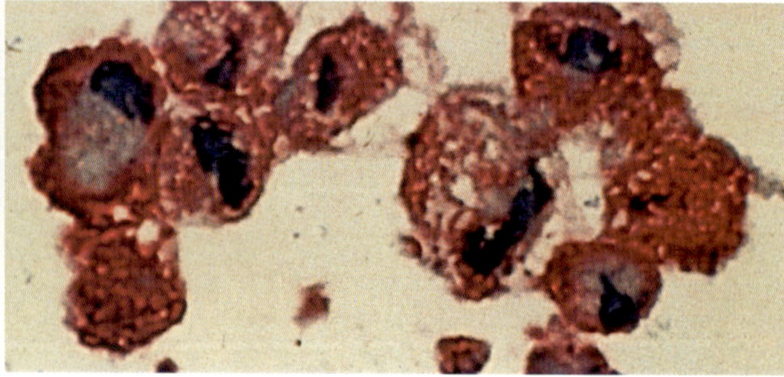

Plate 9.2
Bone marrow collected from a patient with multiple myeloma was cultured with 10% fetal calf and 10% horse serum. The adherent 'stromal' cells were trypsinised and *in situ* hybridisation was performed using a probe for KSHV (HHV-8) demonstrating its presence within these cells. These cells also stained with an antibody to fascin which implies that they are of dendritic cell origin.

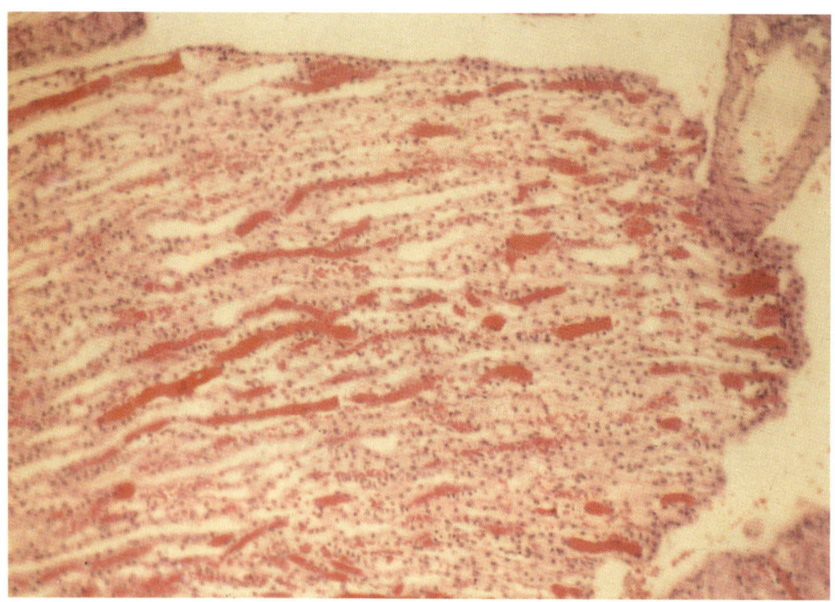

Plate 10.1 Renal medulla of transgenic mice expressing β^{S} and $\beta^{S\text{-Antilles}}$
Notice the extensive obstructive aggregation of sickle red cells in the renal medullary vasculature.

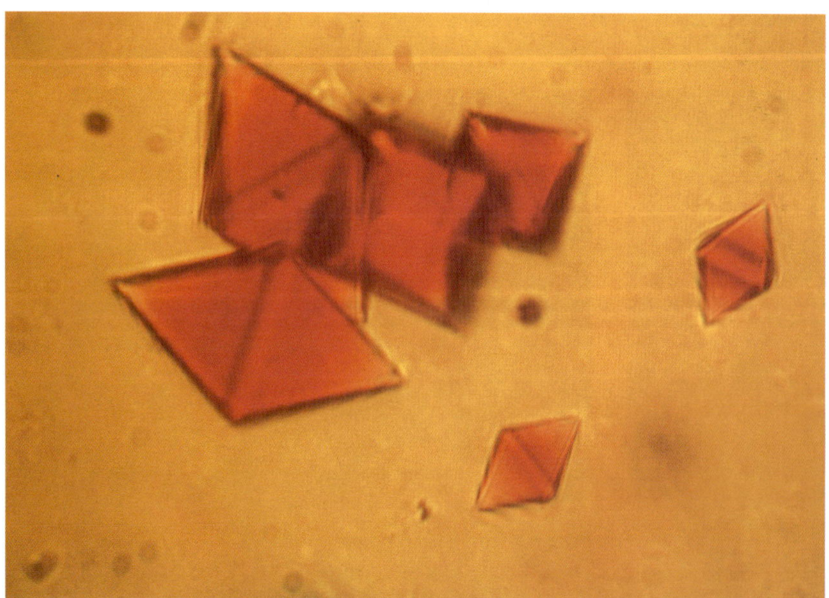

Plate 10.2 Hb C tetragonal crystals

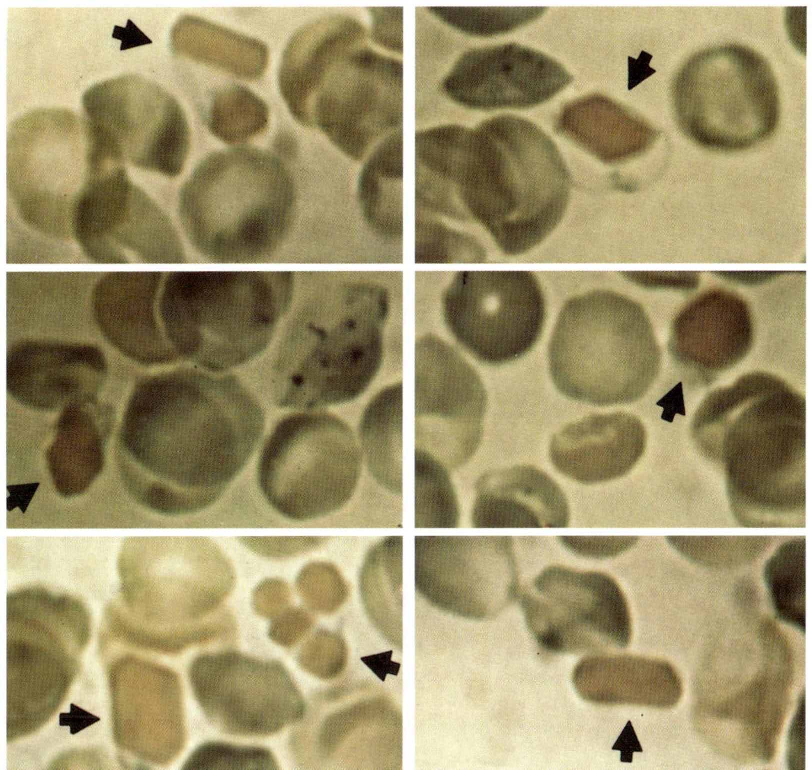

Plate 10.3 SC red cells from a double stained smear
This is a blood smear of a Hb SC patient, stained with Wright's and reticulocyte stain. Notice the flat, thin cells (they generate target cells), folded cells and those with intracellular tetragonal crystals (black arrows).

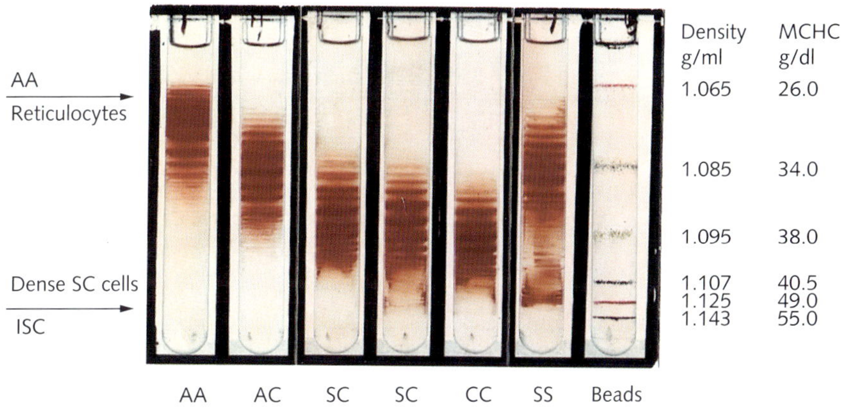

Plate 10.4 Percoll density gradients of AA, CC, SC red cells
This figure depicts the separation of red cells by density. Light-density cells are on top, high-density cells on the bottom. Notice that SS blood has normal density red cells as the largest compartment, then some very dense cells, and some intermediate density cells between the last two. In contrast, all the cells of the CC patients are denser than normal red cells. The SC red cells are intermediate.

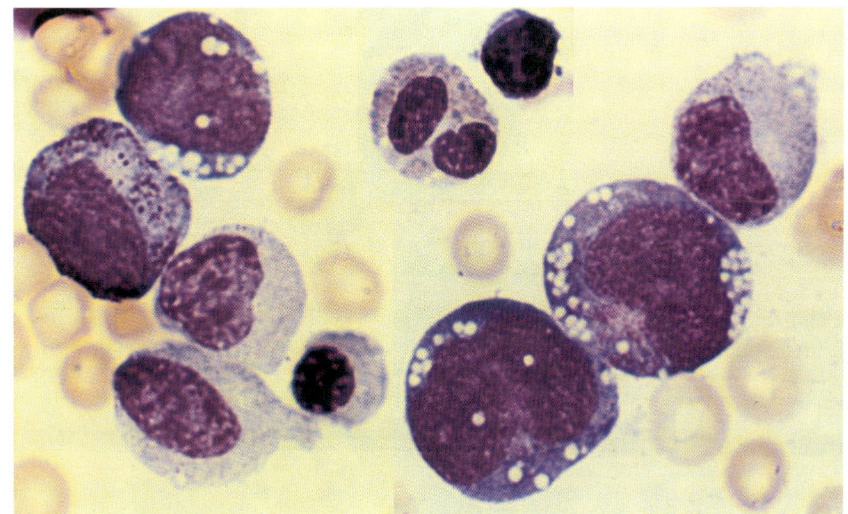

Plate 11.1 Bone marrow findings in Pearson's marrow-pancreas syndrome
The presence of numerous vacuoles in both erythroid and myeloid precursors in an infant is virtually diagnostic of Pearson's marrow-pancreas syndrome. Note also the presence of neutrophils with the Pelger anomaly of the nucleus.

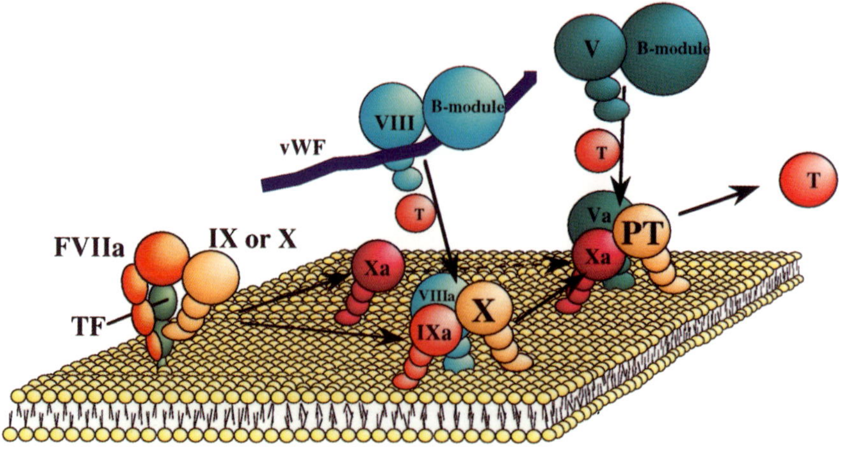

Plate 12.1 Initiation of blood coagulation
Coagulation is activated in response to exposure of tissue factor (TF) to FVII. FVIIa-TF activates FIX and FX. FIXa and FXa bound to their respective cofactors, FVIIIa and FVa, efficiently activate FX and prothrombin, respectively. Thrombin (T) cleaves and activates FVIII and FV in a positive feedback reaction. vWF denotes von Willebrand factor which circulates in a complex with FVIII. The B-modules of FVIII and FV are released upon activation. In the schematic FVIIIa and FVa models, the three larger balls represent the A1, A2 and A3 modules, which are in close contact with each other, whereas the two smaller balls are the C1 and C2 modules.

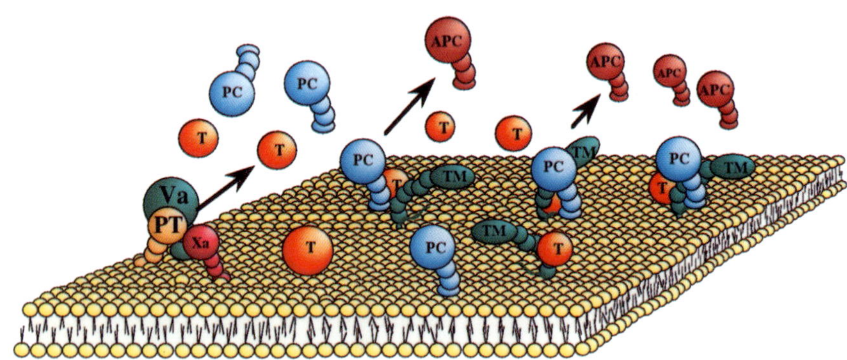

Plate 12.2 Activation of protein C on the surface of endothelial cells
Thrombin, which is generated in the vicinity of endothelial cells, binds to thrombomodulin (TM) and is converted from a pro- to an anticoagulant enzyme. Thrombin bound to TM is highly efficient in activating protein C to activated protein C (APC) but has lost its procoagulant properties.

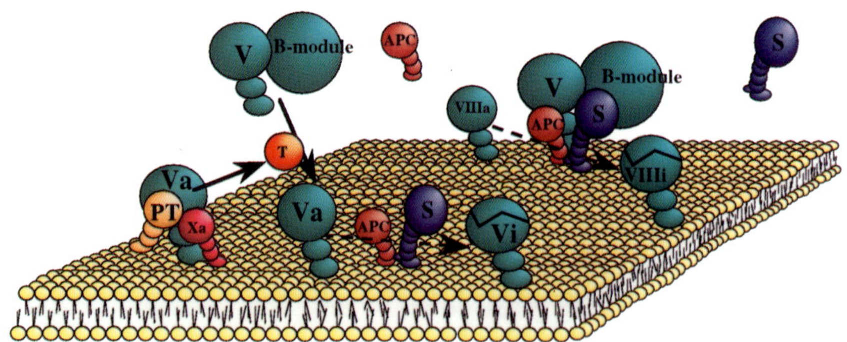

Plate 12.3 Inhibition of coagulation by activated protein C
Membrane bound FVIIIa and FVa are the targets for APC. In the degradation of FVIIIa, the anticoagulant activity of APC is potentiated by both protein S and FV. It is not known whether this synergistic APC-cofactor function of protein S and FV is also involved in the degradation of FVa or if protein S is the only APC-cofactor in this reaction. PT, prothrombin; T, thrombin; V, FV; Va, FVa; Vi, APC-inactivated FVa; VIIIa, FVIIIa; VIIIi, APC-inactivated FVIIIa.

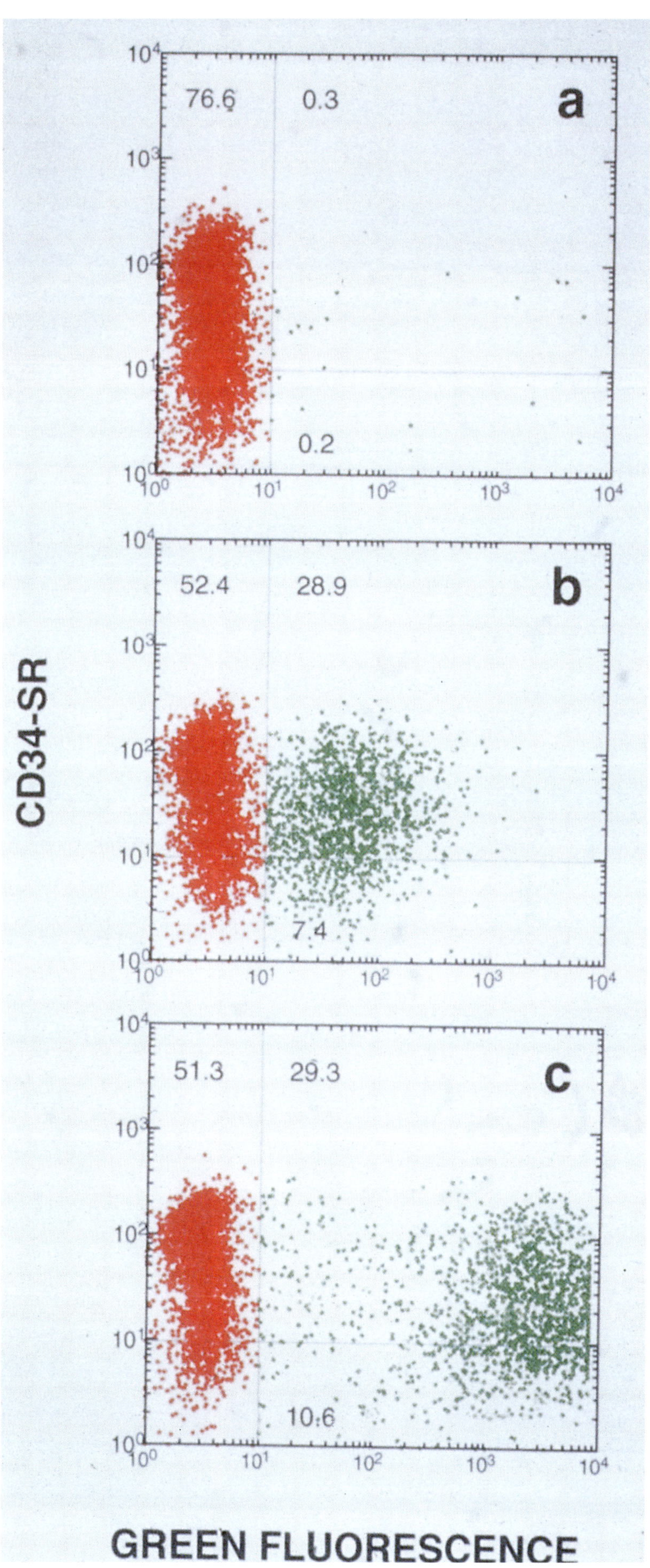

(a)

Plate 16.1
(a) Using a retroviral vector (MSCV) encoding the marker gene green fluorescent protein (GFP), CD34 positive bone marrow stem cells were transduced. The panels show (a) control, (b) MSCV-GFP and (c) MSCV-enhanced GFP. 30% of the cells express the fluorescent marker (*see* Cheng *et al.*, 1997). (b) When grown on methylcellulose the bone marrow progenitors form granulocyte macrophage (1) and erythroid (2) colonies and fluoresce (panels 3 and 4). This system therefore allows for rapid and accurate quantitation of gene transfer (*see* Cheng *et al.*, 1997). Reproduced from Cheng *et al.* (1997), with permission of Stockton Press, UK.

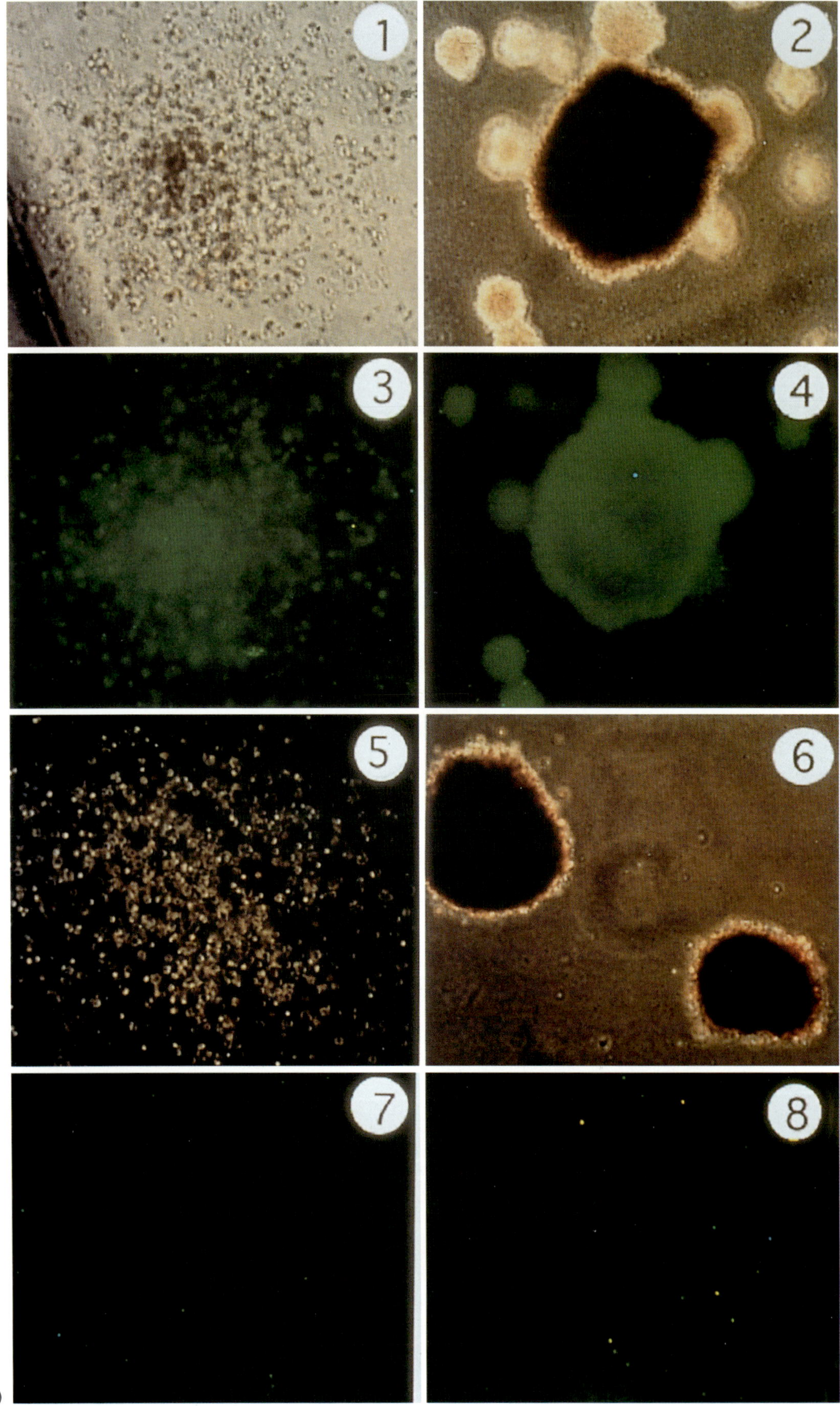

(b)

Plate 16.1 (contd)

volume (MCV) is lower. Retinopathy and osteonecrosis are more common, but autosplenectomy is less common.

The clinical picture of S/β^+ thalassaemia is significantly milder than sickle cell anaemia: less anaemia, lower MCV, lower reticulocyte count but an increased risk of retinopathy and osteonecrosis. The spleen often enlarges during adulthood.

Haemoglobin CC disease

Homozygous CC individuals have a mild haemolytic anaemia which is generally asymptomatic and rarely life-threatening. The anaemia is moderate, the MCV is reduced (50–60 fl), there is minimal reticulocytosis and splenomegaly is common. The peripheral blood film is fairly characteristic and with some training of the observer, diagnostic. The red cells are hypochromic, due to their flatness (rather than low MCH or MCHC—in fact they have a normal MCH and an increased MCHC). Folded and target cells are prominent. Red cells may show intracellular tetragonal crystals of haemoglobin C, best detected in reticulocyte smears, where they retain their red colour.

In terms of the genetics of this disease, the β^C gene (β6 Val $\rightarrow$ Lys), a single base substitution, has a frequency one-quarter that of the β^S gene among African-Americans. The β^C gene most likely originated in Burkina Faso, where we find the highest frequency (up to 50% of the population), decreasing concentrically, and encompassing Mali, Ivory Coast and Ghana, all of which are east of the Niger river.

The pathophysiology of CC disease is dominated by the high tendency of Hb C to produce oxygenated tetragonal crystals (Plate 10.2). The CC red cells are uniformly denser than AA cells. This effect is associated with very high expression of K:Cl co-transport (higher than in SS cells, in spite of lower reticulocyte count), a transport system that, by extruding K^+ and water, can dehydrate red cells. There is evidence that the kinetics of this transport is altered in CC cells, with slower than normal turn-off, when the stimulus for activity, volume increase or low pH, is removed. Whether this alteration is sufficient to explain the pathophysiology of CC cells and the mechanistic basis for the interaction of Hb C with the membrane remains to be determined.

The presence of circulating tetragonal crystal-containing red cells in splenectomised CC patients does *not* result in vaso-occlusion, probably because the CC tetragonal crystals are crystals of oxyHb C, which melt as they approach the capillaries. Deoxy-haemoglobin C has a different crystal form, but not enough to form.

Haemoglobin SC disease

SC disease is genotypically a double heterozygote, i.e. a combination of sickle trait and Hb C trait. Since neither of these trait forms independently has a phenotype, the clinical picture of SC disease requires an explanation (*see below*).

SC disease is milder than sickle cell anaemia, particularly in the first 20 years of life in which the mortality approaches zero. Red cell survival is about 27 days compared to 17 days of sickle cell anaemia red cells. Nevertheless, three complications are inappropriately severe: osteonecrosis, retinopathy and acute chest syndrome. SC patients frequently retain their spleen in adulthood, and have less anaemia lower MCV, lower reticulocyte count, fewer very dense and dense red cells and lower Hb F levels on average than sickle cell anaemia patients. Their survival also seems to be better.

As in CC cells, the blood film in SC disease may be diagnostic. In addition to the cells common to CC disease (flat and apparently hypochromic cells), they exhibit target cells, and more specifically a few ISCs, as well as intracellular tetragonal crystals, better seen in reticulocyte smears (Plate 10.3).

The pathophysiology of SC red cells derives from the contribution that Hb C makes to the red cell: as in CC cells (*see above*), SC cells are denser than AA or most of the sickle cell anaemia red cells (Plate 10.4). The increase in MCHC implicit in this effect promotes the polymerisation of Hb S leading to more sickling than expected for a cell with only 50% Hb S. Interestingly, Hb S in turn favours Hb C crystallisation, which explains, in addition to the differences in splenic activity, why crystals are generally more prominent in SC disease than in CC. Fortunately, for the reasons expressed above, this situation does not lead to an increase in vaso-occlusion beyond that which is predictable from the solubility of the available Hb S with the MCHC for SC cells.

Homozygous Hb E and Hb E/β thalassaemia

The homozygote for Hb E has the phenotype of β thalassaemia trait because this abnormal haemoglobin, common from the Eastern provinces of India to the Philippines, is both a mutation of the sequence of the β chains as well as a thalassaemia, due to the generation of an alternative splicing site by the mutation.

Populations living near to the common border of Cambodia, Laos and Thailand, the Khmer people, have the highest incidence of this abnormal haemoglobin, the selection pressure for which is resistance to infection by *Plasmodium falciparum* malaria.

The clinical syndrome is very mild, with no/minimal anaemia (once the nutritional causes of anaemia are treated), low MCV, with target cells in the smear and hypochromia. Density gradients reveal that although the red cells are small they have a normal MCHC, as a consequence of a diminished MCH, due to the thalassaemic component of this disease. People who inherit Hb E and β thalassaemia trait present a thalassaemia major or intermedia picture (*see Chapter 1*).

Dominant sickle mutations

Dominant sickle mutations refer to β gene mutations that include the β^S mutation, and exhibit a second mutation in the same chain, that turns them into super haemoglobin S that produces symptoms in the heterozygote. Two instances have been characterised. Hb S-Antilles (β6 Glu → Val; 23 Val → Ile) is expressed in the heterozygote at about 40% level, and produces a syndrome resembling a mild sickle cell anaemia phenotype. The mechanism is complex: the second mutation increases the solubility of deoxyhaemoglobin S from 17 g/dl to about 11 g/dl, with the result that Hb S polymerises more readily and more extensively. The second mutation has an oxygen equilibrium effect that favours sickling.

The other dominant Hb S mutation is Hb S-Oman (β6 Glu → Val; 121 Glu → Lys), that generates an even more powerful super haemoglobin S because, even at expression levels of about 20% (resulting from concomitant –α/–α), it has a phenotype very similar to Hb S-Antilles. Since the two dominant Hb Ss have the same solubility in the deoxy state, the more severe phenotype present implies that the 121 second mutation (identical to that in Hb O_{Arab}) must produce pathology of its own. This hypothesis is confirmed by the haemolytic anaemia present in individuals homozygous for Hb O_{Arab} or Hb $G_{Philadelphia}$.

Unstable haemoglobins

There are about 100 mutations that render the haemoglobin molecule unstable, for example Hb Köln, but their incidence is low. They are generally inherited in an autosomal dominant manner. Mutations may render haemoglobin unstable and produce a haemolytic syndrome by four mechanisms:

- When the mutation introduces either a bulky or a charged side chain in the interior of this globular protein.
- When the mutation introduces, in the α-helix portion of the molecule, a side chain that is not α-helix friendly.
- When the mutation destabilises the haem attachment to the globin.
- When the mutation interferes with the stability of the $\alpha_1\beta_1$ contact area, a dimer that normally does not dissociate.

Hb Köln (β 98Val → Met) is the most common of all the unstable haemoglobins, and affects all ethnic groups. It is difficult to diagnose by electrophoresis because of its instability and indistinct electrophoretic pattern. Two light bands are commonly observed because of the severe instability. The best test is isopropanol solubility, in which the haemolysate turns opaque, and a precipitate can be observed after centrifugation.

The patients, who can be of any ethnic origin, exhibit a mild to moderate haemolytic anaemia, and the presence of pigmenturia (mostly dipyrroles). The mechanism of the haemolytic anaemia is the intracellular release of the haems, which leaves very unstable tetramers, the formation of haemochromes and subsequently Heinz bodies, and the recognition of the abnormal red cells with haemoglobin/haemochromes attached to membranes by the spleen and other macrophages. Thrombosis is a recognised complication post-splenectomy.

There is no need for treatment except for folic acid supplement and attention to the possibility of aplastic crises due to parvovirus B19. Rarely, these patients require splenectomy.

High oxygen affinity haemoglobins

The sigmoid curve of the oxygen binding of haemoglobin is the product of the low affinity of the deoxy tetramers (T state), for example Hb Chesapeake, which turn into the R state when two of the four haems are oxygenated. After this molecular switch the haemoglobin acquires high affinity for oxygen. Mutations that stabilise the R state of the haemoglobin and interfere with the switch to T state will tend to have higher affinity than normal. Hence, the receptor mechanism for hypoxia in the kidney will interpret this situation as evidence of the presence of hypoxia and respond with increased secretion of erythropoietin, and stimulate an increase in the number of red cells and haematocrit.

There are around 100 high-affinity haemoglobins which are, on the whole, rare. The first one described was Hb Chesapeake, a mutation of position 92 in the β chain. This mutation destabilises the T state, so the conformational state of Hb Chesapeake is biased to the R state, and hence has increased affinity for oxygen. No serious clinical consequences of this mutation have been found apart from lifelong *erythrocytosis*.

The most common mutations responsible for high-affinity haemoglobins are those that interfere with the R→T transition: mutations in the $\alpha_2\beta_2$ contact area, and in the 'switch region' of the molecule, particularly the C and N terminals, favouring the R state. In addition, mutations that interfere with the 2,3-DPG binding site in the central cavity will tend to increase the affinity of Hb for oxygen.

Low oxygen affinity haemoglobins

Haemoglobins with low oxygen affinity, for example Hb Kansas, Hb Beth Israel, deliver oxygen more efficiently than normal haemoglobin, hence they tend to be detected as generating hyperoxia. The patient becomes anaemic through a correction of the level of erythropoietin secretion. Nevertheless, if the shift to the right is far enough, there is a point at which the delivery of oxygen is normal again and no anaemia exists. However, patients with Hb Kansas and Beth Israel have clinically apparent cyanosis, since they have more than 5 g of circulating deoxyhaemoglobin. Except for cyanosis, no other abnormalities have been found in these patients. The diagnosis is important in order to avoid unnecessary and sometimes invasive investigations. Diagnosis is by electrophoresis (helpful only if the amino acid substitution affects the overall charge of the molecule) and measurement of the oxygen dissociation curve.

The oxygen delivery properties of high- and low-affinity haemoglobins are discussed in Figure 10.7.

Haemoglobin Ms

These haemoglobins are the product of the substitutions of either the proximal or distal histidine by tyrosine. Also a nearby mutation, as in Hb M Milwaukee, may produce a similar picture. The patients appear slate grey in colour, which may be confused with cyanosis (this is really *pseudocyanosis*), due to the increase in deoxyhaemoglobin (>5 g/dl) or methaemoglobin status of the mutated chains as well as the change of the electrical environment, and hence of the visible absorption spectrum (Figure 10.8). The visible spectra of the haemolysate may help confirm the diagnosis, although electrophoresis can be helpful. Differential diagnosis includes genetic or acquired methaemoglobinaemia and sulphaemoglobinaemia.

These mutations have been found worldwide, and they are rare, except in the Iwate prefecture in Japan where they are common.

Conclusions

Genetically abnormal haemoglobins present themselves to the clinician usually in one or more of the following syndromes: (a) the presence of the homozygous or

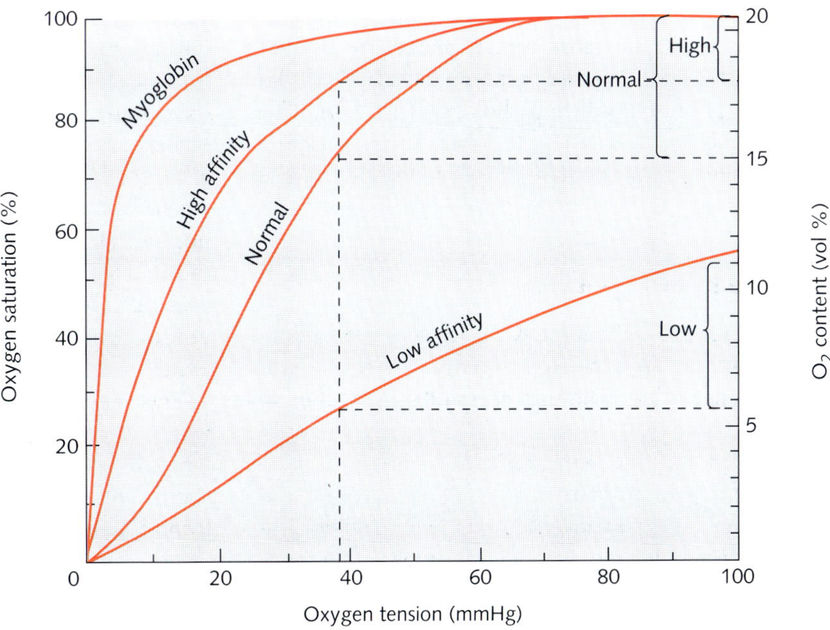

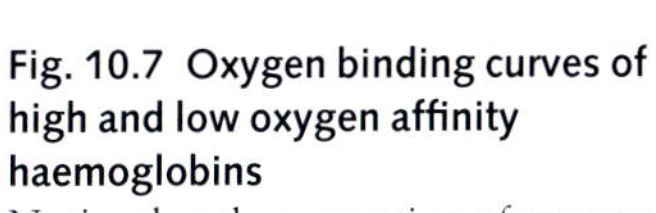

Fig. 10.7 Oxygen binding curves of high and low oxygen affinity haemoglobins
Notice that the extraction of oxygen by the tissues, which is the difference between pulmonary oxygen pressure (100 mmHg) and capillary oxygen pressure (40 mmHg), is lower than normal in high-affinity Hbs (low p50) and higher than normal in low-affinity Hbs. That is why the former have erythrocytosis and the latter (most of the time) anaemia.

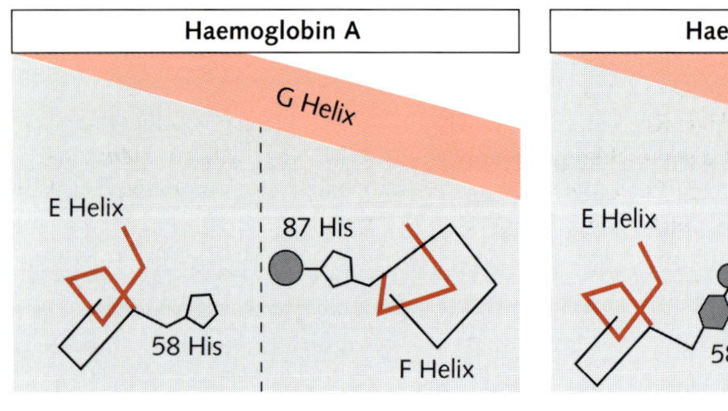

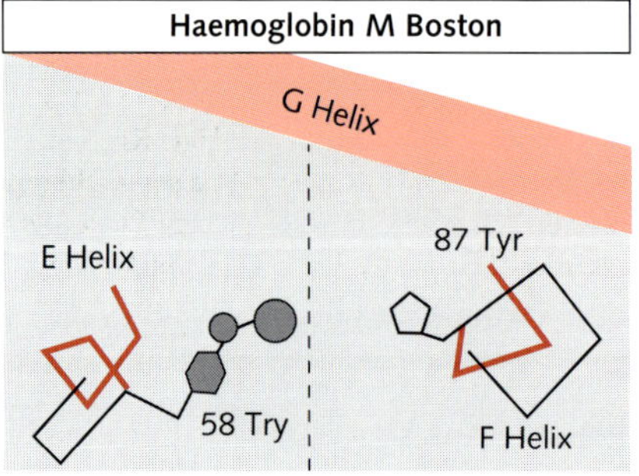

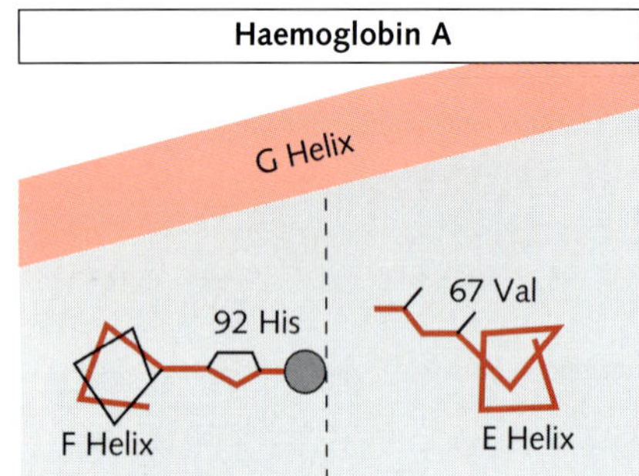

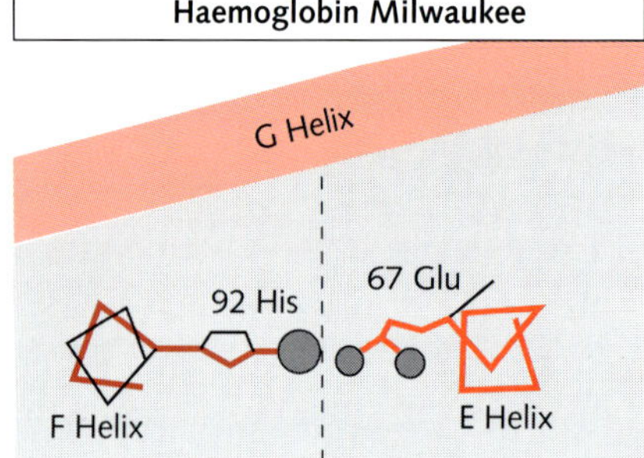

Fig. 10.8 Structure of Hb Ms
Haem environment of two Hb Ms, compared to Hb A. Notice the diverse changes of distal and proximal tyrosines (that have replaced the normal histidines) in each of the Hb Ms. These haemoglobins have a characteristic visible spectra around 610 nm.

double heterozygous state of *Hb S* produces a picture of chronic anaemia, chronic and insidious organ damage punctuated by painful crises and other complications; (b) the presence of *Hb C* in the homozygous state produces a mild chronic haemolytic syndrome; when doubly heterozygous with Hb S (SC disease), a syndrome similar to sickle cell anaemia but milder, and characterised by microcytic anaemia, is seen; (c) the presence of homozygous *Hb E* produces mild microcytic haemolytic anaemia, but in combination with β thalassaemia produces a picture sometimes of very severe thalassaemia intermedia; (d) heterozygotes forms of *unstable haemoglobins* produce variable intensity haemolytic anaemias; (e) heterozygotes for *low oxygen affinity mutant haemoglobins* and *Hb Ms* may produce a mild haemolytic anaemia syndrome, but always with cyanosis or pseudocyanosis as a background; (f) heterozygous forms of *high oxygen affinity mutant haemoglobins* often present with erythrocytosis.

This panoply of clinical syndromes is the product of the following alterations of the haemoglobin molecule:

- The creation of a new property for the haemoglobin molecule (Hb S, polymerisation; Hb C, crystallisation and microcytosis).
- Changes in O_2 affinity (high and low affinity for ligands).
- Changes in the environment of the haem (Hb Ms).
- Changes in the stability of the molecule in solutions (unstable haemoglobins).
- Some mutated haemoglobins are produced at lower rates and generate a thalassaemic syndrome (Hb E).

Of all of these, only Hb S, Hb C and Hb E are frequent in populations at risk due to their selection by malaria; the others are rare and generally represent 'private' mutations.

Further reading

General

Forget, Higgs, Nagel, Steinberg eds. (1999) *Disorders of Haemoglobin*. Cambridge University Press.

Henry ER, Jones CM, Hofrichter J, Eaton WA. (1997) Can a two-state MWC allosteric model explain haemoglobin kinetics? (Review) *Biochemistry*, **36**, 6511–6528.

Nagel RL. (1995) Disorders of hemoglobin function and stability. In: Handon RI, Lux SE, Stossel TP, eds. *Blood: Principles and Practices of Hematology*. Philadelphia: JB Lippincott.

Nagel RL, Roth EF Jr. (1989) Malaria and red cell genetic defects. *Blood*, **74**, 1213–1221.

Thein SL. (1998) Hematological diseases. In: J Larry Jameson, ed. *Principles of Molecular Medicine*. NJ: Humana Press.

Sickle/haemoglobin C

Bunn HF. (1997) Pathogenesis and treatment of sickle cell disease (Review). *New England Journal of Medicine*, **337**, 762–769.

Embury, Hebbel, Mohandas, Steinberg eds. (1994) *Sickle Cell Disease: Basic Principles and Clinical Practice*. Raven Press.

Herrick JB. (1910) Peculiar elongated and sickle-shaped red blood corpuscles in a case of severe anemia. *Archives of Internal Medicine*, **6**, 517.

Kaul DK, Fabry ME, Nagel RL. (1996) The pathophysiology of vascular obstruction in the sickle syndromes. *Blood Reviews*, **10**, 29–44.

Nagel RL, Fleming AF. (1992) Genetic epidemiology of the β^S gene. In: Fleming AF, ed. *Baillière's Clinical Haematology*. London: Harcourt Brace Jovanovich, 5, pp. 331–365.

Nagel RL, Lawrence C. (1991) The distinct pathobiology of SC disease: therapeutic implications. In: Nagel RL, ed. *Hematology/Oncology Clinics of North America*. Philadelphia, PA: WB Saunders, pp. 433–451.

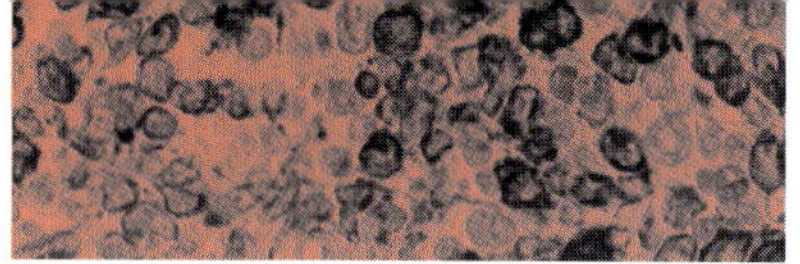

Chapter 11 The molecular basis of anaemia

Lucio Luzzatto & Anastasios Karadimitris

Introduction

The title of this chapter is quite ambitious, and in this respect we beg the readers' indulgence. In fact, as haematologists we *must* have the ambition to explain anaemia at the molecular level; and at the same time we are humbled by the fact that in many cases we are not quite there yet. One major reason is that anaemia is not a disease, but a vast collection of diseases, extremely heterogeneous in terms of aetiology, pathophysiology and clinico-haematological manifestations, as well as in our ability to treat them effectively. Since this book focuses on molecular pathophysiology, it is pertinent particularly to blood diseases that have a genetic basis. There are three main groups of anaemia that qualify in this respect. (a) Hemoglobinopathies, covered in Chapters 1 and 10; (b) red cell membrane cytoskeleton disorders, which are not covered in this book; and (c) inherited haemolytic anaemia due to enzyme abnormalities, covered in this chapter. In addition, considering the space limits allocated to this chapter, we have included several other types of inherited and acquired anaemias: our main inclusion criterion was that, based on current knowledge, we could offer at least some meaningful discussion of their molecular basis.

Megaloblastic anaemia

Megaloblastic anaemia is defined by a highly characteristic set of morphological changes which affect cells of the erythroid, myeloid and megakaryocytic lineage in the peripheral blood and bone marrow. These changes include macrocytosis, Howell–Jolly bodies, hypersegmented neutrophils, giant metamyelocytes and giant platelets. Despite the multitude of these signs, the one pathognomonic feature which we regard as a *sine qua non* for the diagnosis of megaloblastic anaemia is the peculiarly finely stippled chromatin of erythroid cells, combined with a derangement of the normally precisely ordered parallel pattern of maturation of the nucleus and of the cytoplasm. This asynchrony, whereby the maturation of the nucleus lags behind that of the cytoplasm, is the *morphological hallmark* of what we call megaloblastic erythropoiesis.

Aetiology

Megaloblastic anaemia has multiple aetiologies (Table 11.1). Indeed, it is the main haematological manifestation of, on the one hand, classic inherited disorders (e.g. Lesch–Nyhan syndrome, orotic aciduria, transcobalamin deficiency) and, on the other hand, classic acquired disorders such as pernicious anaemia (PA) and nutritional deficiency of either vitamin B_{12} (= cobalamin, Cbl) or folate. In this respect, the acquired (and far more common) conditions can be regarded as *phenocopies* of the much more rare inherited conditions.

Pathophysiology

While megaloblastosis is directly defined by its morphology, the mechanism of the anaemia is complex. In general, anaemia due to excessive destruction of red cells is characteristically associated with a cellular marrow and a high output of reticulocytes, whereas anaemia due to decreased production of red cells is characteristically associated with a hypocellular marrow and a low output of reticulocytes. In megaloblastic anaemia, the marrow is hypercellular, often to an extreme degree, but the output of reticulocytes is low. This contrast is the *pathophysiological hallmark* of megaloblastic anaemia, and it signifies that a large proportion of megaloblasts

Table 11.1 Classification of the megaloblastic anaemias.

Inherited	Acquired
FOLATE DEFICIENCY	
Inherited	**Acquired**
Inborn errors of folate metabolism	*Decreased intake*
Congenital folate malabsorption	Old age, alcoholism
Dihydrofolate reductase deficiency	Haemodialysis
Methylene tetrahydrofolate reductase deficiency	
	Impaired absorption
	Coeliac disease
	Tropical sprue
	Increased requirements
	Pregnancy
	Other increased cell turnover
	Chronic haemolytic anaemia
	Drugs
	Inhibitors of dihydrofolate reductase deficiency
	Anticonvulsants
COBALAMIN DEFICIENCY	
Inherited	**Acquired**
Inborn errors of cobalamin transport	*Impaired absorption*
Imerslund–Grasbeck disease	Gastric causes
Congenital deficiency of Intrinsic Factor	Pernicious anaemia
	Gastrectomy
Inborn errors of cobalamin metabolism disease	Intestinal causes
Methionine synthase deficiency (cblE and cblG)	Blind loop syndrome
cblC and cblD disease	Fish tapeworm
	Pancreatic insufficiency
	Decreased intake
	Vegetarians
	Other
	Nitrous oxide exposure
OTHER	
Hereditary orotic aciduria	
Lesch–Nyhan syndrome	
Thiamine-responsive megaloblastic anaemia	

Modified from Babior BM. (1995) The megaloblastic anemias. In: *Williams Hematology*, 5th edn. New York: McGraw-Hill, p. 471.

fail to mature into viable red cells: in other words, there is a vast component of *ineffective erythropoiesis*.

Molecular pathogenesis

In view of the above, it is clear that any explanation of the pathogenesis of megaloblastic anaemia at the molecular level must, on the one hand, rationalise it as the final common pathway of a variety of underlying lesions and, on the other hand, it must account for the phenomenon of ineffective erythropoiesis. Since the inherited causes of megaloblastic anaemia are defects in the purine or pyrimidine biosynthetic pathways, and folate is the co-enzyme of these pathways, it is natural to focus on this area of metabolism. It has been held for a long time that in megaloblastic anaemia a decreased concentration of nucleotide precursors becomes rate-limiting for DNA synthesis, and as a result cell proliferation is curtailed

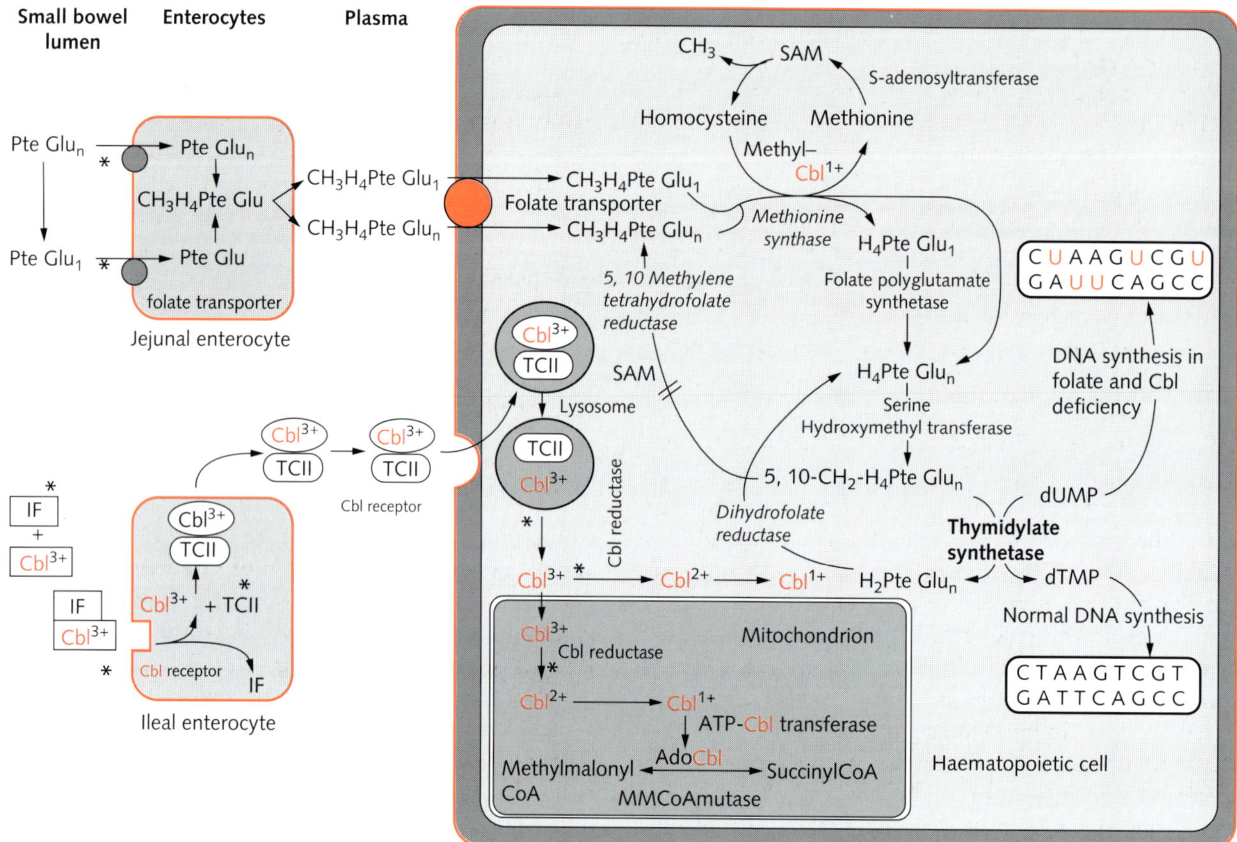

Fig. 11.1 The metabolic basis of megaloblastosis in folate and vitamin B$_{12}$ (cobalamin, Cbl) deficiency
The absorption of folates takes place in the proximal small bowel while vitamin Cbl bound to Intrinsic Factor (IF) is absorbed in the ileum. Folate enters the cells in the form of methyltetrahydrofolate (methylTHF). Cbl is transferred to, and enters the cells bound to transcobalamin II (TCII). In the cytoplasm, Cbl is necessary for the reaction catalysed by methionine synthase, whereby the CH$_3$-group of methylTHF is transferred to homocysteine; THF and methionine are produced, respectively, as a result. The polyglutamated form of THF is converted to 5,10-methyleneTHF which donates the single carbon group CH$_2$- to the reaction catalysed by thymidylate synthetase whereby dUMP is converted to dTMP which is used in DNA synthesis. Under conditions of folate and/or Cbl deficiency there is shortage of 5,10-methyleneTHF and, as a result, on the one hand, dTMP is drastically reduced and not available for DNA synthesis; on the other hand, dUMP is in excess. Strong evidence exists suggesting that, under such circumstances, dUMP is misincorporated in the DNA leading eventually to changes characteristic of megaloblastosis (*see text*). Note also that under Cbl-replete conditions the conversion of 5,10-methyleneTHF to methylTHF is inhibited by S-adenosylmethionine (SAM); by contrast, in Cbl deficiency SAM is in short supply and, as a result, this inhibition is relaxed, diverting the formation of 5,10-methyleneTHF to methylTHF, thus exacerbating further the shortage of dTMP and the accumulation of dUMP. Cbl also plays a significant role in the mitochondrial metabolic pathways necessary for the conversion of the products of propionate metabolism (i.e. methylmalonyl-CoA) into easily metabolised products. As is evident from the metabolic interrelationships of folate and Cbl, in folate deficiency homocysteine levels will increase; in Cbl deficiency, not only homocysteine but also methylmalonyl-CoA (and methylmalonic acid) will be increased: indeed, measurement of the serum and urine levels of homocysteine and methylmalonic acid is used in clinical practice for the diagnosis of folate and Cbl deficiency, especially at early stages.
Explanatory notes:
In the above figure the various forms of Cbl are shown in red. PteGlu$_{1/n}$: mono- or polyglutamated forms of folate; CH$_3$H$_4$PteGlu: methylTHF; 5,10-CH$_2$H$_4$PteGlu$_n$: 5,10-methyleneTHF; H$_2$PteGlu$_n$: dihydrofolate. Enzymes shown in italics are those the hereditary deficiency of which causes megaloblastic anaemia. Asterisks indicate those steps in the folate and Cbl metabolism whose defects can also cause hereditary megaloblastic anaemia.

and therefore few cells are produced. However, since cell proliferation is most active this model can be rejected out of hand: the marrow is hypercellular rather than hypocellular suggesting that the underlying defect may be qualitative and not merely quantitative.

Since the haematological consequences of the deficiency of either folate or Cbl are indistinguishable, it seems reasonable to surmise that there must be at least one point in common in their action, or that one depends on the other (see Figure 11.1). Indeed, Cbl is required for the conversion of methylTHFA (THFA: tetrahydrofolate), the main form of folate in the serum, to THFA, the active form in bone marrow cells. Various derivatives of THFA intervene in several steps of the biosynthesis of purine and pyrimidine nitrogen bases, but when folate is in short supply these steps can be bypassed by using preformed bases (the so-called salvage pathway). The one reaction for which folate (in the form of 5,10-methyleneTHFA) is irreplaceable is the conversion of dUMP to dTMP, for which it is the methyl group donor: as a result, this conversion will be impaired when either folate or Cbl is deficient. This reaction is crucially important because thymidine is, of course, the one base in which normally DNA differs from RNA. In principle, one might have expected that a block of this reaction would prevent DNA synthesis, but we have seen that this is not the case. On the other hand, it is well established that *in vitro* DNA polymerase is able to incorporate dUTP into DNA, especially if the dUTP concentration is much higher than that of dTTP, which will be the case when the conversion of the former to the latter is impeded. Several studies indicate that this also takes place *in vivo*: indeed, the major molecular lesion in megaloblastic anaemia may be this misincorporation of dUridine (dU) instead of T into DNA. The cell's DNA replicating machinery includes an enzyme, uracil glucosidase, which has the specific function to remove dU, should it be occasionally and illegitimately incorporated into DNA. Therefore dU will be retained in newly synthesised DNA only when the capacity of uracil glucosidase to remove it has been exceeded. For this reason, very little dU is actually found in megaloblastic DNA, but even that may have a disruptive effect on chromatin structure. Perhaps more important, if dU incorporation has been rampant rather than occasional, the numerous strand breaks produced by uracil glucosidase may exceed the capacity of other repair enzymes, thus causing the accumulation of damaged DNA, and eventually cell death. Surprisingly, a careful study has not detected in megaloblastic bone marrow features regarded as characteristic of apoptosis. We must therefore presume that cell death takes place by a different pathway or that phagocytosis of dead cells is rapid and highly efficient.

If shortage of dTTP is the fundamental metabolic defect underlying megaloblastic anaemia, since its production is 5,10-methyleneTHFA dependent, the formation of which is in turn Cbl dependent, it is clear that this same mechanism explains why megaloblastic anaemia is the common manifestation not only of nutritional folate and Cbl deficiency, but also of all genetically determined lesions of the transport and metabolism of folate or Cbl (Table 11.1). It is not clear why megaloblastic anaemia should occur in other inherited conditions, such as HPRT deficiency and orotic aciduria, in which it is the salvage pathway rather than the *de novo* pathway of the nitrogen bases that is compromised. At the moment we can only speculate by analogy. Perhaps the metabolic blocks in these conditions also entail serious alterations in the absolute and/or relative pool sizes of the various deoxynucleoside triphosphates. Once again, this could cause misincorporation followed by repair attempts which are not always successful.

Finally, despite the significant advances in the understanding of megaloblastosis, the molecular basis of demyelination that underlies the neurological complications of advanced Cbl deficiency remains elusive.

Congenital dyserythropoietic anaemias

Congenital dyserythropoietic anaemia (CDA) is the current designation for a group of rare inherited disorders that have a common feature: abnormalities in the maturation of the erythroid lineage. It is evident from genetics and from morphology that they are heterogeneous, and it is likely that they may be even more heterogeneous at the molecular level. Of the three 'classical' forms of CDA (Table 11.2), CDA II (or HEMPAS) is the best defined, on account of a pathognomonic serological test; CDA I is defined by characteristic ultrastructural changes in the chromatin of erythroblasts and by autosomal recessive inheritance; CDA III is defined by large, sometimes multinucleated, erythroblasts and by autosomal dominant inheritance. A variety of terms have been used to classify patients who have features of CDA but do not fit neatly in any of these three categories.

As a result of the deranged developmental programme, the mature red cells that are produced in CDA are abnormal, particularly in their membrane, and this often entails a haemolytic component in their anaemia. In addition, and most characteristically, a significant proportion of erythroid cells fail to achieve full maturity, and as a result they are destroyed in the bone marrow. Hence, the pathophysiological hallmark in CDA, just as in acquired megaloblastic anaemias (*see above*), is ineffective erythropoiesis.

The biochemical basis for abnormal maturation has been clarified to a reasonable extent only in the case of CDA II. Sodium dodecylsulphate-polyacrylamide gel electrophoresis (SDS-PAGE) analysis of red cell membrane proteins reveals a characteristically increased sharpness of band 3, the size heterogeneity of which is normally produced by the variable size of its carbohydrate moiety. This finding has focused the attention on the enzymes required for glycosylation of membrane proteins: decreased activity of α-mannosidase and of fucosyl transferase has been reported in individual cases.

Table 11.2 Defining features of CDA types I–III.

	Type I	Type II	Type III
Inheritance	Autosomal recessive	Autosomal recessive	(a) Autosomal dominant (b) Autosomal recessive
Localisation of gene	15q15.1–15.3	20q11.2	15q21–25
Red cells	Macrocytes	Normocytes	
Erythroblasts			
(a) Light microscopy	Megaloblastic; internuclear chromatin bridges	Normoblastic; binuclearity predominates	Megaloblastic; up to 12 nuclei per cell
(b) Electron microscopy	'Swiss cheese' appearance of heterochromatin	Peripheral double membranes	
Serology			
Ham's test	Negative	Positive	Negative
Anti-i agglutinability	Normal/strong	Strong	Normal/strong
SDS-PAGE	Normal	Band 3 thinner and faster	Band 3 slightly faster

Modified from Wickramasinghe SN. (1997) Dyserythropoiesis and congenital dyserythropoietic anaemias. *British Journal of Haematology*, 98, 785–797.

Recently, targeted inactivation of the gene encoding the latter enzyme has produced mice with features of CDA II. However, at least one case of CDA II does not have this lesion, and the gene responsible for the disease, in what is probably the majority of families, maps elsewhere. Thus, variability of clinical expression of CDA II could be due to different underlying genetic lesions, and of course it could be also due to different mutant alleles at the same locus. In fact there is some indirect evidence that alleles causing mild CDA may be relatively common, because two cases have been reported as causing chronic haemolytic anaemia in association with glucose-6-phosphate dehydrogenase (G6PD)-deficient variants which do not, on their own, cause this condition. We do not know whether the CDA mutations present in these patients would have caused clinical manifestations in the absence of G6PD deficiency.

The gene for CDA I has been mapped to chromosome 15 by linkage analysis in a single Swedish family, one of the first from which the concept of CDA developed.

In view of the almost complete restriction of the abnormal phenotype to the erythroid lineage, it is likely that the genes that are mutated in any patient with CDA serve some important role in the programme of erythroid differentiation. Thus, any of these will be of great interest, quite out of proportion to the rarity of CDAs as clinical entities.

It has been recently reported that three patients with CDA I have responded to treatment with interferon-α with near normalisation of the haemoglobin values. Although the clinical data seem convincing, at the moment it is not clear by what mechanism an intrinsic erythroid molecular abnormality can benefit from this treatment.

The sideroblastic anaemias

The term sideroblastic anaemia (SA) encompasses a diverse collection of diseases in which different causes and different mechanisms converge to produce the same rather spectacular feature: accumulation of inorganic iron in the cytoplasm of erythroid cells in sufficient quantities to be easily demonstrated in the form of granules using Perl's Prussian Blue staining. Characteristically, the iron is found in mitochondria positioned around the nucleus—hence the term *ring sideroblast.* SAs are broadly divided into *acquired* and *inherited* forms (Table 11.3). Acquired SAs are the most common and are discussed in *Chapter 6*. Here, we discuss briefly the two inherited forms of SA for which the genetic and biochemical basis have been clarified.

ALAS2 deficiency

Normally, about 90% of the iron (Fe) obtained daily from the diet reaches the erythroblasts, where it is required for the final step of haem biosynthesis, namely the incorporation of iron into the tetrapyrrolic ring of protoporphyrin IX. The first and the last three of the eight steps of the haem biosynthetic pathway take place in the mitochondrion. The first and rate-limiting step consists of the condensation of glycine and succinyl-CoA to δ-aminolaevulinate. This reaction is catalysed by δ-

Table 11.3 Classification of the sideroblastic anaemias.

Mode of inheritance	Chromosomal locus	Gene	Type of mutations	Clinical manifestations other than SA
INHERITED				
X-linked	Xp11.21	*ALAS2*	Missense	None
X-linked	Xq13	Not cloned linked to *PGK1*		Cerebellar ataxia
Autosomal recessive	1q23.2–23.3	Not cloned		Thiamine-responsive megaloblastic anaemia, diabetes mellitus, sensorineural deafness
Autosomal dominant	Not known	Not cloned		None
Mitochondrial e.g. Pearson's MPS	Usually from nt8469 to nt13447 (*see Fig. 11.3*)		Deletions	Pancreatic exocrine dysfunction, cytopenia, metabolic acidosis
ACQUIRED				
Refractory anaemia with ring sideroblasts (RARS)				
Drug induced (e.g. isoniazid, chloramphenicol, ethanol)				
Secondary to systemic, metabolic, malignant disorders				

ALAS2, δ-aminolaevulinate synthase 2; PGK1, phosphoglycerate kinase 1; SA, sideroblastic anaemia; MPS, marrow-pancreas syndrome.

aminolaevulinate synthase (ALAS) and it requires pyridoxal 5′-phosphate (PLP) as a co-factor. Two isoforms of ALAS are known, and both have a homodimeric structure, but they are encoded by different genes. *ALAS1* is a ubiquitously expressed housekeeping gene, whereas *ALAS2* is erythroid-specific.

Genetics of ALAS2 deficiency

The first family with what we now call X-linked SA was reported by T. Cooley in 1945. Subsequently, more families with apparent X-linked SA were described. The X-linked mode of inheritance was further established by the finding that female relatives of the affected males demonstrated red cell mosaicism, i.e. two populations of red cells, hypochromic and normochromic. The observation that some affected males responded to pharmacological doses of pyridoxine focused attention on the erythroid-specific ALAS: indeed, the *in vitro* activity of this enzyme was invariably reduced. The erythroid-specific *ALAS* (*ALAS2*) gene was subsequently cloned (Figure 11.2) and mapped to Xp11.12.

Transcriptional and translational control of ALAS2 expression

The expression of *ALAS2* is regulated both at the transcriptional and the translational level. Transcriptional control is effected through the programmed differentiation of the erythroid lineage, mainly through the erythropoietin-induced transcription factors which include GATA-1, EKLF and NF-E2. In contrast, as one of the few examples of control of gene expression at the translational level, *ALAS2* is involved in the regulation of haem synthesis in relation to Fe availability. Central to this regulatory mechanism is a protein which is able to bind 4 atoms of Fe and also able to bind to an element with a characteristic 'hairpin' secondary structure called iron responsive element (IRE), present within the 5′ untranslated region of the ALAS2 mRNA. When this protein, IRE-binding protein (IRE-BP), is iron replete it does not bind to the IRE, and translation of the ALAS2 mRNA is unimpeded. When iron is in scarce supply, the iron-depleted IRE-BP binds to IRE and the translation of the ALAS2 mRNA is repressed. Interestingly, IRE-BP can also bind to IREs present in the mRNA of the transferrin receptor and of ferritin. When IRE-BP is Fe-replete, it binds to the IRE of transferrin receptor mRNA thus repressing its translation; in contrast, Fe-replete IRE-BP does not bind to the IRE of the ferritin mRNA allowing the translation of ferritin to proceed. Reverse effects are seen when iron supply is low.

Molecular pathology of ALAS2 deficiency

Twenty-one different point mutations have been described in 30 different families (Figure 11.2). They all map to exons 5–11 which are highly conserved across species. Parts of these exons are thought to contribute to the formation of the catalytic site, PLP-binding site and substrate-binding site of ALAS2. The presence of only missense mutations would imply, in an analogy with

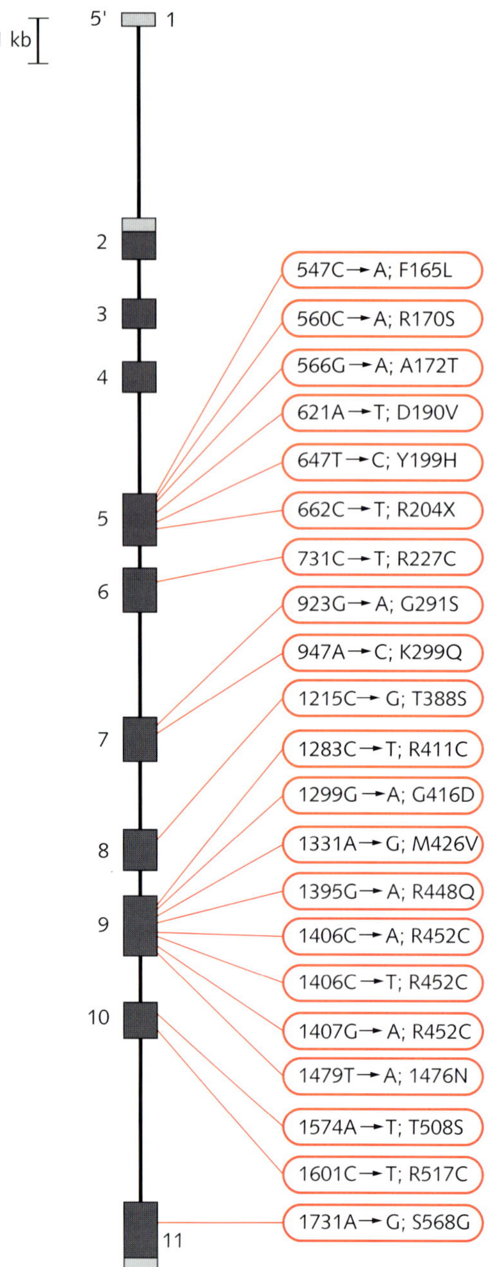

Fig. 11.2 The human *ALAS2* gene and its pathogenic mutations *ALAS2* spans about 22 kb and consists of 11 exons. Two mature forms of mRNA exist: one full length and one shorter as a result of alternative splicing of exon 4. The functional significance of these splicing variants is not known. Exon 1 and part of exon 2 (shown in grey) form the 5′ UTR and contain the iron-responsive element (*see text*). The full-length mRNA (1.95 kb) encodes a protein of 522 amino acids (64.4 kDa). The mature protein derives from the cleavage of the first 49 amino-terminal amino acids (mitochondrial signal sequence) upon entry in the mitochondrion.

another X-linked disorder, G6PD deficiency, that hemizygotes with ALAS2 null mutations would not be viable.

Clinical aspects and treatment of ALAS2 deficiency

The clinical picture of ALAS2 deficiency is that of a hypochromic microcytic anaemia with bone marrow erythroid hyperplasia as a result of ineffective erythropoiesis, and the finding of the characteristic ring sideroblasts, mainly in the late erythroid precursors. There is considerable heterogeneity in the severity of the disease, not only between individuals bearing different mutations but also between related individuals with the same *ALAS2* mutation. Patients at one extreme may present a few months after birth with severe anaemia, severe microcytosis and no response to pyridoxine, or at the other extreme may present in the ninth decade of life with their anaemia being fully responsive to pyridoxine. This variation highlights the fact that ALAS2 deficiency should be considered in any case of SA, irrespective of age. It should also be borne in mind that, because ALAS2-related SA is an X-linked disorder, occasionally females will be afflicted by the disease due to extreme skewing of X-inactivation—indeed such patients have been reported.

Although the anaemia of pyridoxine-responsive SA is treatable, the main complication of the disease is iron overload which, if left untreated, will have the same deleterious results as human leucocyte antigen (HLA)-linked haemochromatosis. Iron overload can be biochemically evident even by adolescence, does not correlate with the degree of anaemia and can affect mildly anaemic females. The importance of effectively treating iron overload cannot be overemphasised for one further reason: excess iron interferes with the function of ALAS2 and patients previously unresponsive to pyridoxine, after effective iron chelation, occasionally become responsive.

The advances in the molecular aspects of X-linked SA make prenatal diagnosis and counselling possible, especially for families with the severe, pyridoxine-resistant forms of the disease.

Pearson's marrow-pancreas syndrome

Pearson's marrow-pancreas syndrome (PMPS) is unique among the SAs because the underlying genetic lesion is not in the nuclear DNA but in mitochondrial DNA (mtDNA).

Note: in early studies of the genetics of various organisms, 'cytoplasmic inheritance' had been recognised, but it remained controversial because of the otherwise overwhelming evidence that genes must be in the nuclear chromosomes. It is now clear that cytoplasmic inheritance does exist, and its physical basis is mtDNA.

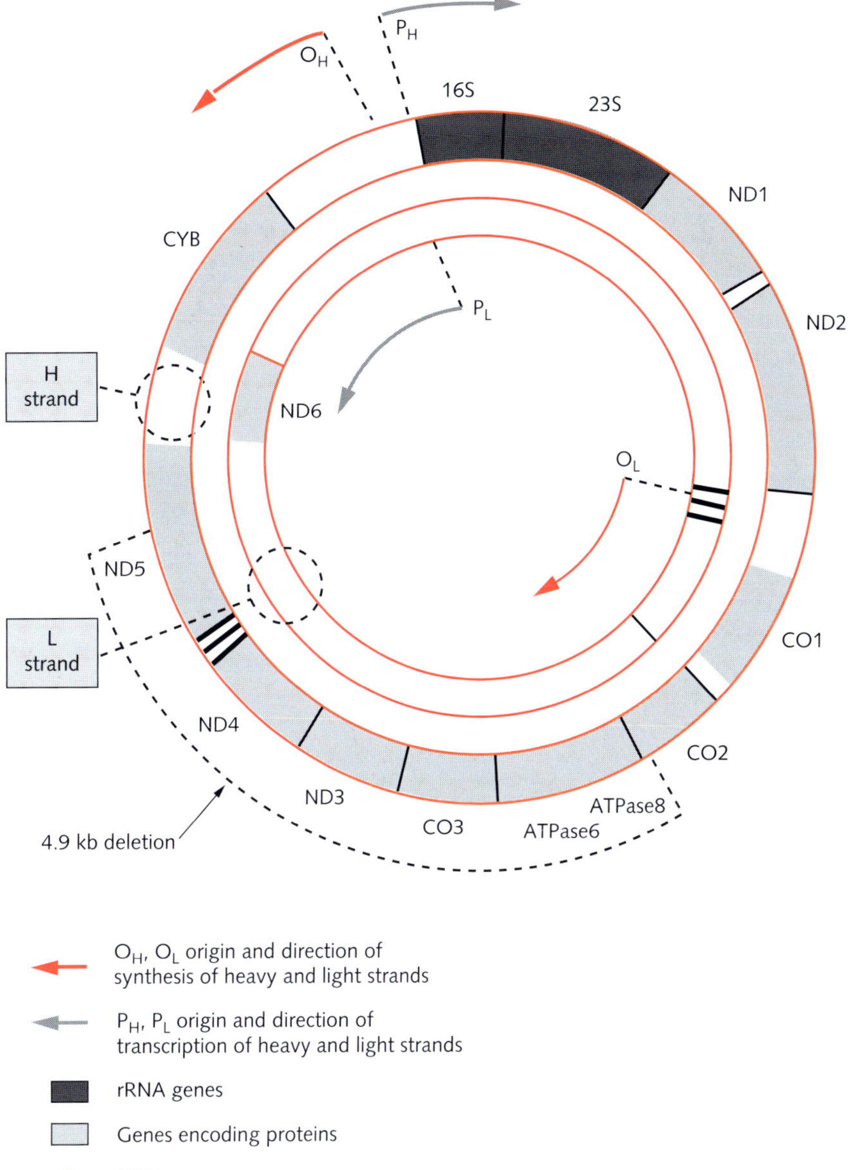

Fig. 11.3 The human mitochondrial genome
Both replication and transcription of the heavy (H) and light (L) strands of mtDNA run in opposite directions as indicated in the figure. The products of transcription are large transcripts which are then cleaved to generate RNAs for individual genes. Note the absence of introns and close apposition of genes. *ATPase 8* and *ATPase 6* overlap. The approximate location of the common 4.9 kb deletion (*see text*) is indicated by the broken line. *πND1–ND6* encode NADH dehydrogenase subunits; *CO1–CO3* encode cytochrome *c* oxidase subunits and CYB encodes cytochrome *b*.
Modified from Strachan T, Read AP. (1996) *Human Molecular Genetics*, 1st edn. BIOS.

Properties of mitochondrial DNA

Each somatic cell has hundreds to several thousand mitochondria, and each mitochondrion contains 2–10 copies of mtDNA. mtDNA consists of a single double-stranded circular molecule, and its 16,569 nucleotides encode 24 structural RNAs (22 tRNAs and 2 rRNAs) required for mitochondrial protein synthesis, as well as 13 protein subunits belonging to four enzyme complexes which are all involved, directly or indirectly, in the generation of adenosine triphosphate (ATP) through oxidative phosphorylation (Figure 11.3). Replication, transcription and translation of mtDNA are all quite distinct from their equivalents of nuclear DNA.

Since mitochondria are abundant in the cytoplasm of the mature oocyte, but absent from that part of the sperm cell that enters it at the time of fertilisation, the hereditary transmission of mtDNA is exclusively through the maternal germline. Therefore, a mitochondrial disease can be transmitted from a mother to all of her children, whether male or female—a non-Mendelian form of inheritance.

mtDNA is estimated to be at least 10 times more vulnerable than nuclear DNA to mutations and to their consequences for various reasons. Firstly, it is constantly exposed to oxygen free radicals generated by oxidative phosphorylation; secondly, mitochondria largely lack effective DNA repair mechanisms; thirdly, because most of the mtDNA sequence is coding, many more mutations will be reflected in the structure of its protein products. On the other hand, since there are so many copies of mtDNA in each cell, mutant mtDNA may co-exist with normal mtDNA, a situation called *heteroplasmy* (the opposite of *homoplasmy*). The phenotype of a particular cell or organ will depend on the relative proportions of normal and mutated mtDNA. Since, unlike nuclear chromosomes, there is no rigorous mechanism for the segregation of mtDNA molecules at either mitosis or meiosis, the inheritance of mtDNA mutations is rather unpredictable, and since heteroplasmy may exist even in oocytes, this further complicates the non-Mendelian inheritance of diseases caused by mtDNA mutations.

Clinical aspects of PMPS

PMPS usually presents within the first few months of life with hypoproliferative SA, variable cytopenias and pancreatic exocrine dysfunction. Bone marrow examination reveals in addition to ring sideroblasts, striking vacuolation of the erythroid and myeloid precursors (Plate 11.1, facing page 128). Metabolic acidosis is another frequent manifestation; renal disease, liver failure, hypoparathyroidism and diabetes mellitus may also occur.

Despite treatment with blood product support, pancreatic enzymes and various vitamins (e.g. co-enzyme Q), about half of the patients do not survive beyond the third year of life. Of the patients who do survive, most develop complications in other organs, particularly ophthalmoplegia, pigmentary degeneration of the retina and cardiomyopathy, i.e. the features originally described as the Kearns–Sayre syndrome (KSS). The overlap between PMPS and KSS is not surprising, since similar genetic lesions are found in both conditions (*see below*).

Molecular pathology

In all but one of the cases that have been adequately investigated, PMPS was due to deletions within mtDNA. The size of the deletion is variable; in one study, 43% of the patients had an identical 4.9 kb deletion which has also been found in patients with other mitochondrial diseases (such as KSS and progressive external ophthalmoplegia: *see* Figure 11.3). In some cases, deletion-dimers and/or deletion-multimers were observed. There is no obvious correlation between the size or location of the deletion and the clinical severity of the disease: rather, what probably largely determines the clinical phenotype is the proportion of mutated mtDNA in a particular tissue. For example, patients with PMPS have mutated mtDNA in all tissues examined, whereas in patients with 'classical' KSS, mutated mtDNA is restricted to muscle and is not found in blood cells. Since the mothers of PMPS patients are invariably unaffected, we can expect that the deletion has taken place *de novo*, and this has been documented in a number of cases.

A difficult practical problem is that of genetic counselling for couples who have had the misfortune of having a child with PMPS. The risk of recurrence depends on whether the deletion is present in most, or only in some, of the mother's gonadal cells. At the moment there is no established methodology for determining this. At an experimental level, it could be achieved by inducing multiple ovulation and polymerase chain reaction (PCR) testing individual oocytes for the deletion previously detected in an affected sib. The same could be done in very early embryos after *in vitro* fertilisation (pre-implantation prenatal diagnosis). Because of the high copy number of mtDNA, testing for mtDNA mutations is much easier than testing for mutations in nuclear genes.

Conditions associated with bone marrow failure (BMF)

The disease entities falling under this heading are quite diverse, but they are grouped on account of a common pathogenesis—the loss of haematopoietic stem cells (HSCs). The pace of HSC depletion varies widely, from weeks (e.g. in idiopathic aplastic anaemia, IAA) to years (e.g. in Fanconi's anaemia, FA). In fact, IAA and FA exemplify two broad classes of BMF syndromes: i.e. *acquired* and *inherited*, respectively (Table 11.4).

Acquired bone marrow failure syndromes

Idiopathic aplastic anaemia

IAA accounts for the majority (~80–90%) of cases of acquired BMF syndromes with an incidence estimated at two cases per million (somewhat higher in the Orient).

Immunopathogenesis of IAA. The most direct evidence that IAA may be an autoimmune disorder has come from the clinical observation that patients with IAA have complete or partial reversion of their pancytopenia when they are treated with antilymphocyte globulin (ALG). Subsequently, it was shown that patients with IAA often have

Table 11.4 Classification of the bone marrow failure (BMF) syndromes.

INHERITED

Disease	Mode of inheritance	Chromosomal locus	Gene	Clinical manifestations
Fanconi's anaemia	Autosomal recessive	FA-A: 16q24.3 FA-C: 9q22.3 FA-D: 3p22–26	*FAA* *FAC* Not cloned	See text
Dyskeratosis congenita	X-linked	Xq28	*DKC1*	See text
Swachman–Diamond syndrome	Autosomal recessive	Not known	Not known	Neutropenia, exocrine pancreatic insufficiency, metaphyseal dysostosis
Amegakaryocytic thrombocytopenia	X-linked? Autosomal recessive?	Not known	Not known	Absent megakaryocytes In bone marrow, late BMF
Pearson's marrow-pancreas syndrome	Mitochondrial	Usually from nt8469 to nt13447	Contiguous genes deleted	Pancreatic exocrine dysfunction, sideroblastic anaemia (*see also text*)
Familial aplastic anaemias	There are numerous reports of family clustering of BMF other than the above. They have shown different patterns of inheritance and a variety of associated clinical manifestations (e.g. malformations), suggesting that this group may be genetically heterogeneous			

ACQUIRED

Idiopathic aplastic anaemia
Secondary
Radiation
Drugs and chemicals
Regular: cytotoxic, benzene
Idiosyncratic: chloramphenicol, NSAIDs, antiepileptics, gold
Viruses
Epstein–Barr virus
Hepatitis
Parvovirus
Human immunodeficiency virus
Immune diseases
Thymoma
Pregnancy
Paroxysmal nocturnal haemoglobinuria

increased numbers of 'activated' CD8+ T-lymphocytes in their blood and bone marrow. In addition, T-lymphocytes from IAA patients can inhibit the growth of autologous *in vitro* haematopoietic colonies, and the growth of colonies from HLA-identical siblings. Based on these observations, a reasonable working hypothesis is that, in IAA, autoreactive T-cells attack HSCs, thus preventing their growth or even causing their demise—hence the pancytopenia and the further complications it entails (i.e. infection and haemorrhage). Unfortunately, the primary event that triggers this aberrant immune response remains elusive: a possible viral cause has been long sought but never proven. The identity of the putative autoantigen on HSCs also remains unknown. There is evidence, however, that the cytotoxic action of autoreactive T-cells is mediated, at least in part, through interferon-γ and TNF-β, which in turn upregulate the Fas receptor on the surface of HSCs, thus facilitating activation of the Fas-dependent apoptotic pathways. The HLA-DR2 alleleis over-represented in patients with IAA of European ancestry, whereas another HLA class II haplotype is overrepresented in Japanese patients with IAA.

Clinical aspects and treatment of IAA. The clinical picture of IAA generally reflects the extent of HSC loss and the subsequent cytopenias. Typically, a patient with severe IAA presents with bruising and mucosal bleeding, anaemia and septic episodes (bacterial or fungal), but without hepatosplenomegaly. The differential diagnosis of IAA includes inherited BMF syndromes, MDS, the aplastic form of childhood ALL, as well as infectious and malignant processes that may infiltrate the bone marrow: thus, the diagnosis of IAA is made eventually by exclusion.

The contemporary treatment of IAA is dictated by the severity of IAA (as determined by the degree of pancytopenia, reticulocytopenia and bone marrow cellularity) and by the patient's age. Bone marrow transplantation (BMT) from an HLA-identical sibling or from an alternative donor is the treatment of choice for younger patients with severe IAA, and offers >65% long-term survival. In the absence of an appropriate donor, or when the patient is older or the disease milder, immunosuppressive treatment (IST: in particular the combination of ALG/ATG and cyclosporin A) results in complete or partial response in the majority of cases. Apart from PNH (*see below*), IAA bears a significant risk of late clonal disorders, especially after IST: the risk of MDS and AML is 17% at 10 years post-IST, and the risk of tumours of other organs brings the total risk to 18% (compared to 3.1% after BMT).

Paroxysmal nocturnal haemoglobinuria

Paroxysmal nocturnal haemoglobinuria (PNH) is a rare acquired haematological disorder with three clinical features which can make its presentation quite protean: *intravascular haemolysis, tendency to thrombosis* and *bone marrow failure* of variable severity. As in IAA, the precise cause for BMF remains unclear; by contrast, the molecular and cellular events responsible for haemolysis are now explained. For this reason, the space devoted here to this condition is out of proportion to its prevalence.

Molecular pathogenesis. The initiating event in the pathogenesis of PNH is a somatic mutation that inactivates the X-linked gene *PIG-A* (see Figure 11.4) in a pluripotent HSC. The protein product of *PIG-A*, although not physically isolated yet, is thought to be one subunit of an enzyme with N-acetylglucosamine transferase activity, which catalyses an early step in the formation of a complex glycolipid molecule called glucosylphosphatidylinositol (GPI). The synthesis of GPI takes place initially on the cytoplasmic surface of the endoplasmic reticulum (ER) and is completed on the luminal surface of ER. Once formed, the GPI molecules (anchors) are attached through a transpeptidation reaction to the carboxyl terminal of a variety of proteins. The GPI-linked proteins, after post-translational modifications in the Golgi apparatus, emerge eventually on the cell surface, to which they remain attached through the GPI anchor. Because GPI synthesis is impaired in the haematopoietic cells of PNH patients, their blood cells are either completely (PNH III) or partially (PNH II) deficient in GPI-linked proteins. Although for the majority of these proteins the functional consequences of this deficiency are not known, some are directly implicated in the pathogenesis of PNH: namely, CD55 and especially CD59, which normally protect the cell from the lytic effect of activated complement. Intravascular haemolysis in PNH (manifesting clinically as haemoglobinuria) is the direct consequence of the fact that CD55- and CD59-deficient PNH red cells are susceptible to complement-mediated lysis. The *in vitro* counterpart of this phenomenon is the Ham–Dacie test, whereby the patient's red cells are lysed by either autologous or ABO-compatible donor acidified serum. As for thrombosis, it seems likely that this may result from complement-mediated activation of platelets deficient in CD55 and CD59, although this has not yet been formally proven; other (as yet unidentified) genetic or acquired factors affecting coagulation and/or fibrinolysis probably have an additive or synergistic effect.

Cellular pathogenesis. Since PNH-HSCs lack GPI-linked proteins, one might expect in principle that they would be poorly competitive in growth with respect to normal HSCs. Instead, PNH-HSCs can expand until they largely supplant normal haematopoiesis. In first approximation this paradox may be explained by invoking an intrinsic proliferative advantage of PNH-HSC(s) over normal HSC, as is the case with leukaemic cells: however, the fact that patients with PNH can live for decades with normal and PNH haematopoiesis co-existing militates against this notion. Lack of competitive growth advantage by the PNH haematopoiesis has also been demonstrated experimentally in a mouse model. *pig-a* null mouse embryonic stem cells can make embryoid bodies which are competent for haematopoietic differentiation in the presence of the appropriate growth factors, but the *pig-a* null colonies are much fewer and grow poorly compared to colonies produced by wild-type embryoid bodies. Furthermore, in mice with conditional targeted disruption of the *pig-a* gene, PNH haematopoiesis reaches its peak at about 20% during fetal life but declines to <5% a few months after birth.

An alternative explanation of the paradox was suggested by the well-known close association between PNH and IAA. As many as 50% of patients with *bona fide* IAA at some stage of their disease develop PNH clones: indeed, in some patients who survive IAA, the clinical picture changes dramatically to PNH. Since IAA and PNH are both rare diseases, it is inconceivable that this succession is due to chance:

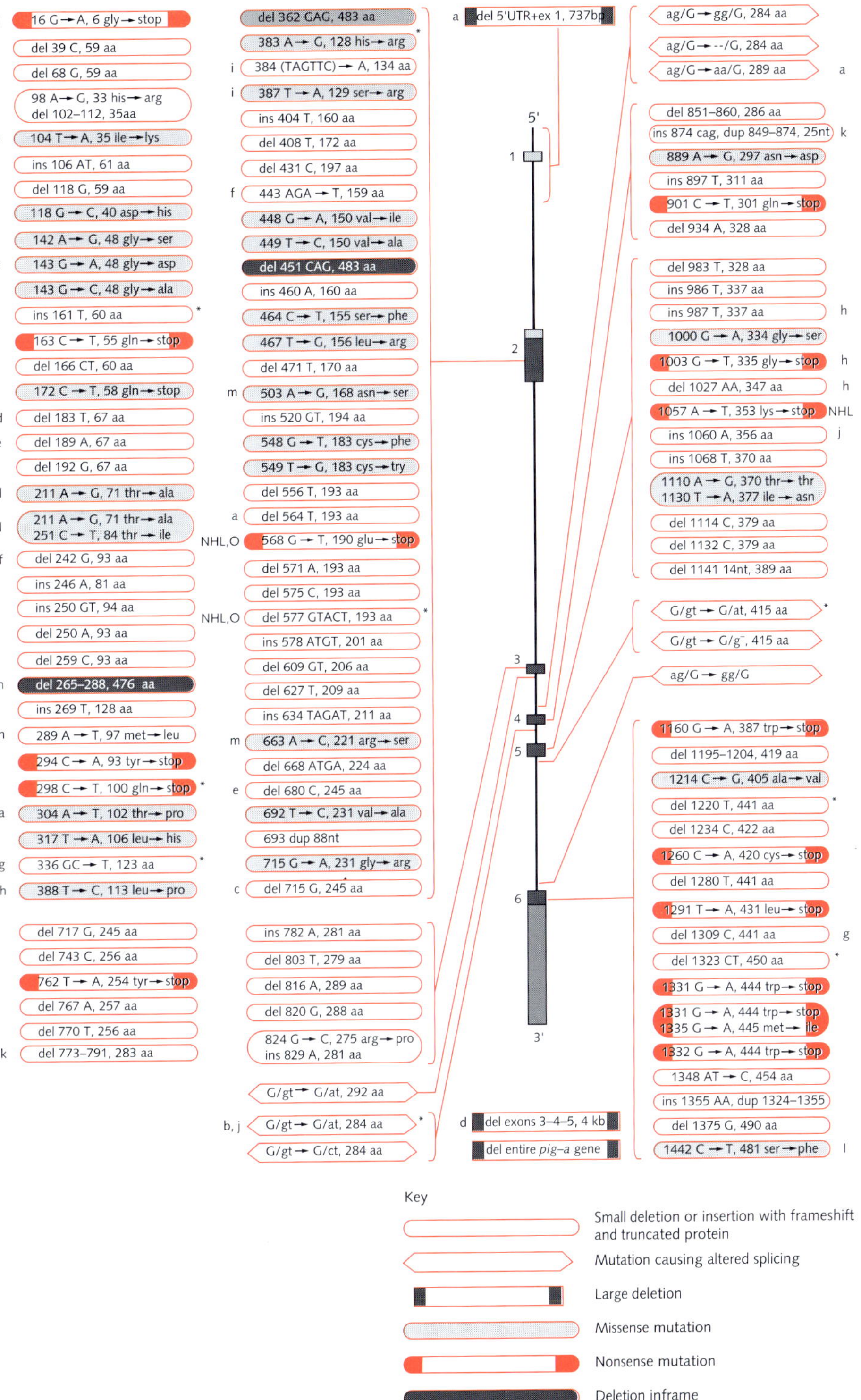

Fig. 11.4 The identity of *PIG-A* and its pathogenic mutations
PIG-A maps to Xp22.1, spans 17 kb and consists of 6 exons with the initiating codon in exon 2. The open reading frame of *PIG-A* is 1.45 kb and encodes a protein of predicted length of 484 amino acids. A small letter outside the box identifies multiple mutations found in a single patient. Only one polymorphism has been described (55 C→T, 19 arg→trp).
*Mutation found in more than one patient.
From Rotoli B, Nafa K. Paroxysmal nocturnal hemoglobinuria. In: Jameson JL (ed) *Principles of Molecular Medicine*. New York, Humana Press, 1998.

rather, we can surmise that stem cells with inactivating mutations of *PIG-A* do not contribute significantly to haematopoiesis under normal circumstances, but they can do so if a process that selectively damages normal HSCs were to spare PNH-HSC(s). Indeed, one might imagine that the PNH-HSC(s) expand and contribute to haematopoiesis (in some cases as much as 90% of it) precisely because the autoreactive T-cells implicated in the pathogenesis of IAA (*see above*) are incapable of damaging PNH-HSC(s), presumably because the damage they can inflict is mediated through a GPI-linked protein.

Molecular pathology. All types of mutations have been observed in the *PIG-A* gene in patients with PNH: a few are large deletions, the majority (~75%) are small insertions or deletions causing frameshifts, and the rest are nonsense and missense point mutations. Interestingly, the nonsense mutations and frameshift mutations are spread throughout the coding sequence (exons 2–6: Figure 11.4), presumably because they cause complete inactivation of the gene product wherever they fall, whereas missense mutations are clustered mainly within exon 2, where we presume that amino acid residues critical for catalytic activity must be located.

Clinical aspects and treatment of PNH. Although in the prototypical PNH patient haemoglobinuria is—by definition—paroxysmal, the brisk intravascular haemolysis is in fact continuous. Additionally, patients with 'florid PNH' (Table 11.5) often experience acute exacerbations of the haemolysis during intercurrent illnesses such as infections (presumably because this is associated with activation of complement through either the classical or alternative pathway), other stressful events, or for no obvious reason.

Haemolytic anaemia with macrocytosis (partly due to reticulocytosis and partly due to BMF), different degrees of thrombocytopenia and leucopenia, iron deficiency and haemosiderinuria should raise the suspicion of PNH. The diagnosis can be confirmed through the Ham–Dacie test (which only detects the PNH abnormality in erythrocytes) and/or flow cytometric analysis of erythrocytes and leucocytes; for this purpose, anti-CD59 is the most reliable antibody. In about 40% of PNH patients, venous thrombosis of small or large vessels (particularly at unusual sites, such as the abdomen or the brain) is a serious and potentially life-threatening complication. If promptlydiagnosed, venous thrombosis may respond to thrombolytic therapy, which must be followed by short- and long-term anticoagulants. Supportive treatment consists of blood transfusions, folic acid and iron supplements.

Long-term therapeutic options for PNH include immunosuppressive agents (e.g. combination of ALG/ATG and cyclosporin A) and, for selected patients, BMT from an HLA-identical sibling.

PNH and other clonal disorders. Patients with PNH have a small risk (<4%) of developing MDS and AML. Because the same risk exists in IAA, it is probably the perturbed marrow environment that allows the emer-

Table 11.5 PNH: clinical heterogeneity and proposed terminology.

Predominant clinical features	Blood findings	Size of PNH clone	Designation
Haemolysis ± thrombosis	Anaemia; little or no other cytopenia	Large	Florid PNH
Haemolysis ± thrombosis	Anaemia; mild to moderate other cytopenia(s)	Large	PNH, hypoplastic
Purpura and/or infection	Moderate to severe pancytopenia	Large	AA/PNH
Purpura and/or infection	Severe pancytopenia	Small	AA with PNH clone
Thrombosis	Normal or moderate cytopenia(s)	Small	Mini-PNH

From Tremml G, Karadimitris A, Luzzatto L. (1998) Paroxysmal nocturnal hemoglobinuria: learning about PNH cells from patients and from mice. *Haema* 1, 12–20.

gence of premalignant (MDS) or malignant (AML) clones, rather than the *PIG-A* mutations *per se* predisposing to MDS and AML.

Inherited bone marrow failure syndromes

Fanconi's anaemia

Fanconi's anaemia (FA) is the most common cause of hereditary BMF. It has long been recognised that the clinical manifestations of FA vary a great deal. This clinical heterogeneity led to the notion that FA may also be genetically heterogeneous, a notion that was confirmed by the identification of as many as eight complementation groups through the use of somatic cell hybridisation. At least three out of the eight predicted FA genes have now been mapped, and two have been cloned and characterised. Despite these major advances in the delineation of the genetic basis of FA and a wealth of data on the respective clinical and cellular phenotypic features, the precise biochemical mechanisms that bring about the disease remain a matter of debate.

The overall frequency of FA mutant genes in the general population is estimated at 1 in 300. In the Ashkenazi Jews and in the Afrikaans of the Republic of South Africa it is much higher (1 in 100 and 1 in 89, respectively), most likely as a result of founder effects.

Clinical aspects of Fanconi's anaemia. Gradual onset of BMF (median age: 7 years, range: birth to 31 years), skeletal abnormalities (most commonly of the radius and thumb), skin lesions (hyperpigmentation, *café-au-lait* spots), renal and urinary tract malformations and gonadal dysfunction are the most common clinical manifestations. However, the clinical spectrum is even wider, as it includes congenital defects of the gastrointestinal system, heart and central nervous system. BMF is often heralded by thrombocytopenia, macrocytosis and increased Hb F levels. Patients with FA have an unusually high risk of developing treatment-resistant MDS and AML, estimated at 52% in total by the age of 40 years. Furthermore, the risk of a variety of solid tumours is several times higher than in normal individuals.

Cellular phenotype. The unique feature of FA cells (which forms the basis of what is now regarded as the most reliable diagnostic test) is their increased chromosomal instability, which is accentuated upon exposure to clastogenic (chromosome breaking) alkylating agents, such as mitomycin C and diepoxybutane (DEB). This chromosomal instability is thought to reflect a defect in DNA repair, which has also been invoked to explain the hypermutability and increased frequency of deletions seen in FA. Other biochemical defects reported include increased sensitivity of the FA cells to reactive oxygen species, defects of the cell cycle and increased tendency to apoptosis.

Molecular genetics of Fanconi's anaemia. FA is an autosomal recessive disorder. The *in vitro* response to DEB has made it possible to test cells from different patients for their ability to cross-correct each other's defect by somatic cell fusion. As discussed earlier, this has led to classifying patients first into four, and recently into eight, complementation groups (*FAA-H*).

FAC was the first *FA* gene to be isolated, and this was achieved by expression cloning in 1992 (Figure 11.5). Four years later, two independent groups reported cloning of *FAA* by two different strategies (i.e. positional and expression cloning, respectively; Figure 11.6). In addition, *FAD* has been mapped to 3p22–26.

FAA and *FAC* encode two novel, ubiquitously expressed proteins of 163 and 63 kDa, respectively. *FAA* and *FAC* do not show any significant homology to other proteins or indeed to each other. Both proteins are primarily localised in the cytoplasm. Their function is not known, but it has been shown recently that FAA and FAC associate physically and, by virtue of the nuclear localisation signal of FAA, the complex can translocate to the nucleus.

Molecular pathology and population genetics. Mutations of *FAA* (Figure 11.6) account for about 60% of FA cases and are spread throughout the gene. None of the mutant alleles is common and few have been encountered more than once. Thus, identifying mutations in newly diagnosed cases of FA is laborious, as the entire coding sequence needs to be scanned.

Mutations in the *FAC* gene account for about 15% of FA cases. The IVS4+A→T and del322 mutations comprise >75% of *FAC* mutations. The IVS4+A→T allele is found in Ashkenazi Jews at a polymorphic frequency (1 in 80), and it is responsible for 85% of the FA cases in this population. Patients with IVS4 or exon 14 mutations tend to have earlier onset of haematological complications (BMF and MDS/AML), and to have a shorter survival compared to patients with exon 1 mutations or patients with non-*FAC*-related FA. This observation is potentially important for the

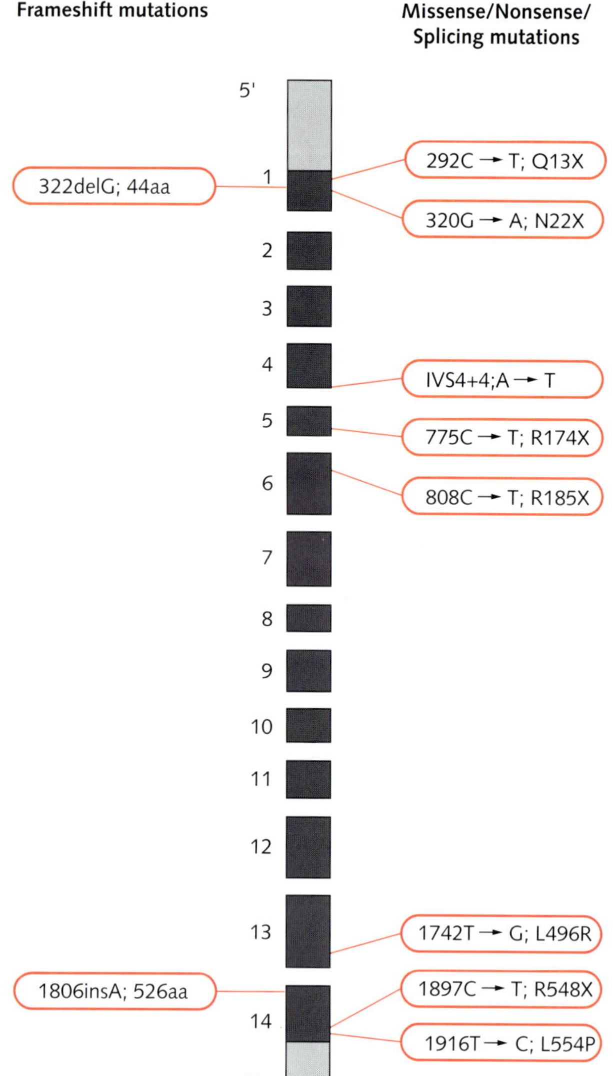

Fig. 11.5 The exon structure of *FAC* gene and its pathogenic mutations
FAC maps to 9q22.3. It spans an area of at least 150 kb and consists of 14 exons. Coding areas are shown in black, the 5′ and 3′ UTRs in grey. Three species of mRNA (2.3, 3.2 and 4.6 kb) have been identified and two of them are the result of alternative exons (exons −1 and −1a) at the 5′ region (not shown). The functional significance of these mRNA variants is not known. *FAC* encodes a protein of a predicted length of 558 amino acids.

functional mapping of *FAC*-and it also has practical implications with respect to management, as it can guide the selection of patients for early BMT.

The cloning of *FAA* and *FAC* has made genetic counselling and prenatal diagnosis possible, at least in principle, for most families with affected children. In areas with a large Ashkenazi Jewish population (e.g. New York City), screening for polymorphic FAC alleles is feasible on a wider basis and can be offered to all couples at risk.

Treatment of Fanconi's anaemia. The conventional management of FA must concentrate on treating the consequences of BMF and includes haematopoietic growth factors, blood product support and androgens. About half of the patients respond to androgens initially, but often suffer from significant side-effects, including androgen-induced hepatic adenomas. Eventually all patients become refractory.

Bone marrow transplantation (BMT) from an HLA-identical unaffected sibling or from alternative sources is currently the only therapeutic approach that can successfully achieve long-term correction of BMF and possible prevention of MDS and AML. Unfortunately, after BMT the patient remains at increased risk of developing solid tumours.

The cloning of *FAC* and *FAA* has opened the way to gene therapy of FA. Three patients with FA-C have been treated in a pilot study but without any apparent clinical benefit. Like in other inherited blood disorders, a major

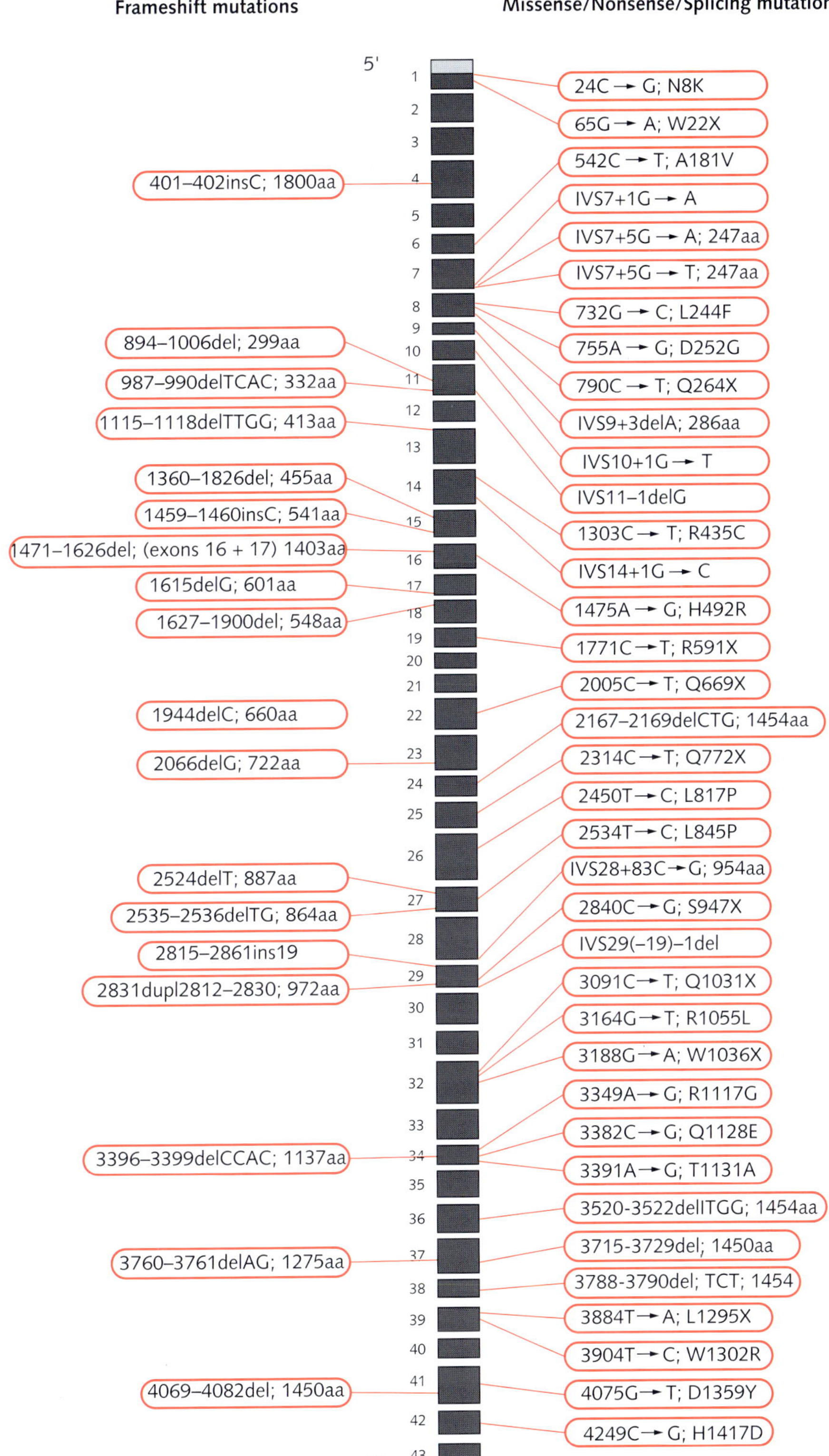

Fig. 11.6 The exon structure of *FAA* gene and its pathogenic mutations *FAA* maps to 16q24.3, spans an area of ~80 kb and consists of 43 exons. The major FAA mRNA transcript is 5.5 kb long with an open reading frame of 4.3 kb. It encodes a protein of a predicted length of 1455 amino acids.

limiting factor to gene therapy through the use of currently available retroviral vectors is that these require DNA replication for integrating into the host cell genome. Haematopoietic stem cells, the ideal targets for gene transfer by these vectors, are out of cycle most of the time.

Dyskeratosis congenita

Dyskeratosis congenita (DC) is another inherited disorder in which BMF is a major component of the clinical picture. The mode of inheritance in the majority of the cases (~85%) is X-linked recessive. In the remaining cases the inheritance is either autosomal dominant or autosomal recessive, again indicating genetic heterogeneity.

The triad of lacy reticulated skin pigmentation, nail dystrophy and BMF classically defines DC. Leucoplakia of the oral mucosa is also common, and similar lesions can occur elsewhere in the gastrointestinal and genital tracts; these lesions account, at least in part, for the increased propensity to solid tumours (12%). Other manifestations include ocular, dental and skeletal abnormalities, hyperhidrosis, hyperkeratinisation of the palms and soles, bullae on minimal trauma, developmental delay, short stature, hair loss and occasionally gonadal failure.

The X-linked form of DC was initially mapped to Xq28, and then more finely to a region of 1.4 Mb; this has led very recently to the successful positional cloning of a gene, now named *DKC1*, which, when mutated, causes DC. The genomic structure of *DKC1* has not yet been defined, but the *DKC1* cDNA is 2465 bp long and encodes a protein (named dyskerin) of 514 amino acids and a predicted molecular weight of 57.6 kDa. The function of dyskerin is unknown, but its high degree of homology with the rat nucleolar protein NAP57 and the yeast nucleolar protein Cbf5p makes it very likely that also in humans dyskerin plays an essential role in ribosome biosynthesis; specifically, in the maturation of the primary transcript of the ribosomal RNA genes (pre-rRNA). If so, DC could be regarded as the first example of a class of human diseases that could be called ribosomopathies.

As for FA, there is no definitive treatment for DC. The disease has certain features of premature ageing, and its natural history is such that most patients die before the age of 30 years, with the main causes of death being complications of BMF, opportunistic infections (cytomegalovirus (CMV), *Pneumocystis carinii*) and malignancy. Few patients have had successful correction of BMF by BMT.

Red cell enzyme deficiencies

Inherited abnormalities of red cell enzymes (*red cell enzymopathies*) are a distinct set of genetic disorders with one important clinical manifestation in common, namely chronic haemolytic anaemia. Most of the enzymes involved are housekeeping enzymes present—by definition—in all cells. Therefore one might expect that a severe reduction in activity of any of these might have generalized clinical manifestations.However, we can identify at least two reasons why red cells are more severely affected: firstly, red cells have a much more limited metabolic machinery than most other somatic cells; if a particular enzyme is deficient, other cells may cope by the use of alternative or surrogate metabolic pathways. Secondly, mature red cells are not competent for protein synthesis: therefore if a particular enzyme is made highly unstable by a mutation, other cells can compensate by increased enzyme synthesis, but red cells cannot. Nevertheless, the fact that enzymopathies are not purely red cell disorders is highlighted by the co-existence, in some cases, of clinical manifestations in other systems; particularly the muscle and the nervous system; indeed, in some enzymopathies neurological damage may dominate the clinical picture.

This section deals with those enzymopathies affecting red cell metabolism for which the molecular basis has been elucidated. We will not discuss conditions in which an enzyme abnormality is expressed also in red cells, but the main clinical manifestations are elsewhere (e.g. the porphyrias, galactosaemia, the Lesch–Nyhan syndrome). For the sake of brevity, most of the enzymopathies will be discussed in groups.

Enzymopathies of glycolysis

Clinical features

All of these defects are rare to very rare (Table 11.6), and all cause haemolytic anaemia with varying degrees of severity. It is not unusual for the presentation to be in the guise of severe neonatal jaundice which may require exchange transfusion; if the anaemia is less severe it may present later in life, or it may even remain asymptomatic and be detected incidentally when a blood count is done for unrelated reasons. The spleen is often enlarged. When other systemic manifestations occur, they involve the central nervous system, sometimes entailing severe mental retardation, or the neuromuscular system, or both.

Diagnosis

The diagnosis of haemolytic anaemia is usually not difficult, thanks to the triad of normomacrocytic anaemia, reticulocytosis and hyperbilirubinaemia. Enzymopathies should be considered in the differential diagnosis of any chronic Coombs-negative haemolytic anaemia. In most cases of glycolytic enzymopathies, the morphological abnormalities of red cells characteristically seen in membrane disorders are conspicuous by their absence. A definitive diagnosis can be made only by demonstrating the deficiency of an individual enzyme by a quantitative assay. For the sake of economy, it is sensible to carry out these rather laborious tests in order of frequency of occurrence of the various enzymopathies (e.g. first PK, then GPI, etc.; see Table 11.6). If a particular molecular abnormality is already known in the family, then of course one could test directly for that at the DNA level, bypassing the need for enzyme assays.

Molecular pathophysiology

Since the main physiological significance of the glycolytic pathway (*see Figure 11.7 for an overview of glycolysis*) in the red cell is to produce chemical energy in the form of ATP, the main consequence of any glycolytic enzymopathy is a shortage of energy supply. Since glycolytic enzymes are apparently present in cells in considerable excess, the 50% residual enzyme activity seen in heterozygotes does not become rate-limiting; thus, heterozygotes do not have haemolytic anaemia, and that is why these enzymopathies show a recessive pattern of inheritance. As seen in Table 11.6, the majority of mutations so far identified in the genes encoding glycolytic enzymes are of the missense type, causing single amino acid replacements. This is important, because the low level of residual enzyme activity can still support some metabolic flow through the glycolytic pathway, and helps explain how red cells survive in circulation, even though their lifespan is reduced. With respect to the precise reason why enzyme activity is reduced, we must consider at the protein level two basic mechanisms. (i) In the majority of cases loss of activity is probably due to a decreased stability of the protein. In such cases we would predict that other cells might be much less affected than red cells, because the former can compensate for decreased stability through increased synthesis of the enzyme. (ii) In some cases the amino acid replacement may affect the active centre of the enzyme which in turn may affect either substrate binding (Km) or the catalytic rate of the enzyme (Kcat), or both: in this case other cells in which the rate of glycolysis is critical will be affected, as well as red cells.

Management

There is no specific treatment for these conditions. Patients with moderate anaemia may require occasional blood transfusion when they experience exacerbations of the anaemia due to increased rate of haemolysis, or to decreased red cell production secondary to infection (the most extreme example being 'aplastic crisis' from parvovirus infection). Patients with chronic severe anaemia may require regular blood transfusion therapy with associated iron chelation. In some patients splenectomy has been beneficial. In severe cases BMT would be a rational form of treatment (for patients who have a suitable donor), provided there are no systemic manifestations other than haemolytic anaemia, and provided it is carried out before there is organ damage (e.g. from iron overload).

Glucose-6-phosphate dehydrogenase (G6PD) deficiency

Epidemiology

G6PD deficiency is distributed world-wide with a high prevalence in populations of Africa, southern Europe, the Middle East, South-East Asia and parts of Oceania, as well as in areas to which migrations from these areas have taken place. The overall geographic distribution of G6PD deficiency and its heterogeneity, together with clinical field studies and *in vitro* culture experiments, strongly support the view that this common genetic trait has been selected by *Plasmodium falciparum* malaria, by virtue of the fact that it confers a relative resistance against this highly lethal infection.

Clinical features

Three types of clinical presentations are well characterised:

1 The vast majority of G6PD-deficient people are asymptomatic most of the time, but they are at risk of developing acute haemolytic anaemia (AHA), which may be triggered by drugs, infections or fava beans.

2 The risk of developing neonatal jaundice (NNJ) is much greater in G6PD-deficient than in G6PD-normal newborns. This is of great public health importance, because untreated severe NNJ can lead to permanent neurological damage.

3 Chronic non-spherocytic haemolytic anaemia (CNSHA). This rare condition is rather similar to CNSHA associated with glycolytic enzymopathies (*see above*) and, again, it is of variable severity. However, it is

Table 11.6 Synopsis of red cell enzymopathies*.

Enzyme (abbreviation)	Isoenzyme[a] characteristic of red cells	Prevalence of enzyme deficiency	Main clinical features associated with enzyme deficiency[b]	Benefit from splenectomy[c]	Chromosomal localisation
Hexokinase (HK)	1	Very rare	HA	Partial	10q22 (q11?)
Glucose-6-phosphate isomerase (GPI)		Rare	HA, NM, CNS	Partial	19q13.1
Phosphofructokinase (PFK)[g]	M	Very rare	HA, myopathy		1cen–q32
	L				21q22.3
Aldolase	A	Very rare	HA, myopathy		16q22–24
Triosephosphate isomerase (TPI)		Very rare	HA, CNS, NM	None	12p13
Glyceraldehyde 3-phosphate dehydrogenase (GAPD)[j]		Very rare	HA		12p13.31–p13.1
Diphosphoglycerate mutase (DPGM)		Very rare	Polycythaemia		7q31–q34
Phosphoglycerate kinase (PGK)	1	Very rare	HA, CNS, NM	Partial	Xq13
Monophosphoglycerate mutase (PGAM-B)	B				10q25.3
Enolase[j]	1 (α)	Very rare	HA		1pter–p36.13
Pyruvate kinase (PK)	R[l]	Rare	HA	Partial	1q21
Glucose-6-phosphate dehydrogenase	B	Common	HA	None	Xq28
Cytochrome *b*5 reductase		Rare	Pseudo-cyanosis, CNS		22q13.31–qter
Adenylate kinase (AK)	1	Very rare	HA, CNS	Partial	9q34.1
γ-Glutamylcysteine synthetase (GLCLC)[j,p]		Very rare	HA, CNS(?)		6p12
Glutathione synthetase (GSS)		Very rare	HA, CNS		20q11.2
Glutathione peroxidase (GSH-Px)		Very rare[q]	?[q]		3q11–q12

* We have listed in the Table all enzymes in the intermediary metabolism of red cells for which, to the best of our knowledge, the corresponding cDNA/gene has been cloned. There are other enzymes the deficiency of which may be associated with HA, but for which no molecular information is yet available, e.g. pyrimidine 5′-nucleotidase.

a. No entry in this column means that there are no known isoenzymes; therefore it is assumed that the same enzyme type is present in all tissues.

b. The following abbreviations have been used: CNS, central nervous system involvement; HA, haemolytic anaemia; NM, neuromuscular manifestations.

c. Data available only on some patients.

d. Including N-terminal methionine which, in fact, is cleaved off in most or all cases.

e. Each individual molecular change, if observed in more than one patient, has been counted only once.

f. The only two HK mutations known were found in the same patient. They were: 529 Leu → Ser and Δ162–193.

g. PFK in normal red cells consists of a mixture of the five tetrameric species that can be formed from random association of the M (muscle) and L (liver) highly homologous subunits (i.e. M4, M3L, M2L2, ML3, L4).

h. The only known aldolase mutation is 128 Asp → Gly.

i. The known mutations of TPI are: 104 Gly → Asp, 122 Gly → Arg, 231 Val → Met, 240 Phe → Leu, 189 Arg → stop.

j. Since no mutations have yet been reported there is no formal proof that HA associated with this enzyme deficiency is due to mutation of the corresponding gene.

characteristically exacerbated by the same agents that can cause AHA in people with the ordinary type of G6PD deficiency.

Diagnosis

The anaemia is usually normocytic and normochromic, and may be from moderate to extremely severe. In AHA the anaemia is due largely to intravascular haemolysis, and hence is associated with haemoglobinaemia and haemoglobinuria. The blood film may show spectacular evidence of haemolysis in the guise of anisocytosis, polychromasia, spherocytes, bite cells, blister cells and hemighosts. Supravital staining reveals the presence of Heinz bodies, consisting of precipitates of denatured haemoglobin. In CNSHA the morphology is less characteristic. The final diagnosis must rely on the direct demonstration of decreased activity of G6PD in red cells by an appropriate enzyme assay.

Genetic basis

G6PD is a homodimeric molecule, and its single subunit is encoded by an X-linked gene. As a result of the phenomenon of X-chromosome inactivation in somatic cells, female heterozygotes are genetic mosaics, in whom

		Number of known mutations[e]							
					Deletion–Insertion				
Number of exons	Number of amino acids[d]	5′ UTR	Missense	Nonsense	In frame	With frameshift	Affecting splice	Total
22	917		1		3–0			4[f]
18	558		16	2			2	20
24	780		7	1		1–0	6	15
22	784							
12	364		2					2[h]
7	249	1	9	2		1–0		13[i]
9	335							
3	259		1		1–0			2[k]
11	417		8		1–0		2	11
	254							
	434							
12	574[l]	1	66	7	2–2	7–3	8	96
13	515		115[m]	1	6–0		1	123
9	276[n]		7	2	2–0		2	13
7	194		2	1				3[o]
	637							
12	474		14		1–0	1–0	1	17
	201							

k. The only two DPGM mutations known were found in the same patient; they were: 89 Arg → Cys and D C205 (or 206). The deletion causes a frameshift resulting in an abnormal protein of 46 amino acids in which only the first 19 N-terminal amino acids are correct.
l. The red cell form of PK called R is produced by the gene encoding the L (liver) subunit. Because a different promoter is used (*see Figure 11.5*) the size of liver PK is 543 amino acids.
m. The 89 missense mutations include two variants with normal activity, A and São Borja. Six variants have two missense mutations each: these include G6PD Santamaria, G6PD Mount Sinai and the three variants which are called G6PD A–, both of which have the mutation of G6PD A plus another mutation; and G6PD Honiara. G6PD Vancouver variant has three different missense mutations (*see Figure 11.6*).
n. The cytoplasmic form of this enzyme, present in red cells, differs from the microsomal form present in other cells because, as a result of an alternative splicing pathway, it lacks the first 25 N-terminal amino acids. Therefore in other cells the size of the enzyme is 301 amino acids.
o. The only AK mutation known is 128 Arg → Trp in exon 6.
p. γ-Glutamylcysteine synthetase consist of two subunits, a catalytic subunit and a regulatory subunit. The data concerning the catalytic subunit are shown here.
q. There is no clear evidence that inherited deficiency of glutathione peroxidase exists.
From L. Luzzatto and Notaro R. *Red Cell Enzymopathies*. In *Principles of Molecular Medicine*, J.L. Jameson (ed), Humana Press, NJ, pp. 197–207, 1998. With Permission.

approximately one-half of the red cells are normal and approximately one-half are G6PD deficient. However, in some cases the ratio is imbalanced. Therefore clinical manifestations, such as favism, can occur in both hemizygous males and heterozygous females, but they tend to be milder in the latter, roughly in proportion to the fraction of red cells that are G6PD deficient.

Molecular pathophysiology

AHA is seen with variants of G6PD whereby red cells retain some 10% of the normal G6PD activity, resulting from the limited capacity of such cells to withstand the oxidative action of an exogenous factor (oxidative haemolysis). By contrast, with other variants the steady-state level of G6PD is so low that it becomes limiting for red cell survival, even in the absence of any oxidant challenge: the result is CNSHA. Numerous point mutations in the *G6PD* gene causing CNSHA have been identified (Figure 11.8). Although we cannot explain the reason for a severe clinical phenotype in every case, a cluster of mutations causing CNSHA in exons 10 and 11 corresponds closely to the region of the molecule where the two subunits interface. It is not surprising that amino acid replacements in this region will interfere with dimer formation or will cause marked instability of the dimer.

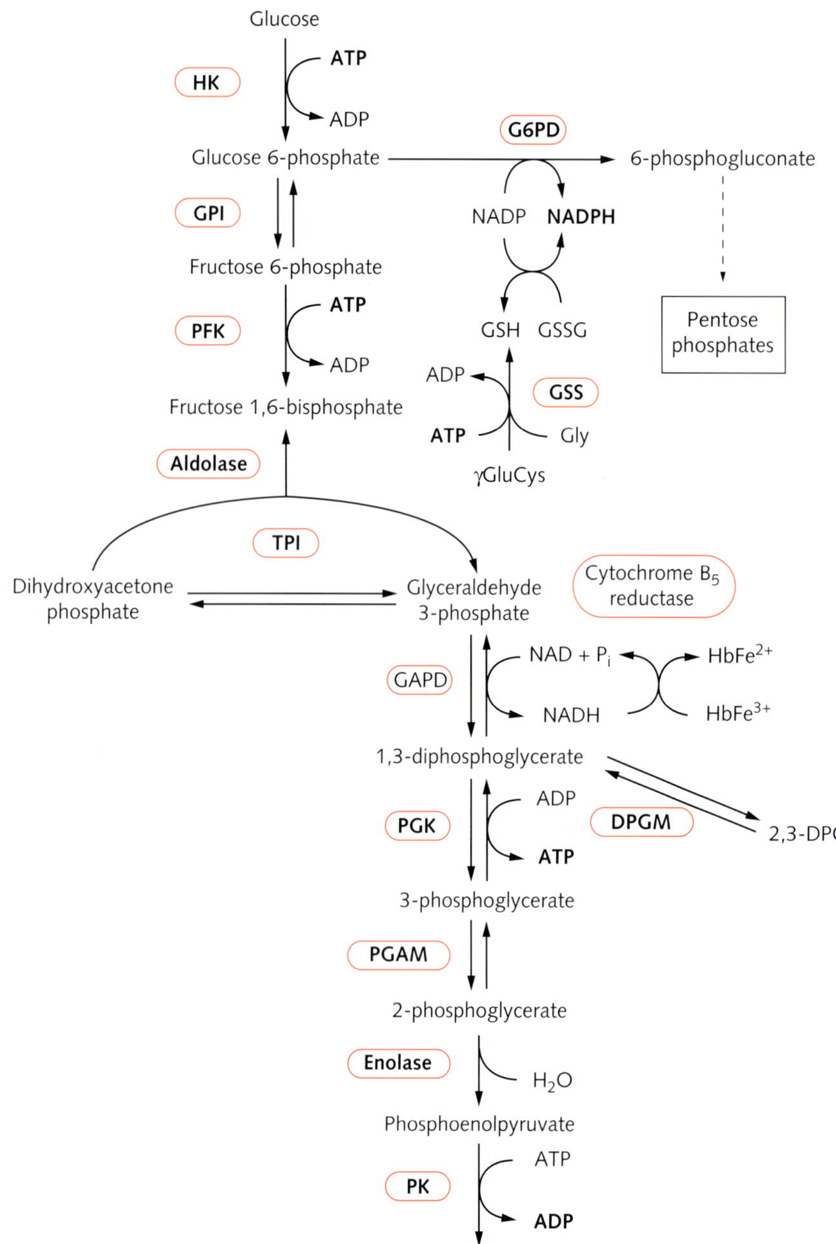

Fig. 11.7 Intermediary metabolism in red cells
The diagram shows the glycolytic pathway and related reactions (not the complete metabolic machinery of the red cells). Enzymes are enclosed in rounded boxes. Abbreviations as in Table 11.6. Additional abbreviations: DPG: diphosphoglycerate; GSH: reduced glutathione; GSSG: glutathione; $HbFe^{2+}$: haemoglobin; $HbFe^{3+}$: methaemoglobin; γGluCys: γ-glutamylcysteine. From Luzzatto L, Notaro R. (1998) Red cell enzymopathies. In: Jameson JL, ed. *Principles of Molecular Medicine*. New York: Humana Press.

Fig. 11.8 (Opposite.) Diagram of selected mutations in the G6PD gene
The G6PD genomic gene spans approximately 18 kb. (⬭) Variant with normal enzymatic activity. (⬭) Variant that causes acute haemolytic anaemia. (⬭) Variant that causes chronic non-spherocytic haemolytic anaemia (CNSHA). (a) In addition to the mutation shown this variant also has the mutation (454 Arg→Cys) of G6PD Andalus. (b) These variants have, in addition to the mutation shown, the mutation (126 Asn→Asp) of G6PD A. (c) This variant has been reported to have three different mutations: two are unique (106 Ser→Lys and 182 Arg→Trp), while one is the mutation (198 Arg→Cys) of G6PD Coimbra. (d) The deletion of the last two nucleotides of intron 10 destroys the acceptor site with unknown effect on the processing of the transcript. From Luzzatto L, Notaro R. (1998) Red cell enzymopathies. In: Jameson JL, ed. *Principles of Molecular Medicine*. New York: Humana Press.

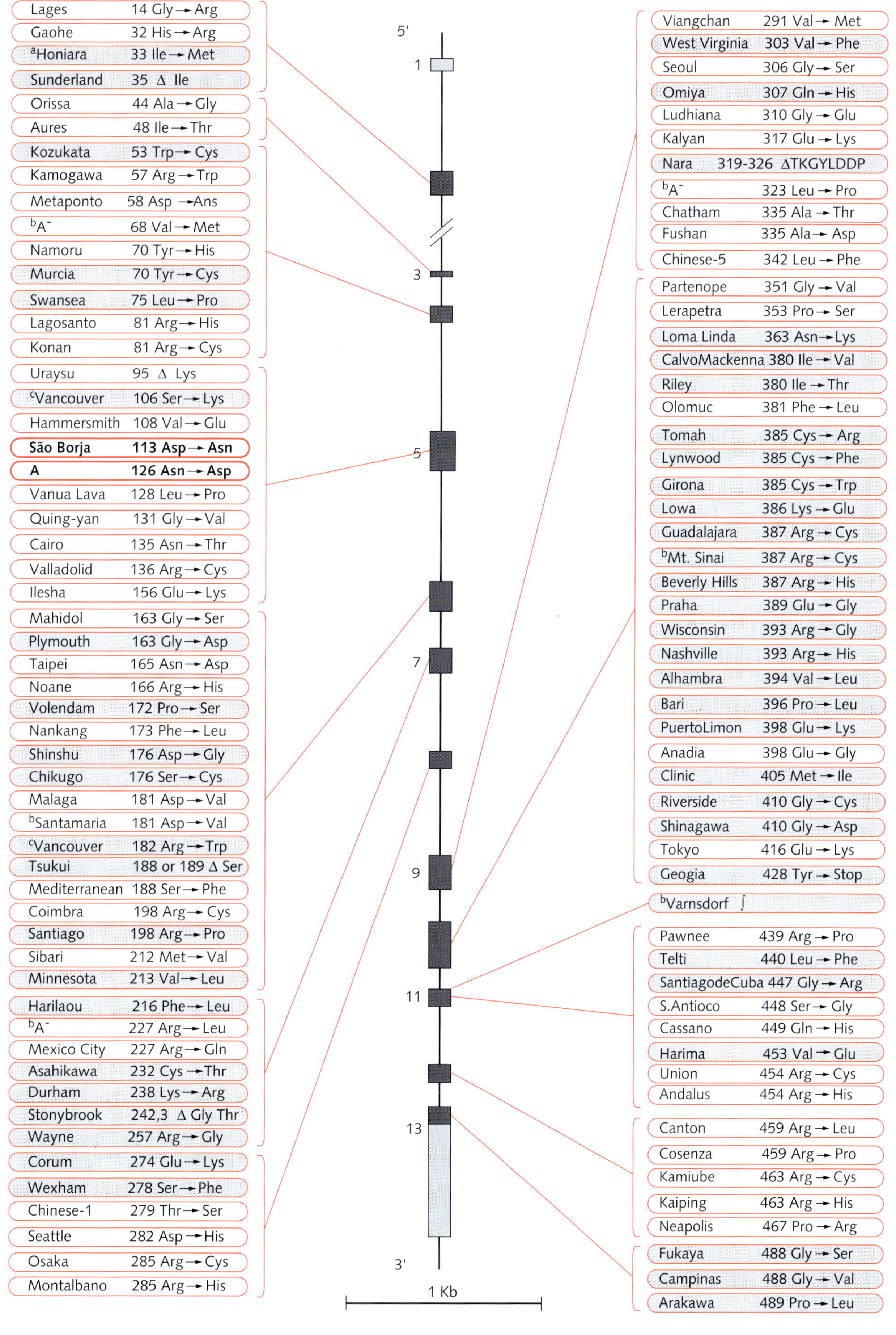

Lages 14 Gly → Arg
Gaohe 32 His → Arg
aHoniara 33 Ile → Met
Sunderland 35 Δ Ile
Orissa 44 Ala → Gly
Aures 48 Ile → Thr
Kozukata 53 Trp → Cys
Kamogawa 57 Arg → Trp
Metaponto 58 Asp → Ans
bA- 68 Val → Met
Namoru 70 Tyr → His
Murcia 70 Tyr → Cys
Swansea 75 Leu → Pro
Lagosanto 81 Arg → His
Konan 81 Arg → Cys
Uraysu 95 Δ Lys
cVancouver 106 Ser → Lys
Hammersmith 108 Val → Glu
São Borja 113 Asp → Asn
A 126 Asn → Asp
Vanua Lava 128 Leu → Pro
Quing-yan 131 Gly → Val
Cairo 135 Asn → Thr
Valladolid 136 Arg → Cys
Ilesha 156 Glu → Lys
Mahidol 163 Gly → Ser
Plymouth 163 Gly → Asp
Taipei 165 Asn → Asp
Noane 166 Arg → His
Volendam 172 Pro → Ser
Nankang 173 Phe → Leu
Shinshu 176 Asp → Gly
Chikugo 176 Ser → Cys
Malaga 181 Asp → Val
bSantamaria 181 Asp → Val
cVancouver 182 Arg → Trp
Tsukui 188 or 189 Δ Ser
Mediterranean 188 Ser → Phe
Coimbra 198 Arg → Cys
Santiago 198 Arg → Pro
Sibari 212 Met → Val
Minnesota 213 Val → Leu
Harilaou 216 Phe → Leu
bA- 227 Arg → Leu
Mexico City 227 Arg → Gln
Asahikawa 232 Cys → Thr
Durham 238 Lys → Arg
Stonybrook 242,3 Δ Gly Thr
Wayne 257 Arg → Gly
Corum 274 Glu → Lys
Wexham 278 Ser → Phe
Chinese-1 279 Thr → Ser
Seattle 282 Asp → His
Osaka 285 Arg → Cys
Montalbano 285 Arg → His
5'
1
3
5
7
9
11
13
3'
1 Kb
Viangchan 291 Val → Met
West Virginia 303 Val → Phe
Seoul 306 Gly → Ser
Omiya 307 Gln → His
Ludhiana 310 Gly → Glu
Kalyan 317 Glu → Lys
Nara 319-326 ΔTKGYLDDP
bA- 323 Leu → Pro
Chatham 335 Ala → Thr
Fushan 335 Ala → Asp
Chinese-5 342 Leu → Phe
Partenope 351 Gly → Val
Lerapetra 353 Pro → Ser
Loma Linda 363 Asn → Lys
CalvoMackenna 380 Ile → Val
Riley 380 Ile → Thr
Olomuc 381 Phe → Leu
Tomah 385 Cys → Arg
Lynwood 385 Cys → Phe
Girona 385 Cys → Trp
Lowa 386 Lys → Glu
Guadalajara 387 Arg → Cys
bMt. Sinai 387 Arg → Cys
Beverly Hills 387 Arg → His
Praha 389 Glu → Gly
Wisconsin 393 Arg → Gly
Nashville 393 Arg → His
Alhambra 394 Val → Leu
Bari 396 Pro → Leu
PuertoLimon 398 Glu → Lys
Anadia 398 Glu → Gly
Clinic 405 Met → Ile
Riverside 410 Gly → Cys
Shinagawa 410 Gly → Asp
Tokyo 416 Glu → Lys
Geogia 428 Tyr → Stop
bVarnsdorf ∫
Pawnee 439 Arg → Pro
Telti 440 Leu → Phe
SantiagodeCuba 447 Gly → Arg
S.Antioco 448 Ser → Gly
Cassano 449 Gln → His
Harima 453 Val → Glu
Union 454 Arg → Cys
Andalus 454 Arg → His
Canton 459 Arg → Leu
Cosenza 459 Arg → Pro
Kamiube 463 Arg → Cys
Kaiping 463 Arg → His
Neapolis 467 Pro → Arg
Fukaya 488 Gly → Ser
Campinas 488 Gly → Val
Arakawa 489 Pro → Leu

Management

The commonest manifestations of G6PD deficiency, NNJ and AHA, are largely preventable or controllable by screening, surveillance and avoidance of triggering factors, particularly fava beans, by G6PD-deficient subjects. When a patient presents with AHA, and once the cause is diagnosed, no specific treatment may be needed if the episode is mild. At the other end of the spectrum, and especially in children, AHA may be a medical emergency requiring immediate blood transfusion. The management of NNJ does not differ from that of NNJ due to causes other than G6PD deficiency and, in order to prevent neurological damage, treatment with phototherapy and/or exchange blood transfusion may be required. The management of CNSHA is similar to that of CNSHA due to glycolytic enzymopathies, but in addition it is important to avoid exposure to potentially haemolytic drugs. Again, although there is no evidence of selective red cell destruction in the spleen (as seen in hereditary spherocytosis), splenectomy has proven beneficial in severe cases.

Conclusions

Haematologists know only too well that anaemia is not a diagnosis, but the recognition of a sign for which we must find the cause and work out the pathogenetic mechanism, which ultimately must be explainable at the molecular level. Overall, in terms of aetiology things are pretty clear with respect to the majority of acquired anaemias, but not necessarily with respect to molecular mechanisms. For instance, although we do understand that iron deficiency limits haem synthesis and consequently haemoglobin synthesis, we do not know exactly how the mean cell volume (MCV) is controlled by the supply of iron (for this reason we have omitted from this chapter a section on the commonest anaemia of all—iron deficiency anaemia). However, it is gratifying that we could at least offer a model for the molecular basis of megaloblastic anaemia; and that the molecular basis of one of the most severe forms of acquired haemolytic anaemia, PNH, has now been elucidated (only in the last 5 years). By contrast, for the majority of congenital anaemias, and certainly for the commonest amongst them, molecular genetics has answered most of the questions with respect to aetiology and pathogenesis. However, lest we become complacent, we must admit that the outlook for patients who have, for instance, a severe chronic haemolytic disease due to PK deficiency has only improved because we can offer better supportive treatment, not because we know the molecular basis. The latter will only become relevant once we learn to correct the PK deficiency by gene addition or by gene replacement. This is a major and worthy challenge for the next decade with respect to all the genetically determined anaemias.

Further reading

Megaloblastic anaemia and congenital dyserythropoietic anaemias

Blount BC, Mack MM, Wehr CM *et al.* (1997) Folate deficiency causes uracil misincorporation into human DNA and chromosome breakage: Implications for cancer and neuronal damage. *Proceedings of the National Academy of Sciences (USA)*, **94**, 3290–3295.

Chanarin I. (1979) *The Megaloblastic Anaemias*, 2nd edn. Oxford: Blackwell Scientific Publications.

Chui D, Oh-Eda M, Liao YF *et al.* (1997) Alpha-mannosidase-II deficiency results in dyserythropoiesis and unveils an alternate pathway in oligosaccharide biosynthesis. *Cell*, **90**, 157–167.

Fukuda MN. (1990) HEMPAS disease: genetic defect of glycosylation. *Glycobiology*, **1**, 9–15.

Ingram CF, Davidoff AN, Marais E, Sherman GG, Mendelow BV. (1997) Evaluation of DNA analysis for evidence of apoptosis in megaloblastic anaemia. *British Journal of Haematology*, **96**, 576–583.

Luzzatto L, Falusi AO, Joju EA. (1981) Uracil in DNA in megaloblastic anemia. *New England Journal of Medicine*, **305**, 1156.

Savage DG, Lindenbaum J. (1995) Folate–cobalamin interactions. In: Bailey L, ed. *Folate in Health and Disease*. New York: Marcel Dekker, pp. 237–285.

Wickramasinghe SN. (1997) Dyserythropoiesis and congenital dyserythropoietic anaemias. *British Journal of Haematology*, **98**, 785–797.

Wickramasinghe SN, Fida S. (1994) Bone marrow cells from vitamin B12- and folate-deficient patients misincorporate uracil into DNA. *Blood*, **83**, 1656–1661.

The sideroblastic anaemias

Sideroblastic anaemia

Bottomley SS, May BK, Cox TC, Cotter PD, Bishop DF. (1995) Molecular defects of erythroid 5-aminolevulinate synthase in X-linked sideroblastic anemia. *Journal of Bioenergetics and Biomembranes*, **27**, 161–168.

Cox TC, Bawden MJ, Martin A, May B. (1991) Human erythroid 5-aminolevulinate synthase: promoter analysis and identification of an iron responsive element in the mRNA. *EMBO Journal*, **10**, 1891–1902.

May A, Bishop DF. (1998) The molecular biology and pyridoxine responsiveness of X-linked sideroblastic anaemia. *Haematologica*, **83**, 56–70.

Pearson marrow-pancreas syndrome

Pearson HA, Lobel GS, Kocoshis SA *et al.* (1979) A new syndrome of refractory sideroblastic anemia with vacuolization of marrow precursors and exocrine pancreatic dysfunction. *Journal of Pediatrics*, **6**, 976–984.

Rotig A, Bourgeron T, Chretien D, Rustin P, Munnich A. (1995) Spectrum of mitochondrial DNA rearrangements in the Pearson marrow-pancreas syndrome. *Human Molecular Genetics*, **4**, 1327–1330.

Bone marrow failure syndromes

Aplastic anaemia

Young NS, Barrett AJ. (1995) The treatment of severe acquired aplastic anemia. *Blood*, **85**, 3367–3377.

Young NS, Maciejewski J. (1997) The pathophysiology of acquired aplastic anemia. *New England Journal of Medicine*, **336**, 1365–1372.

Paroxysmal nocturnal haemoglobinuria

Luzzatto L, Bessler M. (1996) The dual pathogenesis of paroxysmal nocturnal hemoglobinuria. *Seminars in Hematology*, **3**, 101–110.

Miyata T, Takeda J, Iida Y *et al.* (1993) The cloning of PIG-A, a component in the early step of GPI-anchor biosynthesis. *Science*, **259**, 1318–1320.

Rosti V, Tremml G, Soares V *et al.* (1997) Embryonic stem cells without pig-a gene activity are competent for hematopoiesis with the PNH phenotype but not for clonal expansion. *Journal of Clinical Investigation*, **100**, 1028–1036.

Rotoli B, Luzzatto L. (1989) Paroxysmal nocturnal haemoglobinuria. *Baillière's Clinical Haematology*, **2**, 113–138.

Fanconi's anaemia

Alter B, Young NS. (1998) The bone marrow failure syndromes. In: *Nathan and Oski's Hematology of Infancy and Childhood*, 5th edn. WB Saunders, pp. 237–335.

D'Andrea AD, Grompe M. (1997) Molecular biology of Fanconi anemia: implications for diagnosis and therapy. *Blood*, **90**, 1725–1736.

Foe JRLT, Roimans MA, Bosnoyan-Collins L *et al.* (1996) Expression cloning of a cDNA for the major Fanconi anaemia gene, FAA. *Nature Genetics*, **14**, 320–323.

Kupfer GM, Näf D, Suliman A, Pulshipher M, D'Andrea AD. (1997) The Fanconi anaemia proteins, FAA and FAC, interact to form a nuclear complex. *Nature Genetics*, **17**, 487–490.

Levran O, Erlich T, Magdalena N *et al.* (1997) Sequence variation in the Fanconi anemia gene FAA. *Proceedings of the National Academy of Sciences (USA)*, **94**, 13051–13056.

Strathdee CA, Gavish H, Shannon WR, Buchwald M. (1992) Cloning of cDNAs for Fanconi's anaemia by functional complementation. *Nature*, **356**, 763–767.

The Fanconi anaemia/Breast cancer consortium. (1996) Positional cloning of the Fanconi anaemia group A gene. *Nature Genetics*, **14**, 324–328.

Dyskeratosis congenita

Dokal I. (1996) Dyskeratosis congenita: an inherited bone marrow failure syndrome. *British Journal of Haematology*, **92**, 775–779.

Heiss NS, Knight SW, Vulliamy JT *et al.* (1998) X-linked dyskeratosis congenita is caused by mutations in a highly conserved gene with putative nucleolar functions. *Nature Genetics*, **19**, 32–38.

Sirinavin C, Trowbridge AA. (1975) Dyskeratosis congenita: clinical features and genetic aspects. *Journal of Medical Genetics*, **12**, 339–354.

Red cell enzyme deficiencies

Beutler E. (1994) Glucose-6-phosphate dehydrogenase deficiency. *New England Journal of Medicine*, **324**, 169–174.

Luzzatto L, Mehta A. (1995) Glucose-6-phosphate dehydrogenase deficiency. In: Scriver CR, Beaudet AL, Sly WS, Valle D, eds. *The Metabolic and Molecular Basis of Inherited Disease*, 7th edn. New York: McGraw-Hill, pp. 3367–3398.

Mentzer WC. (1998) Pyruvate kinase deficiency and disorders of glycolysis. In: *Nathan and Oski's Hematology of Infancy and Childhood*, 5th edn. WB Saunders, pp. 665–703.

Tanaka KR, Paglia DE. (1995) Pyruvate deficiency and other enzymopathies of the erythrocyte. In: Scriver CR, Beaudet AL, Sly WS, Valle D, eds. *The Metabolic and Molecular Basis of Inherited Disease*, 7th edn. New York: McGraw-Hill, pp. 3485–3491.

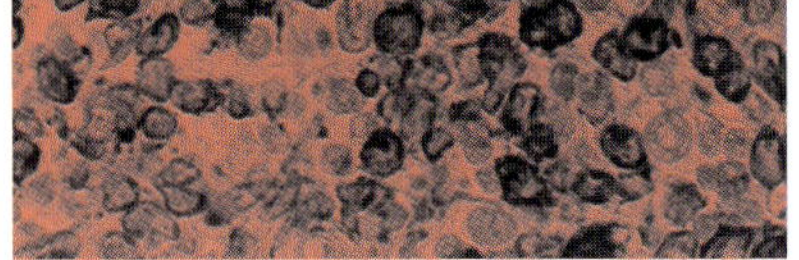

Chapter 12 Molecular coagulation and thrombophilia

Björn Dahlbäck & Andreas Hillarp

Introduction

The risk of venous thrombosis is increased when the haemostatic balance between pro- and anticoagulant forces is shifted in favour of coagulation. If this is caused by an inherited defect, the resulting hypercoagulable state conveys a lifelong increased risk of thrombosis. Inherited resistance to activated protein C (APC-resistance) is the most common hypercoagulable state found associated with venous thrombosis. It is caused by a single point mutation in the factor V (FV) gene, predicting the substitution of Arg^{506} with Gln. The FV gene mutation (FV:Q^{506}) confers a 5–10-fold increased risk of thrombosis and is found in 20–60% of Caucasian patients with thrombosis. Another common inherited risk factor for thrombosis is a point mutation (G20210A) in the 3′ untranslated region of the prothrombin gene. This mutation is present in approximately 1–3% of healthy individuals and is associated with an approximately threefold increased risk of thrombosis. Other less common genetic risk factors for thrombosis are the deficiencies of natural anticoagulant proteins such as antithrombin, protein C or protein S. Such defects are present in less than 1% of healthy individuals and together account for 5–10% of genetic defects found in patients with venous thrombosis. Owing to the high prevalence of FV:Q^{506} and of the G20210A mutation in the prothrombin gene, combinations of genetic defects are relatively common in the general population. As each genetic defect is an independent risk factor of thrombosis, individuals with multiple defects have a highly increased risk of thrombosis, and multiple defects are consequently often found in patients with thrombosis.

Blood coagulation

At sites of vascular damage, circulating platelets adhere to subendothelial structures and undergo a series of reactions which lead to primary haemostasis due to the formation of a platelet plug. Concomitant to these events, the subendothelial membrane protein tissue factor (TF) is exposed to blood. A small amount of activated factor VII (FVIIa) present in circulating blood binds to TF and triggers a series of proteolytic reactions which culminate in the formation of thrombin and the conversion of fibrinogen to insoluble fibrin.

FVIIa bound to TF specifically cleaves and activates the two vitamin K-dependent plasma proteins, factor IX (FIX) and factor X (FX) (Plate 12.1, facing page 128). Activated FX (FXa) activates prothrombin to thrombin, whereas activated FIX (FIXa) activates FX. Both FIXa and FXa are poor enzymes which require protein cofactors, calcium ions and negatively charged phospholipid surfaces for expression of full biological activity. The protein cofactors for FIXa and FXa are the activated forms of factor VIII (FVIIIa) and factor V (FVa), respectively. As a result of multiple protein–protein and protein–phospholipid interactions, enzymatically highly efficient complexes are assembled on the phospholipid surface.

The initiation of blood coagulation by TF is usually referred to as the *extrinsic pathway* or the TF pathway. In association with injury, this is the physiologically most important mechanism of blood coagulation. However, coagulation can also be activated through the *intrinsic pathway* which is triggered by the activation of the contact phase proteins (FXII, FXI, prekallikrein and high molecular weight kininogen) which follows upon exposure of blood to certain negatively charged surfaces.

The intrinsic pathway does not appear to be physiologically important for injury-related coagulation *in vivo* illustrated by the lack of bleeding problems in individuals with deficiency of FXII.

Thrombin generated at sites of vascular injury expresses a number of procoagulant properties. It amplifies the coagulation process by activating FXI and in addition it activates platelets and converts fibrinogen to fibrin. Moreover, in a positive feedback reaction, thrombin converts the procofactors FV and FVIII into their biologically active counterparts (FVa and FVIIIa).

Regulation of blood coagulation

The efficient reactions of the coagulation system have considerable biological potential and strict regulation is required. For this purpose, several plasma proteins and protein–cell interactions are involved in the constant sensoring of the circulation. At each level of the coagulation pathway, membrane-bound molecules expressed on the surface of intact endothelial cells, circulating inhibitors and negative feedback mechanisms provide efficient control.

Antithrombin (AT) is the most important serine protease inhibitor (serpin) involved in the regulation of blood coagulation. AT inhibits thrombin as well as FXIa, FIXa and FXa and, under certain conditions, also FVIIa. AT forms a highly stable complex with the protease and, as a consequence, the protease is trapped and eliminated from the circulation. The activity of AT is stimulated by heparin which accelerates the rate of formation of the AT-protease complexes. Under normal physiological conditions, heparan sulphate proteoglycans present on the endothelial cell surface stimulate the activity of AT, whereas heparin injections are used in clinical situations. During inhibition of thrombin, an important role of heparin is to function as a bridge between thrombin and AT. In addition, heparin induces conformational changes in AT which are associated with the generation of a more efficient inhibitor. In the inhibition of FXa, the conformational change appears to be more important than the bridging mechanism.

The TF pathway is regulated by the tissue factor pathway inhibitor (TFPI). TFPI is composed of three protease inhibitory domains belonging to the Kunitz type of inhibitors. TFPI has the unique capacity to inhibit the FVIIa–TF–FXa complex and is therefore highly efficient in turning off the TF pathway. The inhibition mediated by TFPI occurs in two steps, the first being inhibition of FXa by the middle Kunitz domain and the first Kunitz domain then binds and inhibits FVIIa. The majority of TFPI is bound to glucosaminoglycans on endothelial cells (approximately 80%) and only a minor fraction of TFPI is present in plasma where it is mainly associated with low density lipoproteins.

The highly efficient procoagulant reactions of thrombin are physiologically adequate at sites of vascular injury and are instrumental for efficient haemostasis. However, the same reactions pose a threat to the organism as uncontrolled coagulation leads to thrombus formation. Nature has solved this dilemma in intricate and fascinating ways, one of which is the transformation of thrombin into an efficient initiator of a natural anticoagulant pathway, the protein C system. The conversion of thrombin from a procoagulant into an anticoagulant enzyme depends on the presence of intact endothelium. Thus, thrombin generated at sites of intact vasculature binds to the endothelial membrane protein thrombomodulin, which is a potent modulator of thrombin activity and a cofactor to thrombin in the activation of protein C (Plate 12.2). APC inactivates membrane-bound FVa and FVIIIa by limited proteolysis in a reaction which is potentiated by a cofactor protein designated protein S and also by the non-activated form of FV (Plate 12.3).

Under physiological conditions, pro- and anticoagulant mechanisms are balanced in favour of anticoagulation, whereas the anticoagulant system is downregulated and procoagulant forces prevail at sites of vascular damage. Defects in this ingenious system are associated with increased thrombin generation, a hypercoagulable state, leading to an increased risk of thrombosis.

The protein C anticoagulant system

Protein C is a vitamin K-dependent plasma protein which is synthesised mainly in the liver. It is homologous to FVII, FIX and FX and shares with them a common modular organisation. From the N-terminus, these proteins contain a vitamin K-dependent γ-carboxy glutamic acid (Gla)-rich module, two epidermal growth factor (EGF)-like modules and a serine protease (SP) module. The Gla-domains bind calcium ions and provide the vitamin K-dependent clotting proteins with phospholipid-binding properties. Upon activation by the thrombin–thrombomodulin complex, the SP module is converted to an active enzyme. APC is highly specific in its proteolytic activity cleaving a limited number of peptide bonds in FVa and FVIIIa.

Intact FV is a high molecular weight protein and shares with the homologous FVIII molecule the modular arrangement: A1, A2, B, A3, C1 and C2. Upon activation of FV by thrombin or FXa, peptide bonds surrounding the B-module are cleaved and the B-module is not part of FVa. FVIII is activated by thrombin in a similar fashion which leads to release of the B-module. APC cleaves three peptide bonds in FVa at Arg^{306}, Arg^{506} and Arg^{679}, whereas FVIIIa is cleaved at Arg^{336} and Arg^{526}. As a consequence of the APC-mediated cleavages, FVa and FVIIIa lose their procoagulant properties.

APC alone has poor anticoagulant activity and it is only in the presence of its two cofactors protein S and FV (but not FVa) that efficient anticoagulant function is expressed. In an experimental system based on the degradation of FVIIIa, FV loses its APC-cofactor activity upon proteolysis by thrombin. Concomitantly, it gains procoagulant properties as a cofactor to FXa. Thus, FV is similar to thrombin in being able to express both pro- and anticoagulant effects. The mechanism by which FV functions as an APC-cofactor remains to be elucidated.

Protein S is also a vitamin K-dependent plasma protein, but unlike the other vitamin K-dependent coagulation proteins it is not an SP. It is a multimodular protein containing a Gla-module, a thrombin-sensitive module, four EGF-like modules and a large module homologous to sex hormone-binding globulin (SHBG) (*see Figure 12.4*). Protein S also has functions outside the protein C system and 60–70% of protein S in plasma circulates bound to C4b-binding protein (C4BP), a regulator of the complement system. The Gla-module of protein S provides the protein S-C4BP complex with phospholipid-binding ability which may be important for the localisation of the complement regulatory activity of C4BP to certain cell surfaces.

During the degradation of 'free' FVa (i.e. not bound to FXa) by APC, the cleavage at Arg^{506} is faster than that at Arg^{306}. The cleavage at Arg^{506} leads only to partial loss of FVa activity, whereas the cleavage at Arg^{306} leads to efficient inactivation of FVa. Protein S appears to serve as cofactor for the cleavage at Arg^{306} but not for the Arg^{506} cleavage. This, taken together with a specific protection of the Arg^{506} site exerted by FXa, indicates that the Arg^{306} site is the most important site for regulation of FVa activity in the prothrombinase complex. On the other hand, FVa which is not part of a prothrombinase complex is first cleaved at the Arg^{506} site, because the kinetics of this cleavage are more favourable than those for the cleavage site at Arg^{306}. Protein S also expresses APC-independent anticoagulant activity due to inhibition of prothrombin activation through direct interactions with FVa, FXa and the phospholipid membrane. Regardless of its mode of action, protein S is an important anticoagulant protein *in vivo* as demonstrated by animal studies and by the association between protein S deficiency and venous thrombosis.

Molecular genetics of venous thromboembolism

The annual incidence of venous thrombosis in Western societies is approximately 1–2 per 1000. Thrombotic episodes tend to occur in conjunction with surgery, fractures, pregnancy, the use of oral contraceptives and immobilisation. In addition, genetic defects are frequently involved and many patients report positive family histories. Genetic defects known to predispose for thrombosis include inherited APC resistance due to a single point mutation in the FV gene leading to replacement of Arg^{506} with Gln, a point mutation in the prothrombin gene (G20210A) and deficiencies of anticoagulant protein C, protein S or AT.

Factor V gene mutation (FV:Q^{506}) causing APC resistance

In 1993, APC resistance was described as a cause of inherited thrombophilia and it was soon demonstrated to be highly prevalent (20–60%) among thrombosis patients. In APC resistance, APC does not give a normal prolongation of the clotting time. In more than 95% of cases the molecular defect associated with APC resistance is a single point mutation in the FV gene. The mutation is a G $\rightarrow$ A substitution at nucleotide position 1691 in the FV gene, which predicts replacement of Arg^{506} with a Gln (Figure 12.1). The mutant FV is known as $FVR^{506}Q$, FVLeiden or FV:Q^{506} (R and Q are one-letter codes for Arg and Gln, respectively).

The FV:Q^{506} allele is found only in Caucasians, and the prevalence of the mutant FV:Q^{506} allele in the general population of Western societies demonstrates considerable variation. High prevalence (up to 15%) is found in southern Sweden, in Germany, Greece and Israel. In The Netherlands, UK and USA around 3–5% of the population carry the mutant allele. Lower prevalence (around 2%) is found in Hispanics. Within the same country there exist major differences, for example 1% carry the allele in Lille whereas the corresponding number in Strasbourg is 10%. The prevalence in a population depends upon a number of factors including the prevalence of the mutation among individuals who founded the society (*founder effect*). The high prevalence of the FV:Q^{506} allele in certain populations suggests a possible survival advantage associated with the mutation, for example a reduced bleeding risk after delivery in women carrying the mutation. In the history of mankind, the slightly increased thrombosis risk associated with the FV:Q^{506} allele has presumably not been a negative survival factor because thrombosis develops relatively late in life and does not influence fertility. In addition, many

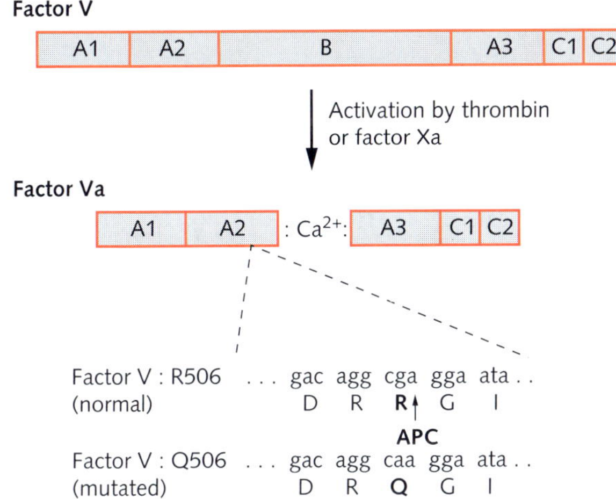

Fig. 12.1 APC resistance due to a mutation in factor V
FV is a large single chain glycoprotein with the modular organisation A1–A2–B–A3–C1–C2. FV is converted to FVa via limited proteolysis by thrombin or FXa. The FVa molecule is composed of a heavy chain (A1 and A2 domains) and a light chain (A3, C1 and C2 domains), which are linked by Ca^{2+}-dependent bonds. The nucleotide and the translated amino acid sequences around the APC cleavage site at position 506 in the A2 domain are shown. In the mutated FV:Q^{506} molecule, a single guanine (g) to adenine (a) mutation at nucleotide position 1691 in the *FV* gene predicts the replacement of arginine 506 (R) by a glutamine (Q). This substitution prevents the APC-mediated inactivation of FVa at this cleavage site.

of the circumstantial risk factors for thrombosis such as a sedentary life style, surgery and the use of oral contraceptives did not affect our ancestors.

The high prevalence of the FV:Q^{506} allele in Western societies is the result of a founder effect. It has been estimated that the mutation event was around 30,000 years ago, i.e. after the 'Out of Africa March' which took place 100,000 years ago and also after the separation of the Asians from the Europeans. This explains why the mutant FV allele is common among European populations, but not present among Japanese, Chinese or in the original populations of Africa, Australia or America.

A large number of studies have demonstrated relationships to exist between the presence of APC resistance (FV : Q^{506} allele) and an increased risk of venous thrombosis. Differences in selection criteria of patients and in the prevalence of the mutant allele in the general population, explain the wide variation in results obtained from different studies. However, the general consensus is that the FV : Q^{506} allele is the most common genetic risk factor for venous thrombosis in Western societies. The odds ratio, describing the increased risk of thrombosis in affected individuals, has been calculated to be six- to eightfold for those carrying the defect in a heterozygous form, whereas homozygous individuals are at 30–140-fold increased risk of thrombosis. The FV : Q^{506} allele does not appear to be a strong risk factor for arterial thrombosis, such as myocardial infarction. However, under certain circumstances it still appears that the FV mutation may be a risk factor for myocardial infarction. For example, it has been found that the FV mutation increases the risk of myocardial infarction in young female smokers.

Two different mutations affecting the Arg^{306} site have recently been found in thrombosis cases but such mutations appear to be extremely rare, and it is still uncertain whether they result in APC resistance and if they are risk factors for thrombosis.

The FV : Q^{506} allele is associated with a hypercoagulable state which is reflected by increased levels of prothrombin activation fragments in plasma of individuals with inherited APC resistance. Two molecular mechanisms are involved: one is that an APC cleavage site in FVa is lost, which impairs the normal degradation of FVa by APC; the other surprising observation is that FV : Q^{506} is a poor APC-cofactor in the degradation of FVIIIa.

In the degradation of normal FVa, the APC cleavage at Arg^{506} has favourable kinetics as compared to cleavages at other sites. The Arg^{506} cleavage is approximately 10-fold faster than the cleavage at Arg^{306} and the activity of FVa : Q^{506} is therefore inhibited at approximately 10-fold lower rate than FVa : R^{506}. Generated FVa persists longer and can form active prothrombinase complexes with FXa. However, degradation of 'free FVa' (i.e. FVa not bound to FXa) is different from that of FVa which is part of the prothrombinase complex. In the prothrombinase complex, the Arg^{506} site is protected by FXa from degradation by APC. In addition, protein S functions as an APC-cofactor primarily for the Arg^{306} cleavage and not for the one at Arg^{506}. As a consequence, APC-mediated degradation of FVa which is part of the prothrombinase complex follows a different pathway compared to that of free FVa. Therefore, when FVa : R^{506} and FVa: Q^{506} are part of assembled prothrombinase complexes, the rates of their degradation by APC plus protein S are similar.

Laboratory investigation of inherited APC-resistance due to the FV : Q^{506} allele can be done both with a functional APC-resistance test and with molecular biology assays. A modified APC-resistance test involving dilution of the patient's plasma in FV-deficient plasma is highly sensitive and specific for the presence of the FV : Q^{506} allele. The most commonly used molecular biology assay for FV : Q^{506} involves polymerase chain reaction (PCR) amplification and restriction enzyme digestion.

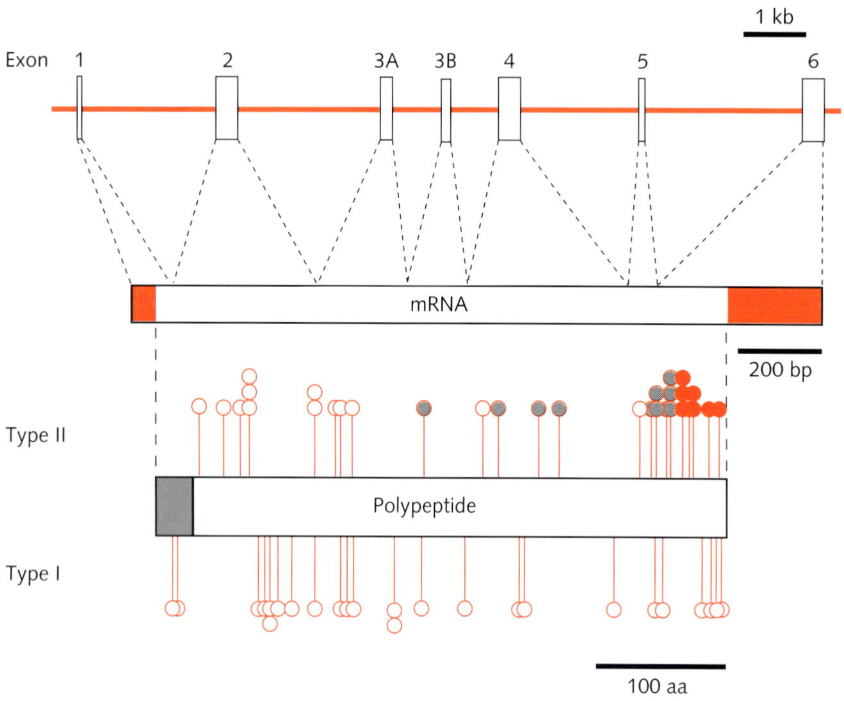

Fig. 12.2 Structure of the human antithrombin gene *AT3* and location of detrimental missense mutations in the antithrombin molecule
The gene for AT is localised to chromosome 1 (1q23–q25) and spans 13.4 kilobases (kb) of DNA (upper part). It is comprised of seven exons and results in an mRNA of 1.7 kb (middle part). The AT molecule (lower part) is synthesised as a single polypeptide chain composed of a 432 amino acid residue mature protein and a signal peptide (shaded) of 32 amino acid residues. Many mutations of different types causing AT deficiency have been described. Shown here are only missense mutations leading to amino acid substitutions associated with type I deficiency (○ indicated below the polypeptide chain) or type II deficiency (open, shaded and filled circles denote type II HBS, type II RS and type II PE variants, respectively).

Deficiency of antithrombin

Heterozygous AT deficiency is found in between 1 per 2000 and 1 per 5000 of the general population and in 1–2% of thrombosis patients suggesting the genetic defect to be associated with a 10–20-fold increased risk of thrombosis, i.e. somewhat higher than estimated for APC resistance. AT deficiency may be of either type I or type II. Type I deficiency is characterised by low levels of both immunological and functional AT, whereas type II denotes functional defects. Type II cases are divided into three subtypes, RS (reactive site mutants), HBS (heparin-binding site mutants) or PE (mutants giving pleiotropic effects). A large number of AT deficiencies have been analysed genetically (Figure 12.2). In the majority of cases, the genetic defect is either a point mutation, a small deletion or an insertion. Partial or whole gene deletions are relatively uncommon causes of AT deficiency. Type II RS variants are defective in protease inactivation and mutations in the vicinity of the reactive site have been found. The type II HBS deficiency carries mutations in the heparin-binding site and type II PE AT variants are caused by a limited number of mutations between amino acids 402 and 429.

Protein C deficiency

Heterozygous deficiency of protein C is identified in 2–5% of thrombosis patients. The prevalence of protein C deficiency in the population is estimated to be approximately 1 per 300. The 10-fold higher prevalence of protein C deficiency in thrombosis cohorts suggests that carriership is associated with a 10-fold increased risk of venous thrombosis, i.e. essentially similar to the risk associated with APC resistance. Protein C deficiency is not a risk factor for arterial thrombosis. Two types of protein C deficiency have been described. In type I, there is a parallel reduction in protein C antigen and functional activity. Type II is characterised by a functional defect in the protein, and its plasma concentration may be normal. The majority of reported cases of protein C deficiency are of type I. Homozygous or compound heterozygous protein C deficiency is a rare condition (1 per 200,000–1 per 400,000) which leads to severe and fatal thrombosis in the neonatal period. The clinical picture is that of purpura fulminans and the symptoms include necrotic skin lesions due to microvascular thrombosis. Other major symptoms are thrombosis in the brain and disseminated intravascular coagulation. Several cases have been successfully treated with fresh frozen plasma or with protein C concentrates.

Genetic analysis has been performed in a large number of cases with protein C deficiency (160 different mutations known). Most genetic defects are missense mutations located within the region coding for the mature protein, which lead to single amino acid substitutions

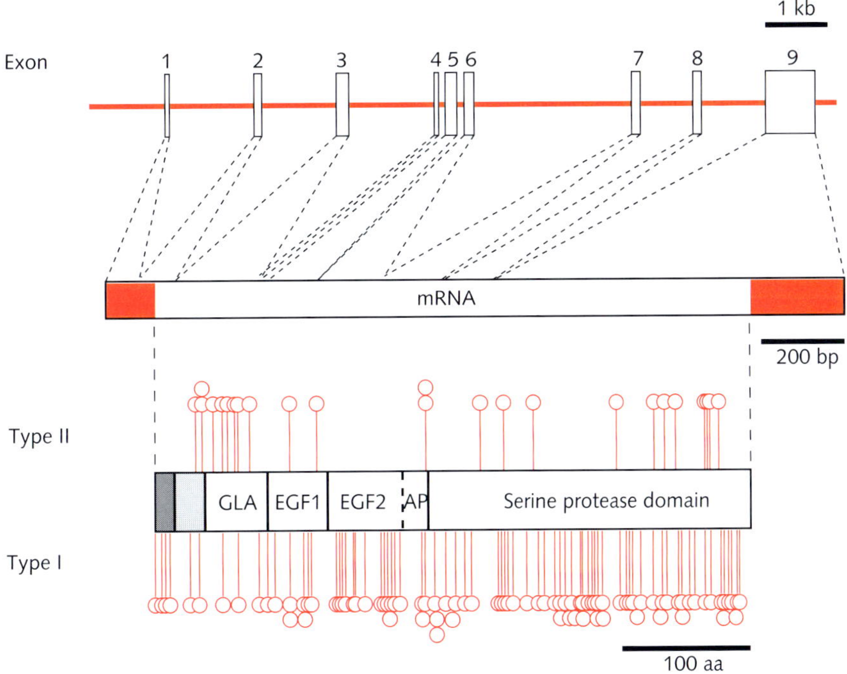

Fig. 12.3 Structure of the human *PROC* gene and location of detrimental missense mutations in the protein C molecule Human protein C is encoded by the *PROC* gene, localised to chromosome 2 (2q13–q14), which spans approximately 11 kb of DNA (upper part). The gene comprises nine exons which yield a ~1.8 kb mRNA transcript (middle part). The protein C mRNA encodes a 461 amino acid residue long pre–pro protein C sequence (lower part). The pre-sequence (shaded) serves as a signal peptide and the pro-sequence (light shading) functions as signal for proper γ-carboxylation of the protein. The mature protein consists of 419 residues and can be divided into a γ-carboxy glutamic acid (Gla) domain, two epidermal growth factor (EGF) domains and a serine protease domain. During processing of the protein, an internal dipeptide is removed from the protein and the mature protein circulates as a covalently linked two-chain molecule. Between the second EGF domain and the protease part of the molecule is an activation peptide (AP) region, which is released upon protein C activation. The circles indicate the localisation of known missense mutations, leading to amino acid substitutions associated with type I deficiency (indicated below the polypeptide chain) or type II deficiency (above).

and type I deficiency (Figure 12.3). Mutations in the promoter region of the gene which affect the plasma protein concentration and mutations affecting RNA splicing have also been found. In a minority of cases, the genetic defects lead to a type II deficiency. Mutations leading to type II deficiency have been found in almost all the modules of protein C, including the propeptide, the Gla-module, EGF1, the activation peptide and the SP module.

Protein S deficiency

Heterozygous protein S deficiency is present in 2–5% of thrombosis patients. The prevalence of protein S deficiency in the population is not known, but family studies suggest that the associated risk of venous thrombosis is similar to that of protein C deficiency and APC-resistance. The level of free protein S discriminates better between those with and without protein S deficiency than the level of total protein S. This is because the concentrations of protein S and C4BPβ+, which is the protein S-binding isoform of C4BP, are equimolar in protein S-deficient individuals and most of the protein S is bound to C4BPβ+. Protein S deficiency with low levels of both free and total protein S is called type I, whereas protein S-deficiency with low free protein S and normal total protein S has been believed to constitute a separate genetic type (type III). However, co-existence of the two types in many protein S-deficient families demonstrates that they represent different phenotypic variants of the same genetic disease. Mutations in protein S leading to functionally defective molecules are referred to as type II deficiency. To date, very few type II deficiencies have been found, which presumably is related to the poor diagnostic performance of available functional protein S assays. Homozygous protein S deficiency is extremely

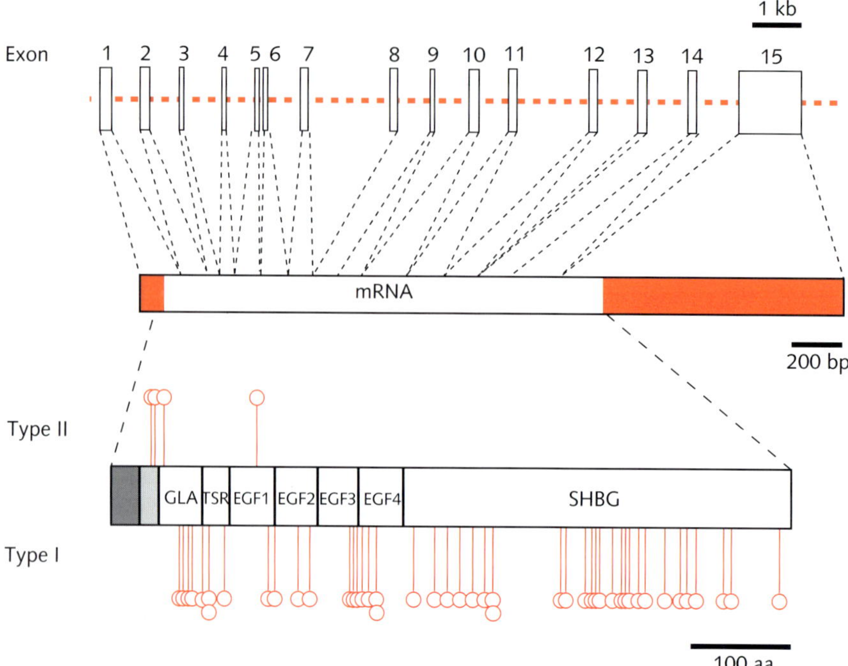

Fig. 12.4 Structure of the human *PROS1* gene and location of detrimental missense mutations in the protein S molecule
The gene for human protein S (*PROS1*) comprises 15 exons (upper part) and spans over 80 kb of DNA and is localised to chromosome 3 (3p11.1–q11.2). Exons are denoted by open bars and introns by lines. Introns denoted by dashed lines between exons indicate gaps and are not drawn to scale. The PROS1 mRNA is approximately 3.5 kb in size (middle part). The mRNA is translated into a 676 amino acid residue pre–pro protein S (lower part). The polypeptide chain can be divided into a signal peptide (dark grey), a pro-peptide (light grey), a thrombin-sensitive region (TSR), a γ-carboxy glutamic acid (Gla) domain, four epidermal growth factor (EGF)-like domains and a large carboxy-terminal domain homologous to sex hormone-binding globulin (SHBG). The circles indicate the localisation of known missense mutations, leading to amino acid substitutions associated with type I deficiency (indicated below the polypeptide chain) or type II deficiency (above).

rare, but appears to give a similar picture to homozygous protein C deficiency with purpura fulminans in the neonatal period. To date, approximately 70 defects in the protein S gene have been reported, most of which are missense or nonsense mutations and mutations affecting splicing or insertion/deletion defects are less common (Figure 12.4).

Prothrombin mutation

A point mutation in the prothrombin gene (nucleotide 20210 G → A) has been identified as the second most common independent risk factor for venous thrombosis. The mutation is located in the 3′ untranslated region, and the mechanism by which this mutation leads to an increased risk of thrombosis is not fully understood even though the mutation is associated with increased plasma levels of prothrombin (Figure 12.5). The prevalence of the mutation in the general population is 1–2% and the mutation is associated with an approximately threefold increased risk of thrombosis.

Severe thrombophilia is a multigenetic disease

Venous thrombosis is a typical multifactorial disease involving one or more environmental and/or genetic risk factors. In Western societies, many individuals carry more than one genetic risk factor because the FV:Q^{506} allele is so common. In contrast, in countries where the FV:Q^{506} allele is rare, few individuals carry more than one genetic defect. This may explain the difference in incidence of thromboembolic disease between Japan and China on the one hand and Europe and USA on the other. The frequency of individuals carrying two or more genetic defects can be calculated on the basis of the prevalence of the individual genetic defects in the general population. In a country where the prevalence of

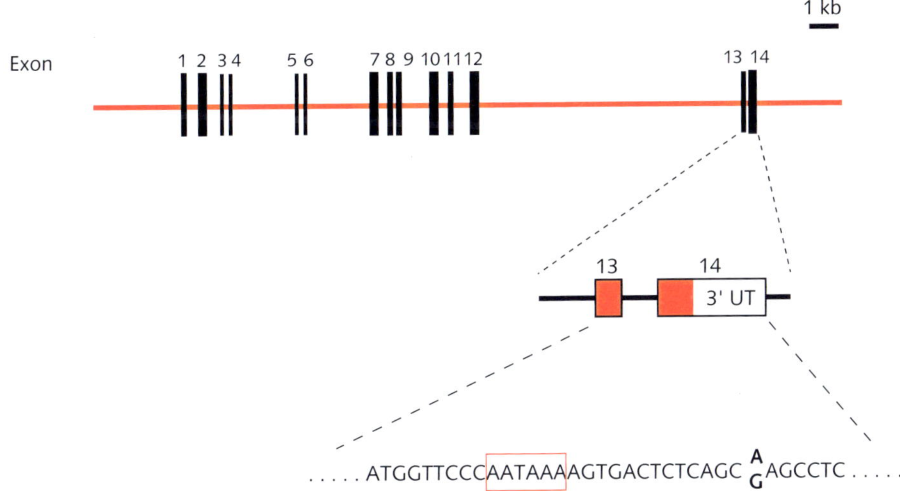

Fig. 12.5 Structure of the human *F2* gene and localisation of the prothrombin 20210 G → A mutation
The human gene for prothrombin (*F2*) comprises 14 exons and spans approximately 20 kb of DNA on chromosome 11 (11p11–q12). The nucleotide sequence flanking the G → A transition at nucleotide 20210 (indicated in bold) in the 3′ untranslated region of the *F2* gene is shown below. The putative polyadenylation signal is boxed. The 20210 A allele was recently described to be associated with elevated levels of plasma prothrombin and an increased risk of venous thrombosis.

FV:Q506 is 10%, combinations of protein C deficiency and FV:Q506 are expected to be present in between 1 per 3–10,000 individuals. A similar calculation for the combination of the prothrombin mutation and FV:Q506 allele suggests the prevalence of combined defects to be 1–2 per 1000 individuals. Thus, a large number of people carry more than one genetic defect and such individuals have considerably increased risk of thrombosis. The FV:Q506 allele is thus found to be an additional genetic risk factor in certain thrombophilic individuals with deficiency of protein C, protein S or AT as well as in cases with the prothrombin mutation (Figure 12.6).

The thrombotic tendency in individuals with inherited genetic defects is highly variable and some individuals never develop thrombosis, whereas others develop recurrent severe thrombotic events at an early age. This depends on the particular genotype, the co-existence of other genetic defects and the presence of environmental risk factors such as oral contraceptives, trauma, surgery and pregnancy. Thus, women with heterozygosity for the FV:Q506 allele who also use oral contraceptives have been estimated to have a 35–50-fold increased risk of thrombosis, whereas those with homozygosity have a several hundred-fold increased risk.

Management of thrombophilia

Decisions about medical intervention due to the presence of one or more genetic defects should be based on careful consideration of the clinical picture, including the patient's family history. The impact of the medical history on the use of oral anticoagulants is perhaps even more important in individuals with APC resistance (FV:Q506) or the prothrombin mutation than in those with the more rare deficiencies of protein C, protein S or AT. The risk of bleeding complications due to anticoagulant therapy must always be weighed against the benefits of the anticoagulation effect, especially if an oral anticoagulant is used for periods exceeding 3 to 6 months when the risk of thrombotic recurrence probably declines. New clinical data are continually emerging and no general consensus regarding screening, prophylaxis and the treatment of symptomatic patients has yet been established.

When the FV:Q506 allele is present in homozygous form, or heterozygosity is combined with a second genetic defect, prophylactic treatment with heparin or oral anticoagulants is recommended in situations known to be associated with a high risk of thromboembolic complications, such as surgery or pregnancy, even if the patient has never experienced any thrombosis or has no family history of such complications. For heterozygous, asymptomatic carriers lacking a family history of thrombosis, short-term prophylaxis has been recommended in high-risk situations, but it remains to be established whether prophylaxis should be given in all situations associated with a risk of thrombosis.

Symptomatic heterozygous patients should be

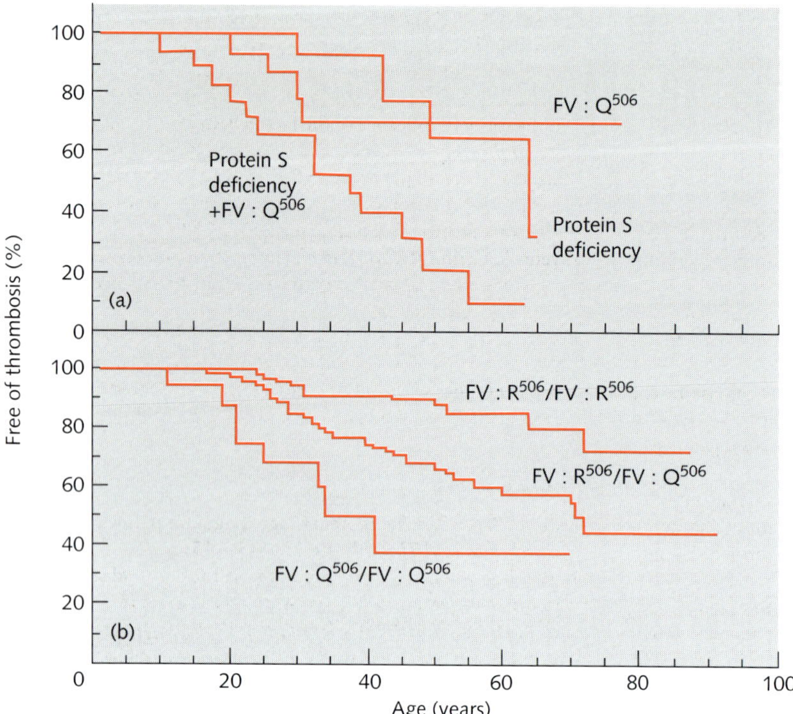

Fig. 12.6 Thrombosis-free survival curves for individuals with different FV genotypes and co-inherited protein S deficiency
(a) The increased risk of thrombosis with combined defects is illustrated with thrombosis-free survival curves for 21 individuals with single defects, FV:Q^{506} or protein S deficiency, and 18 individuals with both defects. There was no significant difference between those with single defects, whereas differences between individuals with the FV:Q^{506} allele or protein S deficiency and those with combined defects were significant.
(b) Probability of being free of thrombotic events at a certain age for 146 normal individuals, 144 heterozygotes and 18 homozygotes for the FV:Q^{506} allele presented by Kaplan–Meier analysis. Highly significant differences were observed between normals and heterozygotes and between heterozygotes and homozygotes.

managed in the same way as any other patient with thrombotic events until more specific recommendations are established. It is not known whether the presence of a genetic defect is associated with an increased risk of recurrence, even though most studies on APC resistance tend to suggest that this is indeed the case. Patients with combined defects, and probably also patients with single gene defects, may be at increased risk of recurrence and should accordingly be given long-term anticoagulation therapy beyond 6 months, even after an isolated thromboembolic event. However, more data are needed before these recommendations can be considered generally applicable.

The potential benefits of general screening for APC resistance and/or the FV : Q^{506} allele prior to thrombotic events or in the presence of such circumstantial factors as oral contraceptive usage, pregnancy and surgery are obvious, but more prospective data are needed, not least in terms of cost–benefit ratios before any general recommendations can be made.

Conclusions

Inherited APC resistance, caused by the $Arg^{506}Gln$ mutation in the FV gene, is the most common genetic risk factor for thrombosis identified to date. The mutated FV (FV : Q^{506}) has normal procoagulant properties, but the loss of the APC cleavage site at position 506 in FV results in impaired regulation of coagulation and a hypercoagulable state. The prevalence of FV:Q^{506} in Caucasian populations varies between 2 and 15%. A genetic variant in the prothrombin gene (G20210A) is another common prothrombotic risk factor with a prevalence of approximately 2% in the general population. Other less common independent genetic risk factors include abnormalities in the genes for antithrombin, protein C and protein S. Families with thrombophilia present with variable penetrance of thrombosis explained by different combinations of genetic defects and environmental risk factors. Patients with combined genetic defects are at higher risk of thrombosis than those with single gene defects. Thus, evaluation of patients with thrombosis must be performed in order to fully estimate the risk for thrombosis in each case.

Further reading

Blood coagulation: introduction and regulation

Dahlbäck B. (1995) The protein C anticoagulant system: inherited defects as basis for venous thrombosis. *Thrombosis Research*, 77, 1–43.

Mann KG, Lorand L. (1993) Introduction: blood coagulation. *Methods in Enzymology*, 222, 1–10.

Rapaport SI, Rao LVM. (1995) The tissue factor pathway: How it has become a 'prima ballerina'. *Thrombosis and Haemostasis*, **74**, 7–17.
van Boven HH, Lane DA. (1997) Antithrombin and its inherited deficiency states. *Seminars in Hematology*, **34**, 188–204.

Molecular genetics of venous thromboembolism

Bauer KA. (1995) Management of patients with hereditary defects predisposing to thrombosis including pregnant women. *Thrombosis and Haemostasis*, **74**, 94–100.
Bertina RM, Koeleman BP, Koster T *et al.* (1994) Mutation in blood coagulation factor V associated with resistance to activated protein C. *Nature*, **369**, 64–67.
Dahlbäck B. (1997) Resistance to activated protein C as risk factor for thrombosis: molecular mechanisms, laboratory investigation, and clinical management. *Seminars in Hematology*, **34**, 217–234.
Dahlbäck B, Carlsson M, Svensson PJ. (1993) Familial thrombophilia due to a previously unrecognized mechanism characterized by poor anticoagulant response to activated protein C: prediction of a cofactor to activated protein C. *Proceedings of the National Academy of Sciences (USA)*, **90**, 1004–1008.
Greengard JS, Sun X, Xu X *et al.* (1994) Activated protein C resistance caused by Arg506Gln mutation in factor Va. *Lancet*, **343**, 1361–1362.
Griffin JH, Evatt B, Wideman C, Fernandez JA. (1993) Anticoagulant protein C pathway defective in majority of thrombophilic patients. *Blood*, **82**, 1989–1993.
Koster T, Rosendaal FR, de Ronde H *et al.* (1993) Venous thrombosis due to poor anticoagulant response to activated protein C: Leiden Thrombophilia Study. *Lancet*, **342**, 1503–1506.
Lindqvist PG, Svensson PJ, Dahlbäck B, Marsal K. (1998) Factor V R506Q mutation (activated protein C resistance) associated with reduced intrapartum blood loss—a possible evolutionary selection mechanism. *Thrombosis and Haemostasis*, **79**, 69–73.
Reitsma PH, Bernardi F, Doig RG *et al.* (1995) Protein C deficiency: a database of mutations, 1995 update. On behalf of the Subcommittee on Plasma Coagulation Inhibitors of the Scientific and Standardization Committee of the ISTH. *Thrombosis and Haemostasis*, **73**, 876–889.
Rosendaal FR. (1997) Risk factors for venous thrombosis: prevalence, risk, and interaction. *Seminars in Hematology*, **34**, 171–187.
Svensson PJ, Dahlbäck B. (1994) Resistance to activated protein C as a basis for venous thrombosis. *New England Journal of Medicine*, **330**, 517–522.
Vandenbroucke JP, Koster T, Briet E *et al.* (1994) Increased risk of venous thrombosis in oral-contraceptive users who are carriers of factor V Leiden mutation. *Lancet*, **344**, 1453–1457.
Varadi K, Rosing J, Tans G *et al.* (1996) Factor V enhances the cofactor function of protein S in the APC-mediated inactivation of factor VIII: influence of the factor VR506Q mutation. *Thrombosis and Haemostasis*, **76**, 208–214.
Voorberg J, Roelse J, Koopman R *et al.* (1994) Association of idiopathic venous thromboembolism with single point-mutation at Arg506 of factor V. *Lancet*, **343**, 1535–1536.
Zivelin A, Griffin JH, Xu X *et al.* (1997) A single genetic origin for a common Caucasian risk factor for venous thrombosis. *Blood*, **89**, 397–402.
Zoller B, Svensson PJ, He X, Dahlbäck B. (1994) Identification of the same factor V gene mutation in 47 out of 50 thrombosis-prone families with inherited resistance to activated protein C. *Journal of Clinical Investigation*, **94**, 2521–2524.

Protein C system

Esmon CT. (1992) The protein C anticoagulant pathway. *Arteriosclerosis and Thrombosis*, **12**, 135–145.
Rosing J, Tans G. (1997) Coagulation factor V: an old star shines again. *Thrombosis and Haemostasis*, **78**, 427–433.
Shen L, Dahlbäck B. (1994) Factor V and protein S as synergistic cofactors to activated protein C in degradation of factor VIIIa. *Journal of Biological Chemistry*, **269**, 18735–18738.

Protein S system

Aiach M, Borgel D, Gaussem P *et al.* (1997) Protein C and protein S deficiencies. *Seminars in Hematology*, **34**, 205–216.
Simmonds RE, Zoller B, Ireland H *et al.* (1997) Genetic and phenotypic analysis of a large (122-member) protein S-deficient kindred provides an explanation for the familial coexistence of type I and type III plasma phenotypes. *Blood*, **89**, 4364–4370.
Zoller B, Garcia de Frutos P, Dahlbäck B. (1995) Evaluation of the relationship between protein S and C4b-binding protein isoforms in hereditary protein S deficiency demonstrating type I and type III deficiencies to be phenotypic variants of the same genetic disease. *Blood*, **85**, 3524–3531.

Prothrombin gene mutation

Poort SR, Rosendaal FR, Reitsma PH, Bertina RM. (1996) A common genetic variation in the 3′-untranslated region of the prothrombin gene is associated with elevated plasma prothrombin levels and an increase in venous thrombosis. *Blood*, **88**, 3698–3703.

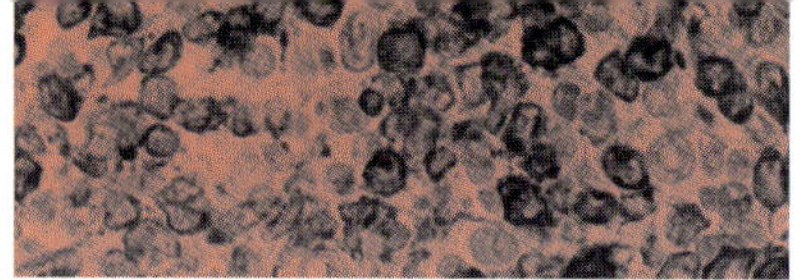

Chapter 13 Molecular basis of haemophilia

Paul L F Giangrande

Introduction: clinical features of haemophilia

Haemophilia is a congenital disorder of coagulation and affects approximately 1 in 10 000 males worldwide, with approximately 5000 patients with haemophilia in the United Kingdom. Haemophilia A is due to a deficiency of factor VIII in the circulating blood, and haemophilia B (also known as Christmas disease) is a clinically identical disorder caused by factor IX deficiency. Typical laboratory findings in haemophilia include a normal prothrombin time (PT) but prolonged activated partial thromboplastin time (APTT). The platelet count and bleeding time are normal. A specific factor assay is required to confirm the diagnosis. The severity of clinical manifestations depends upon the level of factor in the blood (Table 13.1).

Severe haemophilia is defined by a clotting factor level of <2 iu/dl. The hallmark of severe haemophilia is recurrent and spontaneous haemarthrosis. Typically, hinge joints such as the knees, elbows and ankles are affected but bleeds may also occur in the wrist or shoulder. Bleeding into the hip joint is unusual. The affected joint is swollen and warm, and held in a position of flexion (Figure 13.1), with no external discolouration or bruising around the joint. It is unusual for an infant to suffer spontaneous haemarthroses in the first few months of life, and the first joint to be affected tends to be the ankle as the child learns to crawl. The first sign of a haemarthrosis in an infant will often be obvious discomfort and distress, accompanied by limping or reluctance to use a limb. Recurrent bleeds into a joint lead to synovitis and joint damage resulting in crippling arthritis (Figure 13.2). Bleeding into muscles is also a feature of haemophilia, but this is usually a consequence of direct injury, albeit often minor (Figure 13.3). Bleeds into certain areas are particularly dangerous because of the risk of compression of neighbouring structures. Patients with inhibitory antibodies are particularly at risk in this regard, as bleeds may be more difficult to control. Bleeds in the tongue can obstruct the airway, and retroperitoneal bleeding within the ilio-psoas muscle may result in femoral nerve compression, causing weakness and wasting of leg muscles (Figure 13.3). Bleeding from the gastrointestinal tract (melaena) and bleeding into the urinary tract (haematuria) may also occur. There is also a significant risk of intracranial haemorrhage in severe haemophilia which was a significant cause of mortality in the past when treatment was not so readily available.

Approximately 15% of patients with severe haemophilia A can be expected to develop inhibitory antibodies to factor VIII at some stage. Inhibitor development in haemophilia B is, by contrast, very rare. The development of such antibodies poses considerable problems in treatment as these immunoglobulins (IgG) are capable of rapidly inactivating infused factor VIII, and furthermore the antibody titre may rise dramatically after a course of factor VIII. Very occasionally, acquired haemophilia may arise in a previously normal individual, due to the formation of autoantibodies directed against factor VIII, and both males and females may be affected. Haemarthrosis is unusual in acquired haemophilia, and the principal manifestations are usually extensive superficial purpura and muscle bleeds. Acquired haemophilia arises most often in the elderly, and there is an association with underlying malignant or autoim-

Table 13.1 The relation of blood levels of factor VIII (or IX) to the severity of haemorrhagic manifestations.

Level (iu/dl)	Haemorrhagic manifestations
50–100	Normal level, no bleeding problems
25–50	Tendency to bleed after major surgery
5–25	Mild haemophilia. Bleeding only after minor injury and occasional spontaneous haemarthroses
<2	Severe haemophilia with spontaneous and recurrent bleeding into muscles and joints

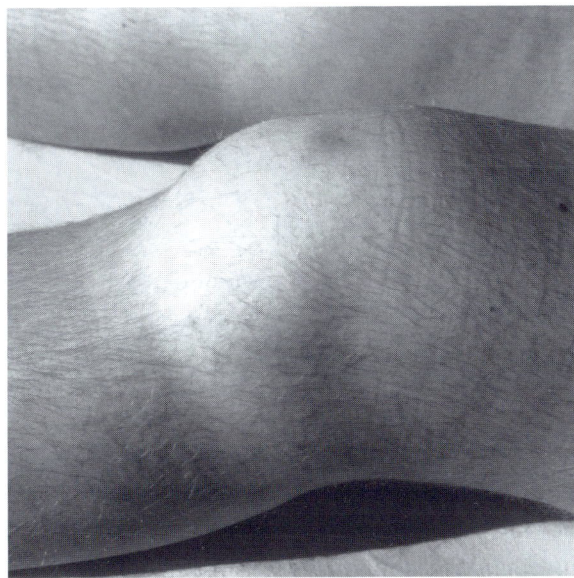

Fig. 13.1 Acute haemarthrosis in severe haemophilia
This usually arises in the absence of injury. The joints most frequently involved are the knees, elbows and ankles. The joint is swollen, warm and tender but there is no external bruising or discolouration.

mune diseases. Treatment of bleeding episodes involves the intravenous injection of coagulation factor concentrates; the total dose and frequency of treatment will also be determined by the severity and site of bleeding.

The great majority of joint bleeds will resolve with a single infusion of material, if the bleed is recognised early and treated promptly. There is an increasing move to prophylactic therapy, in which the patient gives himself injections of coagulation factor concentrate two or three times a week to prevent bleeds rather than just treating on demand when bleeds occur. Patients on prophylactic therapy experience few or even no spontaneous bleeds,

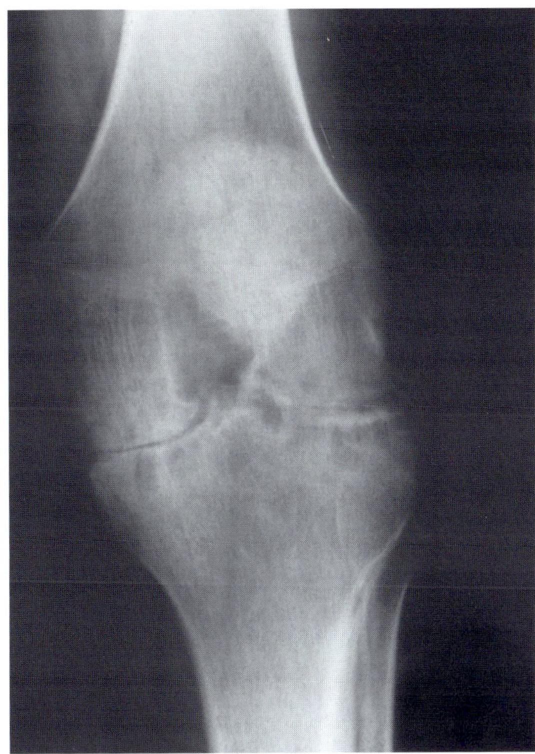

Fig. 13.2 Radiograph of the knee of a patient with severe haemophilic arthropathy
Joint replacement surgery was subsequently carried out in this case.

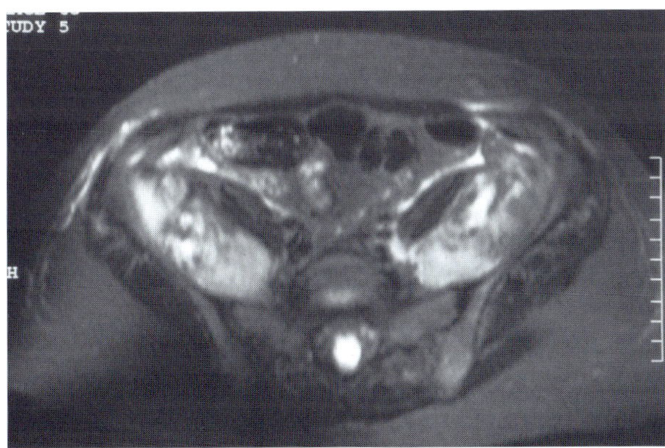

Fig. 13.3 Magnetic resonance imaging (MRI) scan showing bilateral ilio-psoas haemorrhage
This bleed was associated with a complete but transient paralysis in both legs, as the femoral nerve is located on the anterior surface of the muscle and may be compressed in such cases.

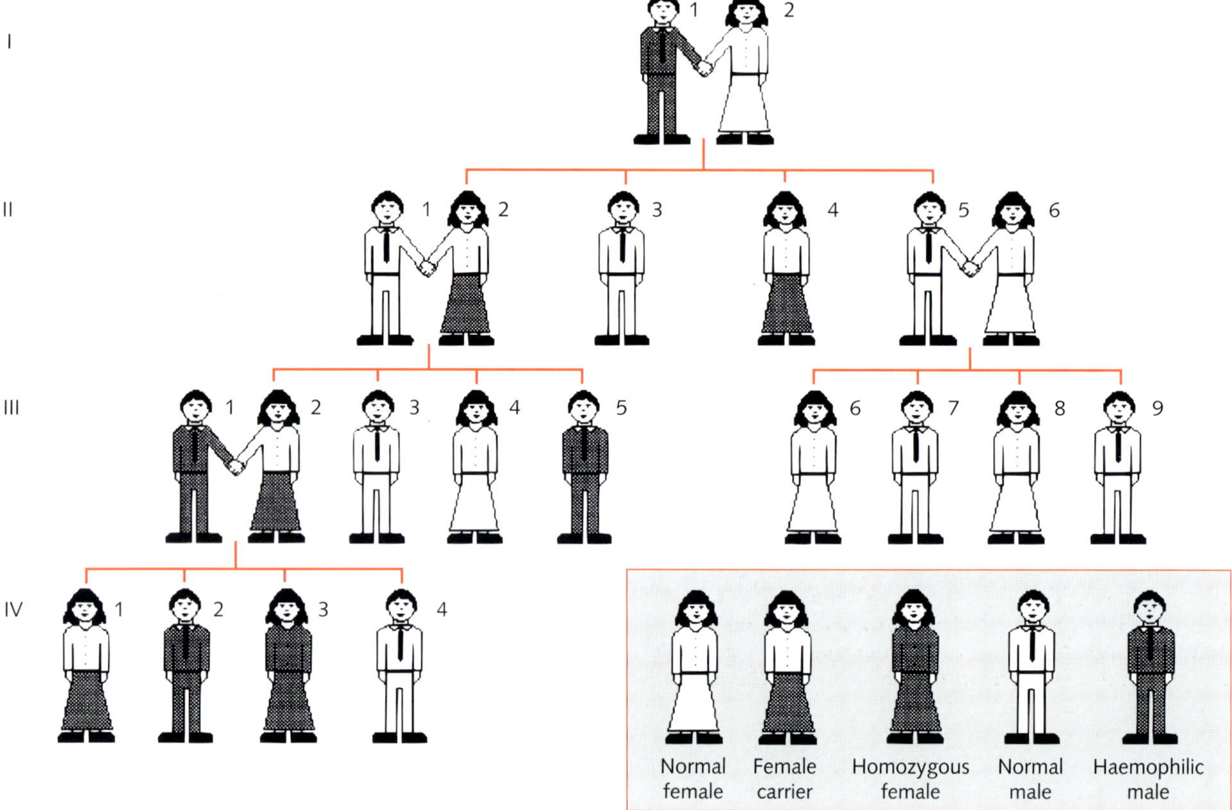

Fig. 13.4 The inheritance of haemophilia
The gene for factors VIII and IX are both encoded on the X chromosome, and inheritance is thus sex-linked. The daughter of a man with haemophilia is an obligate carrier, but the son of a haemophiliac will not be affected. Haemophilia may thus be transmitted to a grandson via a carrier daughter. Colour blindness and Duchenne muscular dystrophy are other examples of conditions which are X-linked disorders.

and thus progressive joint damage and arthritis can be avoided.

Inheritance of haemophilia

The genes for factors VIII and IX are both located at the telomeric end of the X chromosome and thus haemophilia is inherited as an X-linked recessive condition (Figure 13.4). The daughters of affected males are obligate carriers but the sons are normal. The phenotype remains constant within a family, so the daughter of a man with only mild haemophilia may be reassured that she will not pass on a severe form of the condition. However, approximately one-third of all cases of haemophilia arise in the absence of a previous family history and are due to a new mutation. The most famous example is that of Queen Victoria, who had a haemophilic son (Leopold) and also two daughters who turned out to be carriers. There are instances of haemophilia affecting females due to inheritance of the defective gene from both parents, and there are also case reports of haemophilia in females with Turner's syndrome (XO karyotype) and androgen insensitivity syndrome (testicular feminisation, XY karyotype).

Molecular basis of haemophilia A

Factor VIII is an essential cofactor for the activation of factor X by activated factor IXa. Factor VIII must itself undergo proteolytic cleavage at two distinct sites through the action of thrombin before it becomes physiologically active. It circulates in plasma as a large glycoprotein bound non-covalently to the larger protein, von Willebrand factor. The factor VIII gene was first cloned in 1984. It is 186 kb in length and is situated on the long arm of the X chromosome at Xq28 (Figure 13.5). The factor VIII gene consists of 26 exons, of which

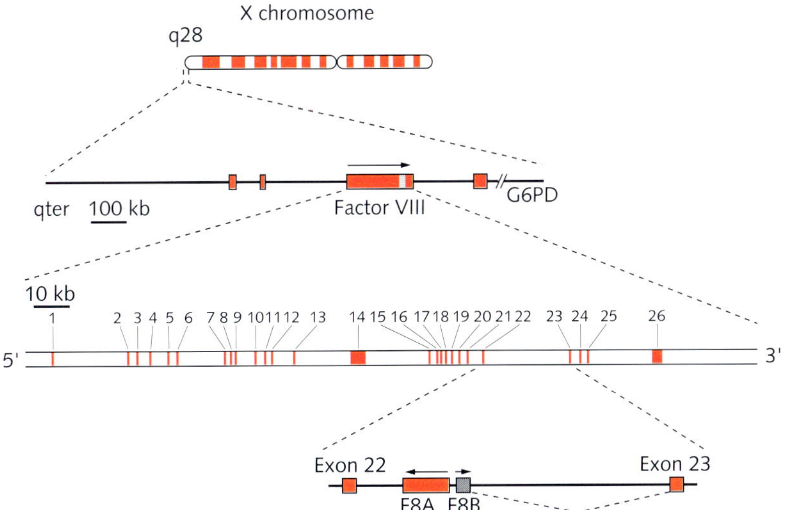

Fig. 13.5 The factor VIII gene
The factor VIII gene was cloned in 1984, and is encoded towards the telomeric end of the long arm of the X chromosome (Xq28). It maps distal to the gene encoding glucose-6-phosphate dehydrogenase (G6PD) at about 1 Mb from the Xq telomere. The gene is composed of 26 exons, of which exon 14 is the largest. The large intron 22 contains a nested intronless gene termed F8A (the function of the gene and its transcript are unknown). There are two further copies of F8A located ~400 kb telomeric to the factor VIII gene. The spliced factor VIII mRNA is ~9 kb in length and the mature factor VIII molecule is composed of 2332 amino acids.

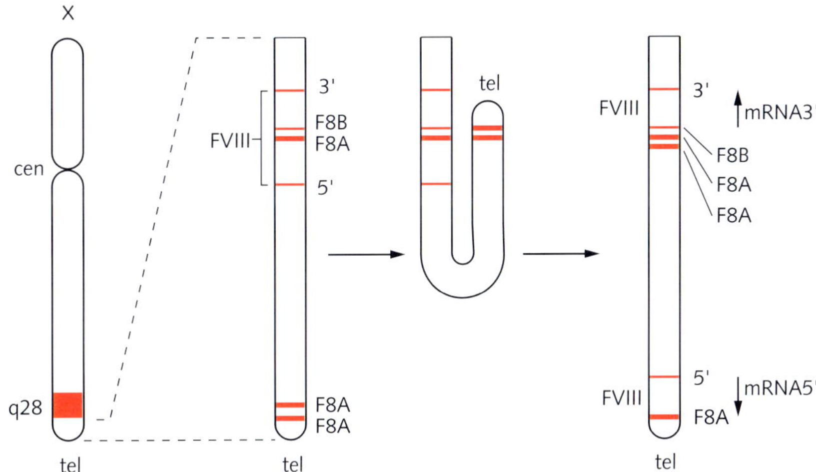

Fig. 13.6 'Flip tip inversion'
This unique inversion of the tip of the X chromosome is now recognised to be responsible for about half of all cases of severe haemophilia in all ethnic groups. Cross-over occurs between a copy of F8A within the factor VIII gene and one of the two telomeric copies. Cross-over with the distal copy is more common, occurring in approximately 80% of cases where an inversion is identified.

exon 14 is the largest, and 25 introns. The mature factor VIII protein is made up of 2332 amino acids.

By far the commonest single genetic defect causing severe haemophilia is an inversion in intron 22, which is encountered in as many as 45% of people with severe haemophilia in all ethnic groups (Figure 13.6). The inversion mechanism involves an intronless gene of unknown function, designated F8A. Two copies of this gene are located near the tip of the X chromosome and there is another copy within intron 22 of the factor VIII gene itself. During meiosis, either of the two telomeric copies may cross over with the intronic copy, resulting in a division of the gene into two halves facing in opposite directions and separated by approximately 500 kb. Cross-over with the distal copy is much more common than cross-over with the proximal copy, and accounts for approximately 80% of all inversions. It is now recognised that inversion almost always forms during a male meiosis. It is believed that the presence of a large region of non-homology between the X and Y chromosomes

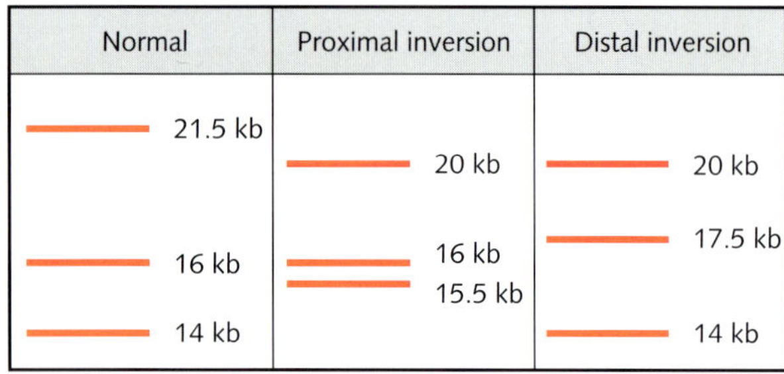

Fig. 13.7
Inversions within intron 22 of the factor VIII gene are by far the commonest cause of severe haemophilia, and are detected in almost half of all cases. This figure shows the results of Southern blot analysis using the Bcl I restriction enzyme. The normal pattern is shown on the left. A female carrier with an inversion will show a combination of the normal and either the proximal or distal inversion pattern.

during meiotic pairing may favour a misalignment and the presence of a second X chromosome with a complementary region may act as a stabilising factor. An important clinical consequence of this observation is that, when an apparently new and spontaneous case of haemophilia is diagnosed in which the gene inversion is identified, it is likely that the defect arose in the maternal grandfather's allele and thus the mother can generally be assumed to be a carrier and at risk of having another affected male child. The resulting truncated protein product is presumably unstable, resulting in severe haemophilia. The inversion is not found in individuals with mild forms of haemophilia.

The inversion is easily detected and the identification of this defect as the commonest cause of severe haemophilia has simplified both screening for carriers and antenatal diagnosis of haemophilia (Figure 13.7). Using the restriction enzyme Bcl I, three bands are identified in normal individuals. The 21.5 kb band is contributed by intron 22, and the 14 and 16 kb bands are derived from the proximal and distal repeats, respectively. The inversion may be identified and classified according to the appearance of abnormal bands representing the products of recombination (Figure 13.7).

Developments in molecular biology have permitted the more rapid identification of defects in haemophilia. Southern blotting has been superseded by methods involving polymerase chain reaction (PCR) amplification of either patient DNA or material derived from the reverse transcription of mRNA (RT-PCR). Although automated sequence analysers have been developed, gene sequencing of the entire factor VIII gene is both expensive and labour intensive. Methods have been developed to identify restricted areas of abnormal DNA in patients with haemophilia, which may then be targeted for specific attention. These methods include *amplification and mismatch detection* (AMD), *conformation sensitive gel electrophoresis* (CSGE) and *denaturing gradient gel electrophoresis* (DGGE).

Approximately 4% of cases of haemophilia are the consequence of gene deletions, which have been reported throughout the gene and which are very variable in size. As with the intron 22 inversion, most deletions are associated with a severe clinical phenotype. Frameshift mutations resulting from insertions or small deletions have also been identified as a cause of severe haemophilia. Most other cases of both severe and mild haemophilia are associated with single point mutations, and approximately 200 missense mutations have been identified as causing haemophilia A. A full list is outside the scope of this chapter, but a *Further reading* list is provided at the end. Such mutations affect RNA processing, mRNA translation or the fine structure of factor VIII itself. Nonsense mutations result in the formation of stop conditions and the production of truncated factor VIII molecules devoid of any functional activity, for example TGG(Trp)→TGA(Stop) at nucleotide 255 in exon 7, and CGA(Arg)→TGA at nucleotide 1941 in exon 18. Missense mutations that involve critical sites will also result in haemophilia A, for example Arg^{372}→His or Cys and Ser^{373}→Leu mutations involving a thrombin cleavage site. Approximately 40% of all missense mutations arise at CG dinucleotide sites, resulting in a change to TG or CA sequences. It is generally believed that CG nucleotides represent genomic 'hotspots'. Cytosine is predominantly methylated in human DNA, but this is relatively unstable and 5-methylcytosine is prone to spontaneous deamination to yield a GT mismatch which is inefficiently repaired. It is also of interest that a missense mutation may be associated with varying degrees of clinical severity. Thus a C→T mutation at nucleotide 1689 has been reported in association with both severe and moderately severe phenotypes. Similarly, a Val^{326}→Leu substitution has been reported in individuals with either a severe or moderately severe phenotype.

Molecular basis of haemophilia B

The factor IX gene is also located on the long arm of the X chromosome at band Xq27, and is encoded by a stretch of DNA approximately 34 kb long which contains eight exons (Figure 13.8). The basic structure of the gene is similar in organisation to those of protein C and coagulation factors VII and X, and it is likely that they all originated in the distant past from a common

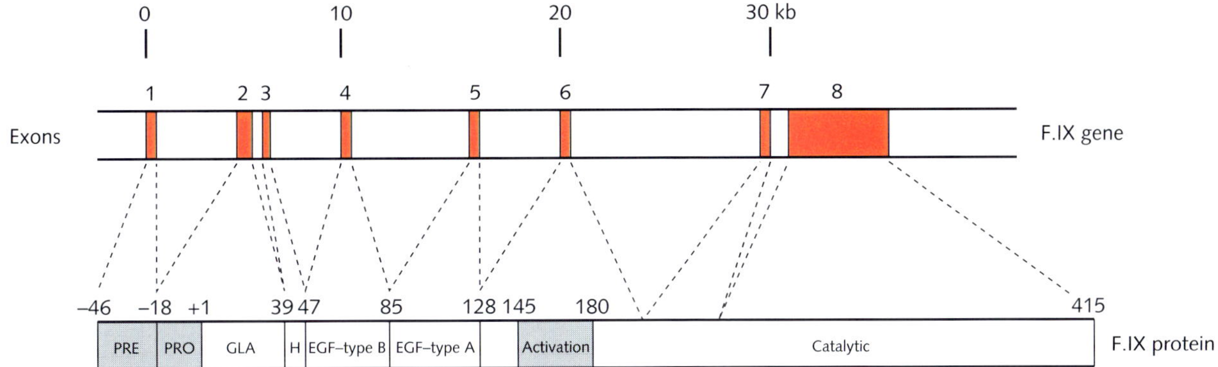

Fig. 13.8 The factor IX gene
The factor IX gene was first cloned in 1982. It is located on the long arm of the X chromosome at band Xq27. The gene spans 34 kb and encodes eight exons (exons are shown as dark boxes, and dotted lines between the gene and protein indicate protein domains encoded by each exon). The signal peptide and propeptide sequences are cleaved during processing and activation of factor IX.

ancestral gene by duplication. Factor IX is a polypeptide of 415 amino acids, and is made up of a glutamic acid-rich sequence (Gla domain) and two epidermal growth factor (EGF)-like domains separated from the serine protease domain by an activation region. The 12 glutamic acid residues in the Gla domain undergo post-translational γ-carboxylation which is necessary for binding of calcium, and exon 2 encodes a recognition site for the carboxylase. Exon 1 encodes the signal peptide necessary for transport into the endoplasmic reticulum. Exon 6 encodes the activation peptide that is cleaved off during the activation of factor IX by either factor XI or a complex of tissue factor and factor VII. Exons 7 and 8 encode the catalytic regions of factor IX, which are responsible for subsequent activation of factor X in the coagulation cascade. The gene is controlled by a promoter.

The gene for factor IX which was cloned in 1982 is considerably smaller than that of factor VIII, and patients with haemophilia B have been studied more extensively than those with haemophilia A. The first defects identified in haemophilia B were gross deletions, detected by Southern blotting. However, it is now recognised that gene deletions account for only approximately 3% of all cases of haemophilia B. No equivalent of the factor VIII gene inversion has been encountered in haemophilia B and it is now clear that point mutations account for the vast majority of cases of haemophilia B, and over 500 have been described from families from around the world. The great majority involve single base changes which have been identified in all domains of the protein. The unusually high frequency of mutations at CG dinucleotide sites in haemophilia B probably reflects the high number of CG dinucleotides at critical sites in the factor IX gene.

Mutations involving the glutamic acid residues within the Gla domain (residues 1–38) result in severe haemophilia, emphasising their functional importance, for example Glu^{7}→Val and Glu^{17}→Lys. Mutations within exon 6 result in haemophilia through disruption of the activation of the factor IX molecule, for example CGT→TGT at position 20,413 results in Arg^{145}→Cys. The majority of cases of haemophilia B are attributable to mutations within exons 7 or 8, resulting in impaired catalytic activity, for example a change from AGT to AGA at nucleotide 31,216 results in a change from Ser^{365}→Arg within the active site. The original case of Christmas disease has been identified as a TGT→TCT mutation at nucleotide 31,170 resulting in a change from Cys^{206}→Ser within exon 8. The creation of nonsense mutations will lead to severe haemophilia B due to the production of ineffective, truncated proteins, for example CGA(Arg)→TGA(Stop) at nucleotide 30,863 and TGG(Trp)→TGA(Stop) at nucleotide in exon 8.

A few patients with haemophilia B have been described in whom the factor IX level rises significantly after puberty, and this is associated with loss of the bleeding tendency. Several point mutations have been reported in association with this interesting variant, referred to as the haemophilia B Leiden phenotype. All are located in the promoter region of the factor IX gene, for example TTG→TAG at −20 and G→A at nucleotide −6. Most of these mutations have been shown to be located in regions which contain binding sequences for liver-enriched transcription factors which are presumably influenced by androgenic steroids.

Inhibitor formation: aetiology and clinical implications

A minority of patients with haemophilia will develop IgGs directed against infused factor VIII (or IX) after exposure to these blood products for treatment of bleeding episodes. This is potentially serious, as patients will be refractory to conventional doses of coagulation factor concentrates and bleeding will be difficult to control. Inhibitor development in haemophilia B is a very rare event, occurring in probably less than 1% of patients, and these patients often have an underlying large gene deletion. By contrast, inhibitor formation in haemophilia A is much more common, and data from the UK registry show that 14% of all patients with severe haemophilia A have developed antibodies at some time, but it is quite likely that this figure underestimates the true prevalence. The reasons why some patients develop inhibitory antibodies are not clear. Family studies suggest that there is a genetic predisposition but no human leucocyte antigen (HLA) or other linkages have been conclusively identified. There is some evidence that people of Afro-Caribbean origin are more susceptible to inhibitor formation. Certain types of gene defects in haemophilia are undoubtedly associated with a significantly increased risk of inhibitor development, particularly large gene deletions and mutations resulting in stop codons. There is a weaker association between inhibitor formation and the presence of an inversion in intron 22 of the factor VIII gene.

Therapeutic applications of molecular biology to patient care

Carrier testing

Ideally, carriers of haemophilia should be identified before a pregnancy, and offered counselling. Daughters of men with haemophilia are obligate carriers of the condition, with a 50:50 chance of passing on the condition to a son, and there is a similar chance that a daughter of a carrier will also herself be a carrier of the condition. Thus no special genetic tests are required to determine the carrier status of daughters of men with haemophilia, although the results of DNA-based studies are likely to be useful for subsequent antenatal diagnostic procedures. The phenotype of haemophilia remains constant within a family, so that the daughter of a man with only mild haemophilia may be reassured that she can only transmit a similarly mild form of the condition. However, a more common problem is to be confronted with a woman with only a vague history of a bleeding disorder in a distant relative. National patient registers are particularly useful in such circumstances. In the UK a register of people with haemophilia and other bleeding disorders has been held at the Oxford Haemophilia Centre since 1969, and this resource has proved useful in establishing the type and severity of bleeding disorder of an affected relative as a first step in determining which tests need to be carried out.

It may seem logical to initiate carrier testing to determine carrier status as soon as possible in girls with a family history of the condition, as this would facilitate management of pregnancy in the case of an early and possibly unexpected pregnancy. It is clear that there are significant differences of opinion between geneticists and haematologists with regard to the timing of testing of children for genetic disorders. Clinical geneticists in the UK usually take the view that it is unethical to test healthy young children to determine carrier status for inherited disorders for conditions which have no immediate implications for their own health. There are also legal implications in the UK, as testing of young children ignores the rights of children with respect to the Children Act (1989), and testing cannot be considered to have been obtained with the informed consent of the individual child concerned. By contrast, guidelines from the Genetics Working Party of the UK Haemophilia Centre Directors' Organisation (UKHCDO) conclude that carrier testing in young children may be appropriate, but that the issues must be discussed openly with the family.

From a theoretical point of view, the ideal approach would be to characterise the precise genetic defect responsible for haemophilia within a family. Once the molecular defect has been identified in an individual with either haemophilia A or B, direct screening for that defect could be applied in subsequent generations for both carrier testing and also antenatal diagnosis. However, with perhaps the single exception of the intron 22 inversion associated with severe haemophilia A, this is often simply not practical or feasible. In such cases, indirect methods have to be used to determine carrier status. This involves the tracking of intragenic or extragenic polymorphisms in families which act as convenient markers for the molecular defect causing haemophilia within a family. The method is based on the fact that there are some genetic polymorphisms which represent natural variations of the genome sequence, without any adverse impact on the function of the molecule. Ideally, such polymorphic sequences should be intragenic, but closely linked extragenic polymorphisms may also be exploited. If extragenic markers are relied on, the small possibility of recombination may also result in erroneous diagnoses. The polymorphisms are detected by cleavage

Table 13.2 Factor VIII intragenic DNA polymorphisms.

Site	Restriction enzyme	Southern blot alleles	Allelic frequencies
5′ flanking region	Taq I	9.5 kb	72%
		4.0 kb	28%
Intron 18	Bcl I	1.1 kb	29%
		0.88 kb	71%
Intron 22	Xba I	6.2 kb	41%
		4.8 + 1.4 kb	59%
3′ of exon 26	Bgl I	20 kb	10%
		5 kb	90%

of patient DNA with restriction enzymes, which generate fragments of varying size according to the presence or absence of the polymorphism (Table 13.2). The fragments are detected either by PCR-based methods or Southern blotting. Figure 13.9 shows the results of restriction fragment length polymorphism (RFLP) analysis in one family, and illustrates how the method may permit identification of carriers.

Limitations of this approach include the fact that samples have to be taken from several members to permit the tracking of the mutant gene responsible for haemophilia in the family. Blood from an affected family member will be required, and this may not be possible in some cases where early death from complications such as HIV infection has occurred. Furthermore, non-paternity may confound attempts to track the gene in families. It should also be appreciated that there is ethnic variation of the allelic frequencies of the various polymorphisms, more so with factor IX than factor VIII, and this may influence the choice of probes used in some family studies. For example, the allelic frequencies with Bcl I and Hind III are reversed in African-Americans as compared with Caucasians. Bgl I is more likely to be informative in people of Afro-Caribbean origin but it is not likely to be informative in families of Chinese origin. RFLP analysis is likely to be informative in the majority of families, but occasionally carrier status cannot be determined even with multiple probes. The commonest problem is homozygosity for all markers in the proband's mother. However, the recent identification of hypervariable dinucleotide tandem repeats (VNTR) in introns 13 and 22 has also helped to identify a greater proportion of carriers. Once the carrier status has been determined and DNA markers have been identified, it is then possible to offer antenatal diagnosis of haemophilia to pregnant women.

Antenatal diagnosis of haemophilia

As a general rule, it is the practice in the UK to perform antenatal procedures to determine whether or not a fetus has haemophilia *only* where a termination is being contemplated. The general experience in the UK has been that only a minority of women subsequently take up the offer of antenatal diagnosis with a view to termination if an affected fetus is identified. This may well reflect the fact that many women with affected relatives appreciate that major advances in treatment in recent years, such as the introduction of recombinant products for children and the wider adoption of prophylaxis, offer the prospect of an essentially normal life for the younger generation of people with haemophilia.

Amniocentesis was the first technique employed for antenatal diagnosis of haemophilia and other X-linked disorders such as muscular dystrophy. Whilst amniocentesis is both technically simple and safe, an important limitation is the fact that it may only be employed in the second trimester of pregnancy, after approximately 15 weeks' gestation. Chorionic villus sampling (CVS) was first applied to antenatal diagnosis of a number of genetic disorders in the early 1980s, but this technique is now the principal method used for antenatal diagnosis of haemophilia and several other single gene disorders. The principal advantage is that the method may be applied for antenatal diagnosis during the first trimester, so that if termination of the pregnancy is required this is easier to carry out. Furthermore, the results of the test are often available within only a few days of the procedure as (in contrast to amniocentesis) there is no need to culture cells before genetic analysis. A sample is obtained by either a transabdominal or transvaginal route, under ultrasound guidance (Figure 13.10). However, CVS should not be undertaken before 11 weeks of pregnancy in order to minimise the risk of inducing congenital limb abnormalities. A disadvantage of CVS is that the procedure has to be carried out at a time when fetal sexing through ultrasound scanning is not feasible, so that a female fetus is unnecessarily exposed to risks.

Direct fetal blood sampling may be used for antenatal diagnosis of haemophilia but this method is usually only offered as a last resort, either because it was not possible to carry out DNA-based family studies in time or because such studies were carried out but were not informative. In this technique, fetal blood is taken from fetal umbilical vessels under ultrasound guidance. The procedure requires considerable expertise to perform and will thus not be available in all hospitals. It is usually carried out at a minimum of 18 weeks' gestation. The levels of factor VIII and IX in a normal fetus at around 19 weeks'

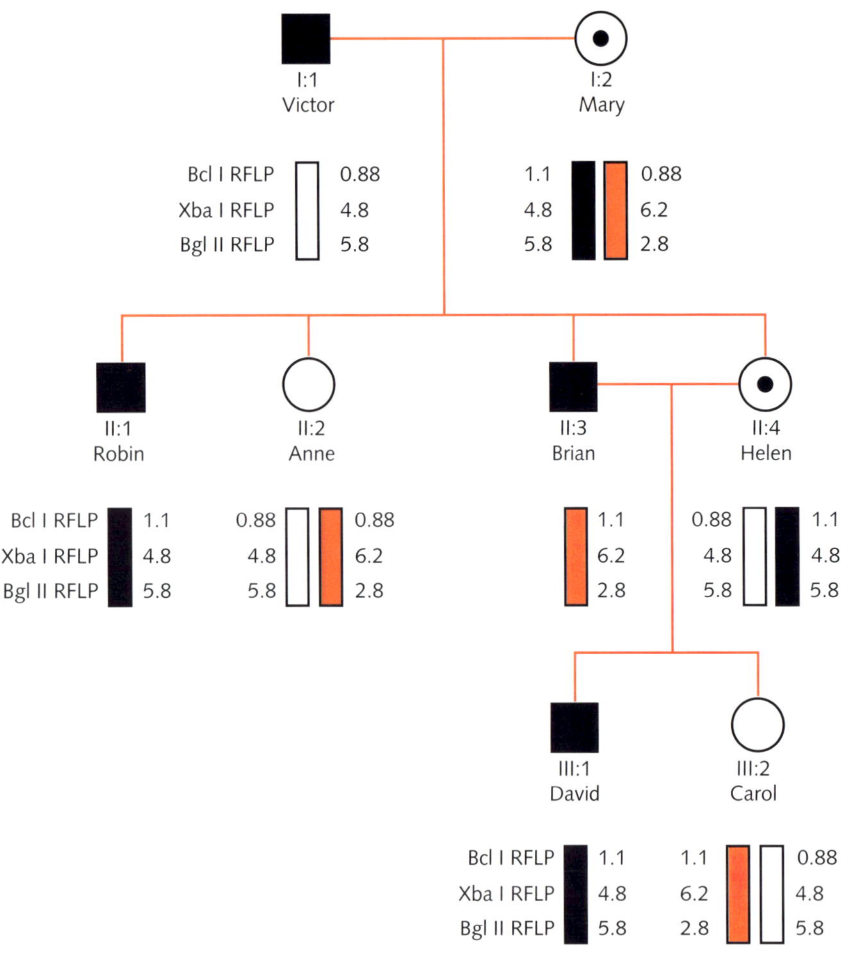

Marker	Probe	Enzyme(s)	Alleles kb
Bcl I RFLP Intron 18	p114.12	Bcl I	1.1 + 0.88
Xba I RFLP Intron 22	p482.6	Xba I + Kpn I	6.2 + 4.8
Bgl II RFLP DXS15	DX13	Bgl II	5.8 + 2.8

Key
- Unaffected female
- Haemophilic male
- Carrier
- Unaffected male

Fig. 13.9 The use of restriction fragment length polymorphism (RFLP) analysis in a family to determine carrier status
Robin and David both have severe haemophilia A. Victor and Brian are normal. It is clear from the family tree that the disorder is associated with the 1.1/4.8/5.8 haplotype, and this permits the identification of Robin's sister, Helen, as carrier. Anne and Carol are not carriers.

gestation are significantly lower than that in an adult, at approximately 40 iu/dl and 10 iu/dl, respectively.

In future, it is likely that antenatal diagnosis of haemophilia (and other genetic disorders) will be based on *isolation of fetal cells from the maternal circulation*. It is well documented that fetal lymphocytes may be isolated from the maternal circulation during pregnancy, and determination of karyotype in the fetal cells has been used to predict fetal sex. However, fetal lymphocytes may persist in the maternal circulation for many years after a pregnancy and this limits use of this method for second or subsequent pregnancies. More recently, fetal normoblasts have been isolated from the maternal circulation with a flow cytometer/cell sorter, and fetal DNA

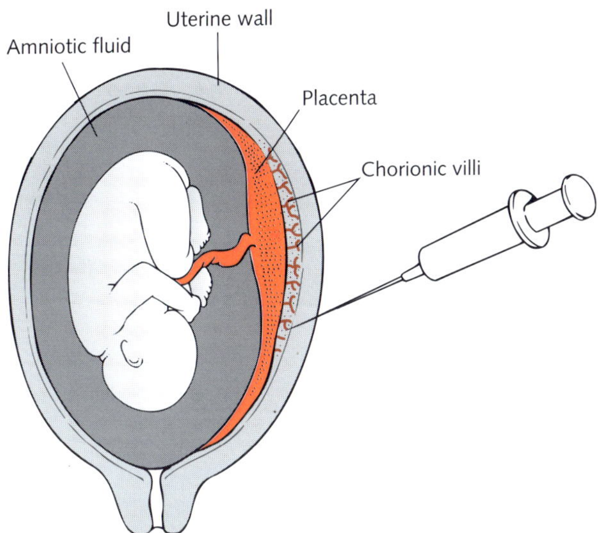

Fig. 13.10 Chorionic villus sampling (CVS)
A sample of trophoblastic tissue from the placental area is aspirated with a fine needle under general anaesthetic. The procedure is usually carried out after 11 weeks' gestation. DNA isolated from the fetal tissue can then be analysed to determine fetal sex and status with regard to haemophilia.

extracted from these in order to probe for markers of hereditary genetic disorders. The attraction of this approach is that it is non-invasive and also offers the prospect of very early diagnosis, even as early as 7 or 8 weeks of gestation. Pre-implantation diagnosis is another technique that has been developed, involving determination of embryonic sex using dual fluorescence *in situ* hybridisation of blastomere cells with labelled probes specific for the sex chromosomes. The method may be particularly attractive to women who would not be prepared to undergo a conventional termination of a well-established pregnancy.

Recombinant blood products

The development of plasma-derived coagulation factor concentrates in the early 1970s dramatically improved both the longevity and quality of life of patients with haemophilia, and the demand for factor VIII and IX has risen steadily. Twenty-five million units of factor VIII were used in the UK in 1975, but consumption had increased to 200 million units by 1996. The growing need for factor VIII cannot be met by products derived from volunteer blood donors. The manufacture of recombinant coagulation factor proteins offers the promise of unlimited supplies, albeit at increased cost. However, the most important advantage of recombinant products is safety with regard to transmission of human pathogens. Many patients with haemophilia were infected with either HIV and/or hepatitis C before the introduction of physical methods of viral inactivation of plasma-derived coagulation factor concentrates in 1985. More recently, there has been concern about the possibility of transmission of new variant Creutzfeld–Jakob disease to haemophiliacs as the prions believed to be the cause of this neurological disorder are extremely resistant to the usual viral inactivation procedures. Recombinant coagulation factor products offer the best possible protection from transmission of human blood-borne viruses and are regarded as the treatment of choice for all patients with haemophilia. However, they cost almost twice as much as conventional plasma-derived products and this has limited availability of these products.

Recombinant coagulation factor concentrates are manufactured by insertion of the human gene into mammalian cell lines (such as Chinese hamster ovary cells or baby hamster kidney cells), which are then grown in culture on an industrial scale. Factor VIII (or IX) is then secreted into the growth medium from which it is subsequently extracted by monoclonal or other immunoaffinity chromatography (Figure 13.11). All currently available licensed recombinant factor VIII products contain added human albumin as a stabiliser, but 'second generation' products are being developed in which albumin has been replaced by alternative stabilisers such as the carbohydrate, polysorbate-80. This will further increase the margin of safety as regards viral and other infections, as will the elimination of all bovine materials from the culture media. Recombinant factor VIII has an identical structure and glycosylation profile to natural, plasma factor VIII. Its pharmacokinetic profile and post-infusion recovery are also identical to that observed in plasma-derived concentrates. There has been controversy as to whether the use of recombinant factor VIII is associated with an increased risk of inhibitor formation. However, it is not possible to give a definitive answer in the absence of prospective, randomised and comparative studies, but most physicians would now agree that the risk is similar to that associated with conventional, plasma-derived products. Recombinant factor IX has become available only more recently. Recombinant factor IX is identical in amino acid sequence to the Ala^{148} (as opposed to the less common Thr^{148}) human polymorphic variant. Plasma factor IX is synthesised in the liver and undergoes post-translation glycosylation of a number of glutamic acid residues, for which vitamin K is a cofactor, which is essential for its activity. Recombinant factor IX is not as

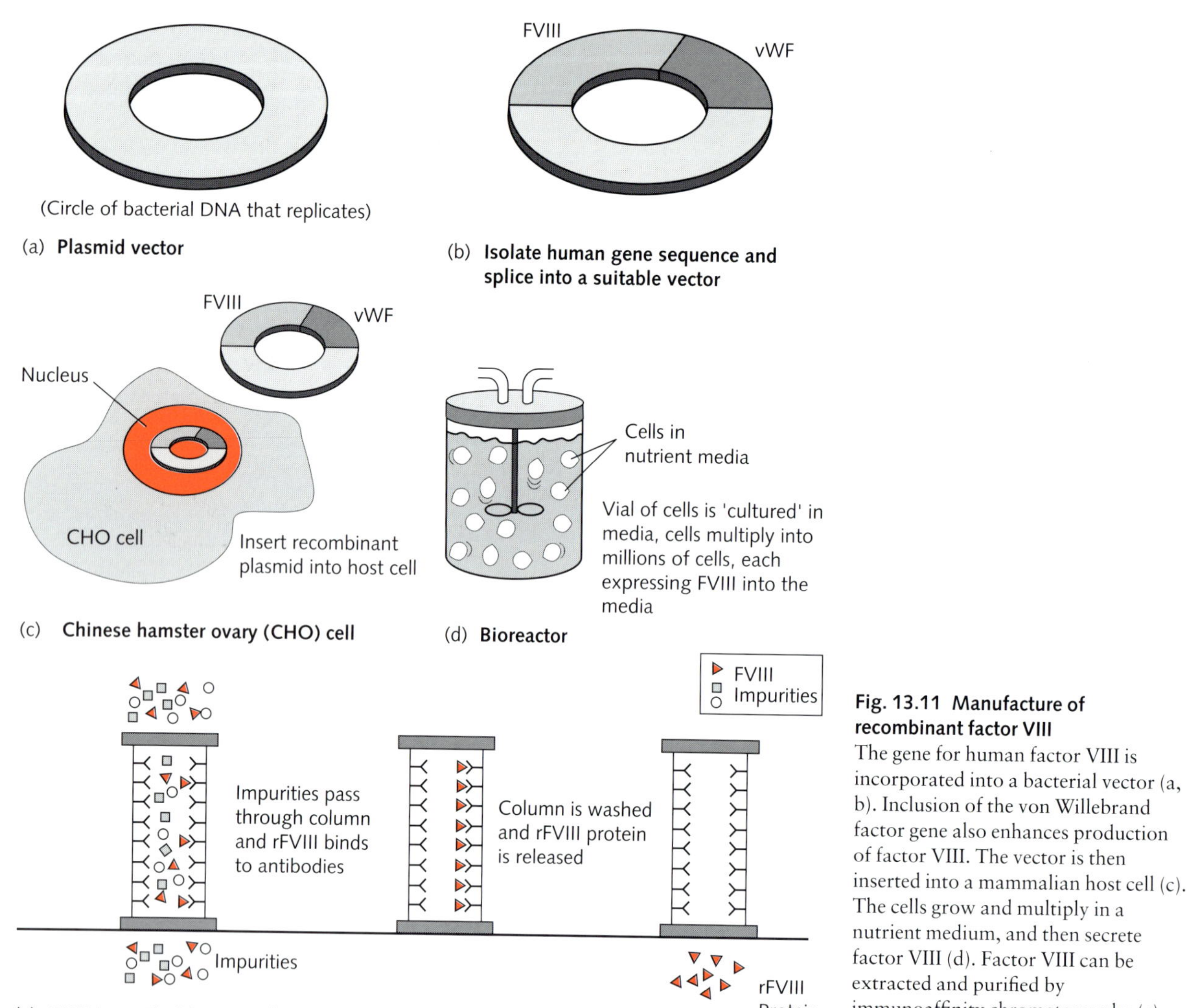

Fig. 13.11 Manufacture of recombinant factor VIII
The gene for human factor VIII is incorporated into a bacterial vector (a, b). Inclusion of the von Willebrand factor gene also enhances production of factor VIII. The vector is then inserted into a mammalian host cell (c). The cells grow and multiply in a nutrient medium, and then secrete factor VIII (d). Factor VIII can be extracted and purified by immunoaffinity chromatography (e). The final product also contains no von Willebrand factor.

effectively carboxylated, but the pharmacokinetic profile is identical to that observed with plasma-derived products. It is a smaller molecule than factor VIII and requires no albumin, or other material, to be added to the final product as a stabiliser. The cell line is grown in media that contain no animal- or human-derived proteins. There is no suggestion of an increased risk of inhibitor development associated with the use of recombinant factor IX.

Another useful recombinant product is recombinant factor VIIa (*Novoseven*, Novo Nordisk). It is now recognised that factor VII plays a key role in the initiation of the coagulation cascade through contact with tissue factor released from damaged tissues, to form activated factor VII (VIIa) (*see also Chapter 12: Molecular coagulation and thrombophilia*). Recombinant factor VIIa is very useful in the clinical management of patients with either haemophilia A or B and inhibitory antibodies, as well as those with acquired haemophilia.

Looking to the future, it is likely that the direction of future research in genetic engineering will increasingly be applied to production of modified molecules, with more favourable properties. For example, it would obviously be useful to produce factor VIII molecules with a longer plasma half-life or reduced propensity to stimulate inhibitor development. Hybrid factor VIII molecules have been developed in which the A2 and C2 domains have been replaced by porcine equivalents. Since almost 90% of inhibitory antibodies bind to these two domains of the human factor VIII molecule, it is hoped that these

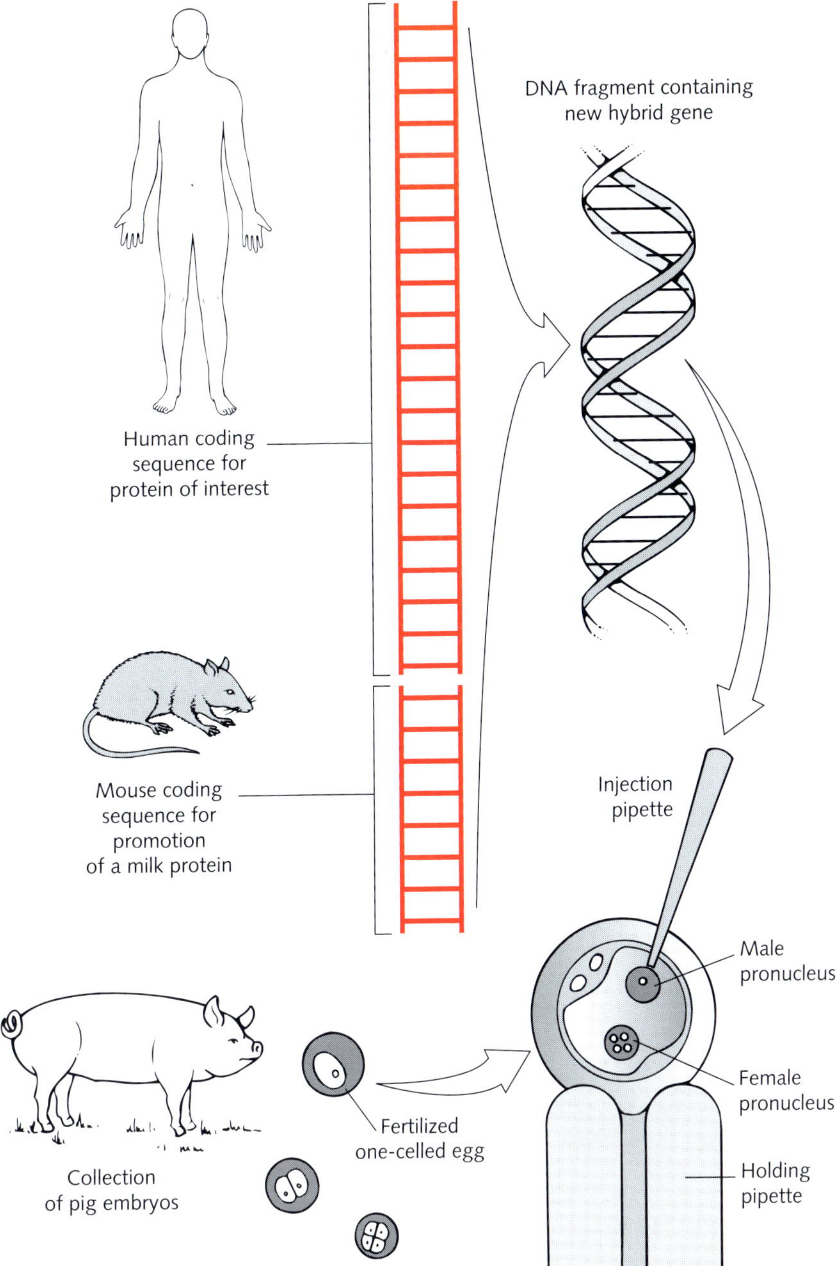

Fig. 13.12 Production of recombinant proteins using transgenic livestock ('pharming')

new constructs may be of clinical use in the treatment of people with inhibitory antibodies. A further development has been the generation of transgenic livestock such as sheep, pigs and goats for production of human coagulation proteins. Transgenic animals which secrete antithrombin, factor VIII or factor IX into their milk have been produced, and this approach is likely to be developed for the widescale production of relatively cheap and unlimited supplies of biologically active products free of the risk of transmission of human pathogens (Figure 13.12). More recently, this work has been extended by successful cloning of sheep. Production of transgenic animals by nuclear transfer will permit the establishment of large breeding colonies of livestock more quickly and efficiently than would be possible through production of individual transgenic sheep by pronuclear microinjection.

Table 13.3 Comparison of adenoviruses and retroviruses as vectors.

Retroviruses	Adenoviruses
• Physical limit to gene cassette (8 kb)	• Accommodate much larger genes
• Relatively low copy number	• More efficient transfer
• Can only infect dividing cells	• Infect non-dividing cells
• Permanent integration: sustained expression of transduced gene and potential for oncogenesis	• Not integrated after infection: transient gene expression only
• Poor immune response of host	• Stimulate immune responses of host

Gene therapy for haemophilia

(*See also Chapter 16: Molecular therapeutics in haematology.*) Gene therapy offers the prospect of a cure for haemophilia in the long term, but work in the field of haemophilia is at an early stage and there is no prospect of clinical trials for some years. Gene therapy poses a number of ethical problems, particularly since effective and safe treatment with recombinant coagulation factors is now available for patients with both haemophilia A and B. The use of viral vectors introduces risks such as oncogenesis and infection, or even modification of patient germlines. Patients will also need to be enrolled in clinical trials of very long duration, so that close follow-up will identify problems. Finally, in contrast to usual clinical studies, it is likely that children will have to be used in initial clinical studies in preference to adults because the limited yield of coagulation proteins from current cell culture systems would not suffice for larger subjects.

There are two basic approaches to gene delivery into cells. The first technique involves the direct injection of transducing vector into the bloodstream or target tissue, with subsequent *in vivo* transformation of the cells which take up the gene. Alternatively, target cells may be modified by removal of cells from a patient, with subsequent modification *ex vivo* of these cells followed by re-infusion.

Retroviruses and adenoviruses have been used extensively as vectors (Table 13.3). The principal advantage of using retroviruses as vectors is that the genetic material is actually integrated into the genome of the target cell, so expression of the transfected gene is permanent. However, integration is random introducing the potential for oncogenesis through disruption of oncogenes. A further problem with the use of retroviruses as vectors is that there is a physical size limit of approximately 8 kb in the size of cassette that can be accommodated within the virus. The factor IX gene may be accommodated, but the full-length factor VIII gene cannot. Adenoviruses permit transfer of larger genes and can transfect non-dividing cells but transferred DNA does not integrate permanently, so expression of the transfected gene is only transient. A further limitation is that immune response to adenoviral proteins, commonly encountered in everyday life, may limit efficiency of transfer.

As there are a number of legitimate concerns relating to the use of viruses for gene transfer, other modes of gene transfer have been sought. For example, liposomes have a number of other advantages in that there is no limit to the size or conformation of the DNA which may be incorporated and the liposomes themselves are composed of non-toxic materials which are easily degraded, thus facilitating repeated treatment. *In vivo* experiments in mice have shown that intravenous injection of liposomes composed of multilamellar egg phosphatidylcholine containing human factor IX DNA can result in expression of the human factor IX in a number of tissues for a limited period. Direct gene injection has also been employed, for example skeletal muscle can take up and express plasmid DNA after injection into muscle, but this is very inefficient and expression is only transient.

It is likely that gene therapy for haemophilia B will be achieved earlier than gene therapy for classical haemophilia A since the smaller size of the factor IX gene compared to the factor VIII gene permits the use of retroviral vectors and, furthermore, factor IX (in contrast to factor VIII) may be absorbed from subcutaneous tissues after local injection. Although the liver is the site of synthesis of factor IX, a number of other cells can produce factor IX very effectively after transfection with the human factor IX gene, even in the absence of vitamin K. Both human fibroblasts and keratinocytes can produce factor IX, but keratinocytes are particularly attractive cells for gene therapy as they are very accessible, grow well in culture and can be grafted with ease. Cultured human keratinocytes transfected with human factor IX grafted on to athymic (nude) mice secrete human factor IX which is detectable at low levels in the blood of the mouse for sustained periods.

Conclusions

Haemophilia is an inherited disorder of coagulation, associated with congenital deficiency of factor VIII (or IX). It is inherited in a sex-linked fashion, so that only males are affected. Approximately one-third of cases arise in families with no previous family history, and represent new mutations. The typical features of severe haemophilia include spontaneous bleeding into joints, but in the absence of treatment more serious complications (such as intracranial haemorrhage) will lead to early death.

The first products used for the treatment of haemophilia were derived from human plasma, but unfortunately the use of pooled plasma products before 1985 resulted in the transmission of serious viral infections such as HIV and hepatitis to many patients. In recent years, the development of recombinant blood products has eliminated the risk of transmission of these infections, and also offers the prospect of unlimited supplies. The life expectancy of the younger generation of haemophiliacs now approaches that of the normal population.

The commonest molecular defect in haemophilia A is an inversion in intron 22 of the factor VIII gene on the X chromosome, which accounts for approximately half of all cases. Genetic testing is now readily available in many centres to document the genetic defect in each family, and identify carriers within families. Antenatal diagnosis is now easily available, facilitating early termination of the pregnancy if haemophilia is identified.

Haemophilia resources on the Internet

- Factor VIII mutation database: europium.mrc.rpms.ac.uk
- Factor IX mutation database: www.umds.ac.uk/molgen/haemBdatabase.html
- World Federation of Haemophilia: www.wfh.org
- Oxford Haemophilia Centre: www.medicine.ox.ac.uk/ohc/

Further reading

Introduction

Potts DM, Potts WTW. (1995) *Queen Victoria's Gene*. Alan Sutton Publishing Ltd.

Rizza C, Lowe G (eds). (1997) *Haemophilia and Other Inherited Bleeding Disorders*. Eastbourne: WB Saunders.

Tuddenham EGD, Cooper DN. (1994) *The Molecular Genetics of Haemostasis and its Inherited Disorders*. Oxford Medical Publications.

Haemophilia A

Kemball-Cook G, Tuddenham EGD, Wacey AI. (1998) The factor VIII structure and function resource site: HAMSTeRS version 4. *Nucleic Acids Research*, **26**, 216–219.

Lakich D, Kazazian HH, Antonarakis SE, Gitschier J. (1993) Inversions disrupting the factor VIII gene as a common cause of severe haemophilia A. *Nature Genetics*, **5**, 236–241.

Lalloz MRA, McVey JH, Pattinson JK, Tuddenham EGD. (1991) Haemophilia A diagnosis by analysis of a hypervariable dinucleotide repeat within the factor VIII gene. *Lancet*, **338**, 207–211.

Rossiter J, Young M, Kimberland ML *et al.* (1994) Factor VIII gene inversions causing severe haemophilia A originate almost exclusively in male germ cells. *Human Molecular Genetics*, **3**, 1035–1039.

Schwaab R, Brackmann HH, Meyer C *et al.* (1995) Haemophilia A: mutation type determines risk of inhibitor formation. *Thrombosis and Haemostasis*, **74**, 1402–1406.

Haemophilia B

Briët E, Bertina RM, Van Tilburg NH, Veltkamp JJ. (1982) Hemophilia B Leyden: a sex-linked hereditary disorder that improves after puberty. *New England Journal of Medicine*, **306**, 788–790.

Crossley M, Ludwig M, Stowell KM *et al.* (1992) Recovery from hemophilia B Leyden: an androgen-responsive element in the factor IX promoter. *Science*, **257**, 377–379.

Giannelli F, Choo KH, Rees DJG *et al.* (1983) Gene deletions in patients with haemophilia B and factor IX antibodies. *Nature*, **303**, 181–182.

Giannelli F, Green PM, Sommer SS *et al.* (1998) Haemophilia B: database of point mutations and short additions and deletions - eighth edition. *Nucleic Acids Research*, **26**, 265–268.

Carrier testing/antenatal diagnosis

Antonarakis SE, Rossiter JP, Young M *et al.* (1995) Factor VIII gene inversions in severe hemophilia A: results of an international consortium study. *Blood*, **86**, 2206–2212.

Clarke A and the Working Party of the Clinical Genetics Society (UK). (1994) The genetic testing of children. *Journal of Medical Genetics*, **31**, 785–797.

Giangrande PLF. (1998) Management of pregnancy in carriers of haemophilia. *Haemophilia*, **4**, 779–784.

Goodeve AC. (1998) Advances in carrier detection in haemophilia. *Haemophilia*, **4**, 358–364.

Peake IR, Lillicrap DP, Boulyjenkov V *et al.* (1993) Report of a joint WHO/WFH meeting on the control of haemophilia: carrier detection and prenatal diagnosis. *Blood Coagulation and Fibrinolysis*, **4**, 313–344.

Recombinant blood products

Lusher JM. (1996) Recombinant clotting factor concentrates. *Baillière's Clinical Haematology*, **9**, 291–303.

Lusher J, Ingerslev J, Roberts H, Hedner U. (1998) Clinical experience with recombinant factor VIIa. *Blood Coagulation and Fibrinolysis*, **9**, 119–128.

Gene therapy

Brownlee GG. (1995) Prospects for gene therapy for haemophilia A and B. *British Medical Bulletin*, **51**, 91–105.

Schnieke AE, Kind AK, Ritchie WA *et al.* (1997) Human factor IX transgenic sheep produced by transfer of nuclei from transfected fetal fibroblasts. *Science*, **278**, 2130–2133.

Velander WH, Lubon H, Drohan WN. (1997) Transgenic livestock as drug factories. *Scientific American*, **276**, 70–74.

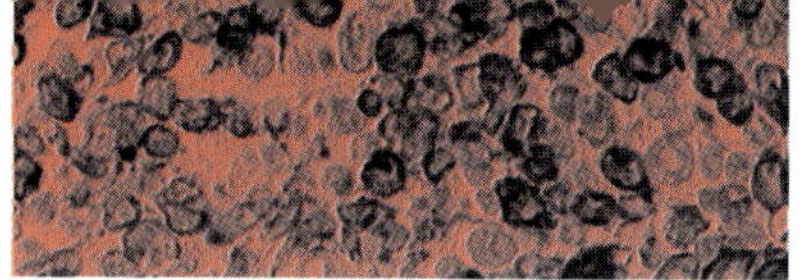

Chapter 14 The molecular basis of blood cell alloantigens

Willem Ouwehand & Cristina Navarrete

Introduction

The transfusion of blood and fetal–maternal haemorrhage during pregnancy have both provided unique models to study the immune response against a plethora of polymorphic blood cell surface markers, including the alloantigens of the human leucocyte antigen (HLA) system. Many blood cell membrane determinants show allelic variation, which can elicit the formation of alloantibodies. In nearly all transfusion situations and pregnancies, the recipient's immune system is challenged by blood cells mismatched for multiple alloantigen systems. As the difference between self and non-self is limited, alloantibodies are only formed by a subset of recipients. Red cell alloantibodies are detected in 1–1.5% of pregnant women and in 2–3% of transfused individuals, and can increase significantly in multitransfused patients. The HLA alloantigens are more immunogenic than red cell ones and 15–25% of multiparous women and 30–40% of patients on long-term prophylactic platelet transfusions are positive for HLA class I antibodies.

Whereas alloantigens were initially defined as polymorphic membrane determinants identified by polyclonal alloantibodies in serum samples from alloimmunised patients or pregnant women, nowadays the molecular basis of most alloantigens has been resolved. Alloantigens can be categorised as those shared between blood cells (e.g. HLA class I) and those unique to one type of blood cell (e.g. Rh on red cells and human platelet antigen (HPA) on platelets) (Table 14.1). When expression is limited to one type of blood cell, destruction of cells in the newborn by maternal blood cell alloantibodies may ensue (immune-mediated anaemia, thrombocytopenia or neutropenia of the newborn). In contrast, HLA class I alloantibodies do not cause cytopenias in the newborn but may compromise the effectiveness of platelet transfusions, complicate organ transplant or cause febrile non-haemolytic transfusion reactions, or on rare occasions precipitate transfusion-related acute lung injury.

The formation of alloantibodies after an incompatible challenge is more the exception than the rule. In contrast to our detailed understanding of the molecular basis of blood cell alloantigens, we remain relatively ignorant about the mechanism of non-responsiveness. We have learned from animal experiments that restriction in the ability to mount an immune response is largely controlled by genes of the major histocompatibility complex (MHC) or HLA. However, the reason why, for example, some 25% of RhD-negative individuals fail to mount an anti-D response on repeated challenge with RhD-positive red cells remains elusive. An exception to this is our detailed understanding of the immune response against the HPA-1a alloantigen on platelets. There is a near complete restriction on the ability to form HPA-1a antibodies by the HLA class II allele DRB3*0101. However, except for the latter example, our ability to identify the genes controlling the risk of alloimmunisation remains limited and further research is needed to identify the genetic basis of this variability in responsiveness.

This chapter aims to review the recent developments in the molecular aspects of blood cell alloantigens, and will highlight their impact on clinical management. Recognising the wide variety of clinical conditions in which the HLA alloantigens play a role, we have placed the main emphasis on:

• Antibody-mediated cytopenias in the newborn by maternal blood cell-specific alloantibodies.

Table 14.1 Antigen expression on peripheral blood cells.

Antigens	Erythrocytes	Platelets	Neutrophils	B-lymphocytes	T-lymphocytes	Monocytes
A, B, H	+++	++/(+)	–	–	–	–
I	+++	++	++	–	–	–
Rh*	+++	–	–	–	–	–
K	+++	–	–	–	–	–
HLA class I	–/(+)	+++	+++	+++	+++	+++
HLA class II	–	–	–/+++**	+++	–/+++**	+++
GPIIb/IIIa	–	+++	(+)#	–	–	–
GPIa/IIa	–	+++	–	–	–	–
GPIb/IX/V	–	+++	–	–	–	–
FcRγIIIb	–	–	+++	–	–	–/+++~

* Non-glycosylated; ** when activated; # inconclusive; ~ when differentiated to macrophages expressing FcγRIIIa.

• The complication of HLA class I alloimmunisation in patients receiving prophylactic platelet transfusions.

The HLA antigens have also been used to introduce the molecular techniques currently applied to identify alleles of genes.

Identification of HLA gene polymorphism

The impact of molecular biological techniques on our ability to scan and identify allelic variation of human genes is best exemplified by the HLA system. For decades the enormous diversity of the alloantigens of the HLA system has been a challenge in both the technical and clinical sense. It is now obvious that the use of molecular techniques, including sequencing-based high-resolution typing, is contributing to improved outcome in transplant patients. Improved matching allows graft maintenance at lower levels of immunosuppression, which is of great importance with the emerging evidence that long-term use of potent immunosuppressive drugs is not without side-effects. In the following paragraphs a number of current molecular techniques used to define alleles of the HLA genes are reviewed. The same techniques may be used to define allelic variation in genes encoding other blood cell alloantigens.

Molecular typing techniques

Traditionally, the definition and characterisation of the HLA molecules and polymorphisms have been carried out using serological and cellular techniques. With the development of gene cloning and DNA-based molecular techniques, it is now possible to perform a detailed analysis of these molecules at the single nucleotide level. The result of this analysis has shown the existence of shared nucleotide sequences between alleles of the same and/or different loci. Similarly, it has been shown that there are certain locus-specific nucleotide sequences in both the coding (exons) and non-coding (introns) regions of the various genes.

The DNA sequencing of a number of alleles at various MHC loci has demonstrated that the majority of the nucleotide substitutions are located in exons 2 and 3 of the HLA class I and exon 2 of the HLA class II molecules. These exons code for the distal membrane domains of the molecules, which form the peptide-binding groove (Figures 14.1a and 14.1b). Based on this information, a number of techniques have been developed to identify this polymorphism using the polymerase chain reaction (PCR) to amplify specific genes or regions to be analysed. These include PCR-SSOP (sequence specific oligonucleotide probing), PCR-SSP (sequence specific priming) and conformational methods including *reference strand conformational analysis* (RSCA) and *sequencing-based typing* (SBT).

PCR-SSOP

In this technique the gene of interest is amplified by PCR using generic primers complementary to highly conserved gene segments. The PCR products are then immobilised onto support membranes, for example nylon membranes, and analysed by probing the membranes with labelled oligonucleotides designed to anneal with polymorphic sequences present in the various alleles. By scoring the probes that bind to specific regions, it is possible to assign an HLA type (Figure 14.2). A recent modification includes the addition of PCR-amplified product to labelled probes immobilised on membranes or plates. This technique does not determine whether the detected sequences are *in cis* or *trans* and, in order to

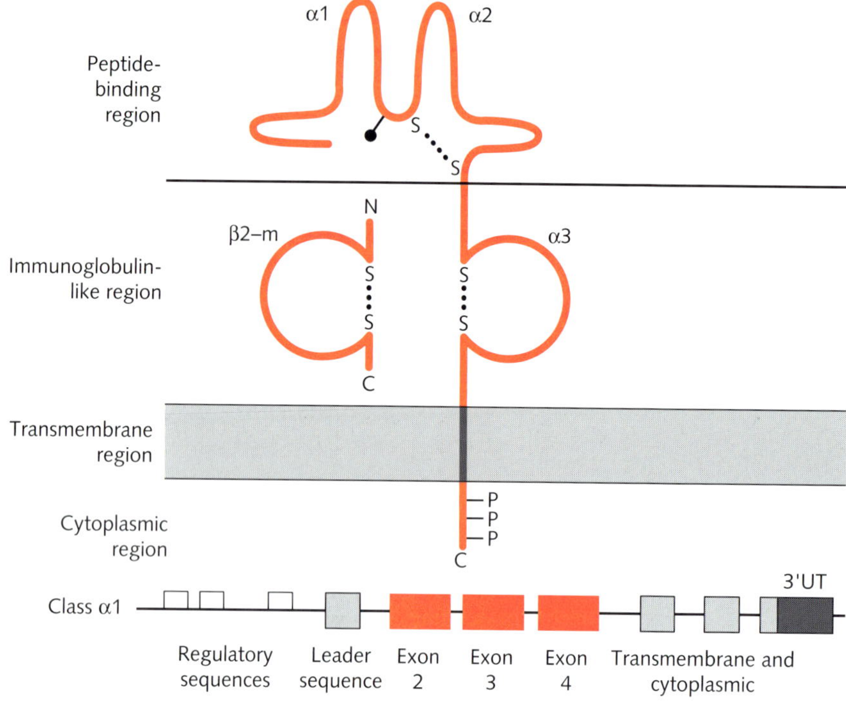

Fig. 14.1a Schematic presentation of HLA class I
The non-covalent association between the HLA class I protein (with three immunoglobulin-like domains, α1, α2 and α3) and β2-m is shown. The three α domains are encoded by three exons of the HLA class I A gene on chromosome 6.

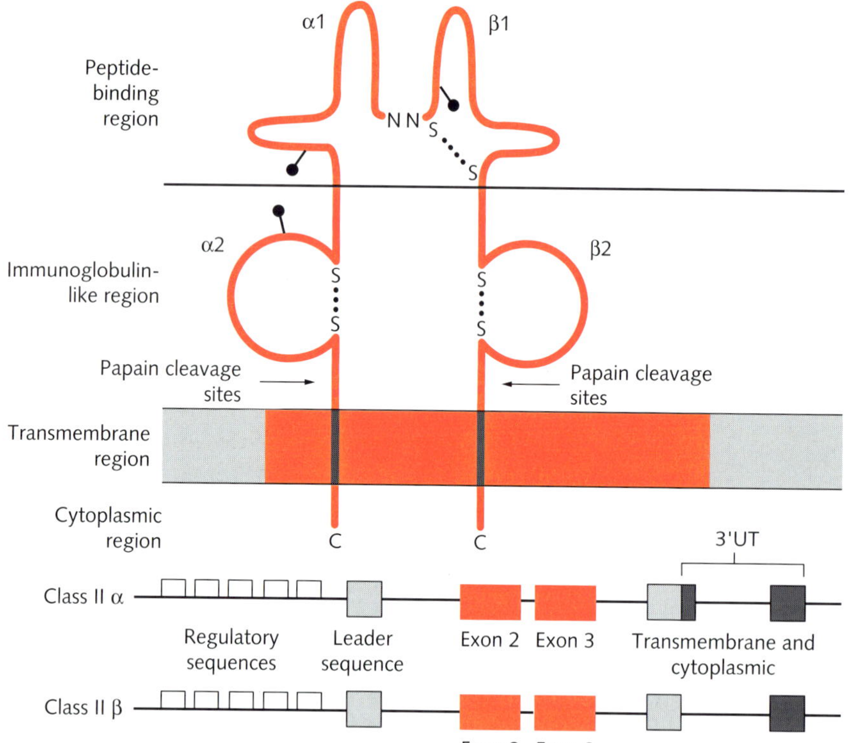

Fig. 14.1b Schematic presentation of HLA class II
The α and β chains of the HLA class II protein (each with two distinct immunoglobulin-like domains, α1 and α2, and β1 and β2) are non-covalently associated. Both domains of each chain are encoded by their respective exons of the α and β class II genes on chromosome 6.

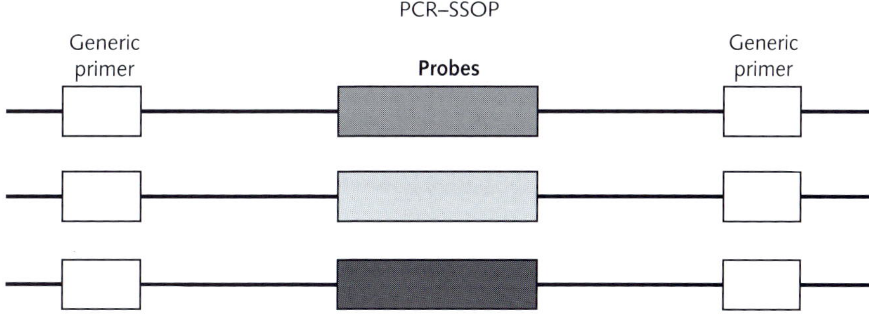

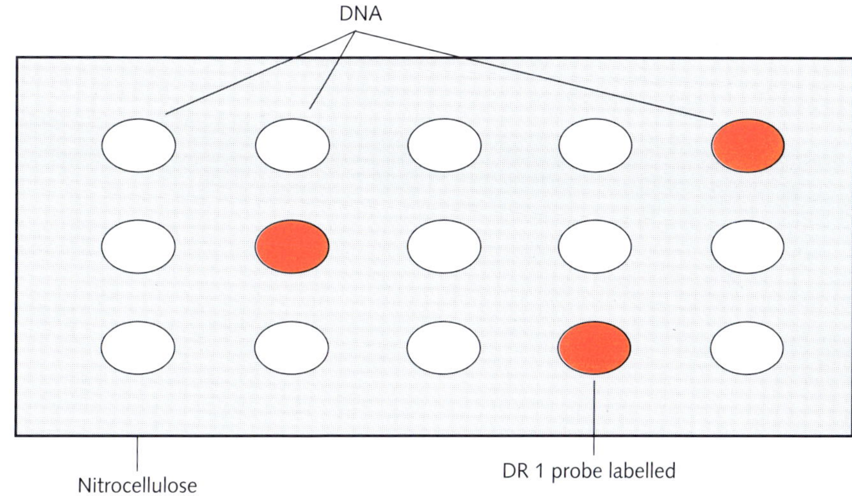

Fig. 14.2 Schematic presentation of PCR-SSOP
A schematic representation of the probing of PCR products with sequence-specific oligonucleotide probes. A segment of the HLA class II DR genes is amplified by PCR with a set of generic primers complementary to highly conserved sequences flanking the polymorphic site. The PCR product is immobilised on a nitrocellulose sheet and probed with sets of allele-specific DR probes. Binding or non-binding of the labelled probes is revealed (red and white spots, respectively).

resolve this ambiguity, PCR-SSP must be used. However, the use of SSOP is useful to screen a large number of samples.

PCR-SSP (Figure 14.3)

This technique involves the use of sequence-specific primers in the PCR. The detection of the amplified DNA is carried out by gel electrophoresis and allows the rapid identification of the HLA alleles in individual samples, since the read-out of this method is the presence or absence of an amplicon for which a specific primer was used. PCR-SSP was first developed to define the various HLA-DRB3 alleles. Although this is a rapid technique, many PCR reactions have to be set up per sample, for example 24 reactions for low-resolution DR typing. An obvious advantage of PCR-SSP is that, as two sequences are detected *in cis*, ambiguities which may arise from PCR-SSOP typing can be resolved. For PCR-SSP typing, however, the target sequence of the alleles must be known, and novel unknown sequences may not always be detected. PCR-SSP is also the technique of choice for HPA typing (*see The molecular basis of platelet-specific or HPA antigens, p. 192*).

Conformational analysis methods

Conformational methods rely on the differential mobility of PCR products in gels. In single-stranded conformational polymorphism analysis or SSCA, PCR-generated DNA products are denatured by heating and rapid cooling to prevent re-annealing of the strands. The products are then run on a polyacrylamide gel, and the mobility depends upon the secondary structure of the single-stranded DNA. The major disadvantage of this technique for HLA typing is the tendency of single-stranded DNA to adopt many conformational forms under the same electrophoretic conditions, resulting in the presence of several bands from a single product.

A modification of this technique, which compares the mobility in polyacrylamide gel electrophoresis of duplex molecules generated by mixing PCR products, is called double-stranded conformational analysis or DSCA. In

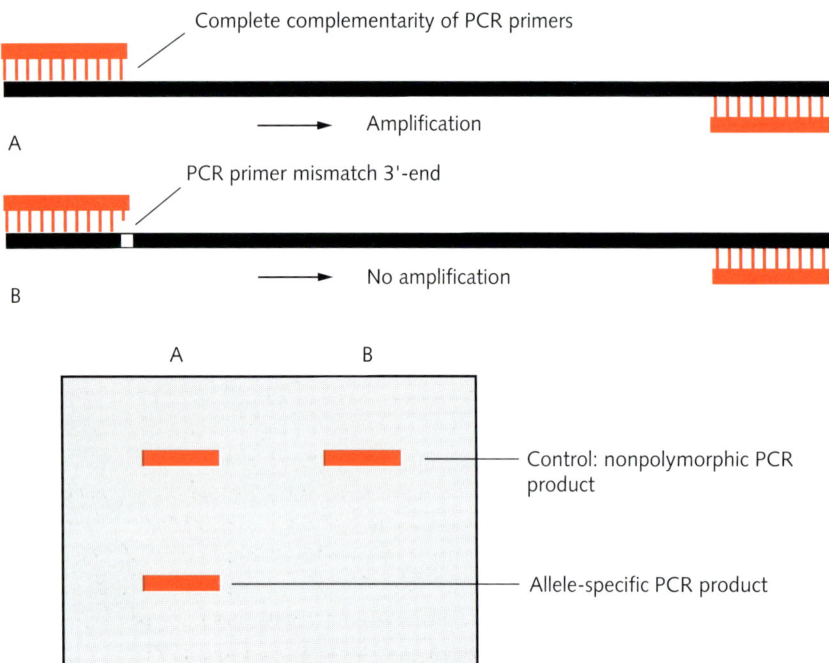

Fig. 14.3a PCR-SSP
With allele-specific PCR specificity is obtained during the PCR. A single nucleotide mismatch at the 3′-end of the allele-specific primer ('B' primer in the figure) will prevent the polymerase from commencing DNA amplification. Therefore, no amplification of template DNA will occur with the 'B' allele primer whilst, with the 'A' allele one, a product is obtained. Ethidium bromide is used to reveal amplified DNA with ultraviolet light after DNA gel electrophoresis. Allele-specific DNA is obtained in the 'A' reaction (lower band) but not in the 'B' reaction. In both reactions a control PCR product is generated by amplification of a segment of the growth hormone gene (upper two bands).

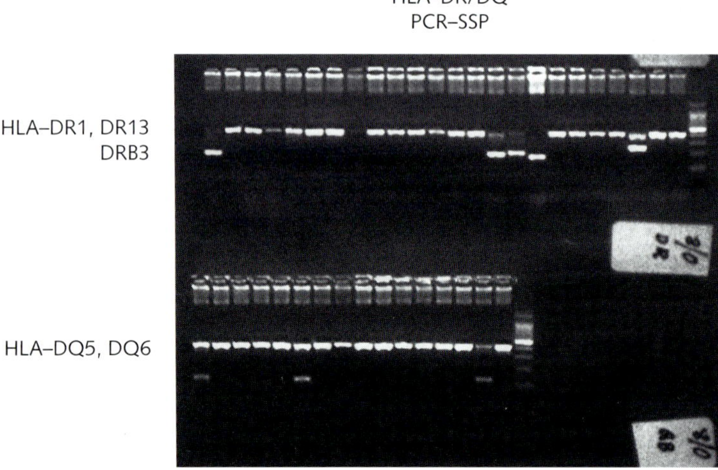

Fig. 14.3b PCR-SSP for DR and DQ alleles
Results of PCR-SSP with template DNA from a single donor. Each lane represents the result of gel electrophoresis of a single PCR reaction with one of the allele-specific DR or DQ primers. From the pattern of positive results, a DR (upper panel) and DQ (lower panel) type can be concluded; in this case DR1, DR13, DRB3 and DQ5, DQ6.

this case, the mobility depends on the mismatching of the sequence and the formation of heteroduplex molecules. A modification of DSCA, known as reference strand conformational analysis or RSCA, has recently been developed and successfully applied to class I and II (DP) typing. In this technique, PCR is carried out on the DNA under test and on a reference DNA sample of known sequence using fluorescently labelled primers for the PCR of the reference DNA. The PCR products of 'tester' and 'reference' are melted and then mixed, re-annealing allowed and then run in an automated DNA sequencer. Only those duplexes containing a labelled strand are detected, i.e. the 'reference DNA' homoduplex and the heteroduplexes of 'reference' and 'tester' DNA. As the mobility of every known allele with the reference DNA has been established, the results obtained with unknown samples can be read. Test samples running at an as yet not observed mobility could represent possible new alleles, whose sequence can be determined by direct sequencing.

Sequencing-based typing

The principle of DNA sequencing is relatively straightforward. It involves the denaturation of the DNA to be analysed to provide a single-strand template; a sequencing primer is then added and the extension is performed by the addition of polymerase in the presence of excess nucleotides. The sequencing mixture is divided into four tubes each of which contains a specific dideoxyribonucleoside triphosphate (ddATP). When this is incorporated into the DNA strand, elongation is interrupted leading to chain termination. In each reaction there is random incorporation of the chain terminators and therefore products of all sizes are generated. The products of the four reactions are then analysed by electrophoresis in parallel lanes of a polyacrylamide–urea gel and the sequence is read by combining the results of each lane using an automated DNA sequencer.

HLA antigens

These are a group of highly polymorphic cell surface molecules, which play a central role in the induction and regulation of immune responses and as such they are involved in the self/non-self recognition, tolerance, rejection of allografts and graft-versus-host disease. The genes coding for these molecules form part of a complex genetic system called the MHC located on the short arm of chromosome 6. This region spans a distance of approximately 4000 kl and is divided into HLA class I, class II and class III. The latter includes a group of non-MHC genes coding for proteins with various immunological functions, such as the complement factor 4 and tumour necrosis factor or TNF-α.

The development of recombinant DNA technology has led to an increased understanding of the genetic complexity, structure and function of the HLA genes and molecules.

HLA class I genes

The HLA class I genes have been classified according to their structure and function as classical and non-classical, or class Ib genes. The classical HLA class I genes HLA-A, B, Cw code for heterodimers formed by a heavy (α) chain of approximately 43 kDa, non-covalently linked to the β2 microglobulin (β2-m) light chain of 12 kDa (Figure 14.1a). The latter is coded for by a gene located outside the HLA region on chromosome 15.

The extracellular portion of the α chain has three domains (α1, α2 and α3) encoded by exons 2, 3 and 4, respectively. Each domain is approximately 90 amino acids in length. The transmembrane and cytoplasmic domains are encoded by exons 5, 6 and 7, respectively. The β2-m which confers stability to the molecule is non-covalently linked to the α3 domain (Figure 14.1a).

The α1 and α2 domains are the most polymorphic regions of these molecules and form a groove consisting of two α helices with an anti-parallel running β pleated sheet forming the floor of the groove. This groove, which is approximately 25 Å long and 10 Å wide, can accommodate a variety of antigen-derived peptides of about 8 to 10 amino acids long to be presented to T-cells.

In addition to the classical HLA class I genes, the non-classical HLA class I genes are also located in this region. They include HLA-E, F and G and their exon/intron organisation is similar to the classical class I genes, but they have a more restricted polymorphism. The HLA class I genes are expressed on the majority of tissues and blood cells including T- and B-lymphocytes and platelets (Table 14.1). The non-classical class I genes, HLA-E and F, are expressed on most tissues tested so far.

HLA class II genes

The HLA class II genes DR, DQ and DP are all located within the HLA class II region. There is one non-polymorphic DRA and nine highly polymorphic DRB genes, of which DRB2, B6 and B9 are pseudogenes. The number of DRB genes expressed in each haplotype varies depending upon the DRB1 allele expressed, for example HLA DR1, DR103, DR8 and DR10 haplotypes only express the DRB1 gene. DR15 and DR16 haplotypes additionally express the DRB5 gene, which codes for the DR51 product. HLA DR17, DR18, DR11, DR12, DR13 and DR14 haplotypes also express the DRB3 genes, which code for the DR52 specificity, whilst the HLA DR4, DR7 and DR9 alleles also express the DRB4 gene, which encodes the DR53 product. There are few exceptions to this gene distribution, for example a DRB5 gene has been found linked to a DR1 haplotype and 'null' DRB5 and DRB4 genes have been identified.

In contrast, there are two DQA and three DQB genes of which only A1 and B1 are expressed, and both are polymorphic. Similarly, there are two genes, A1 and B1, for DPA and DPB, and both are polymorphic.

In addition, a number of HLA-related genes are located within the MHC class II region. These include the LMP2, LMP7, TAP1 and TAP2 genes which are involved in the transport and processing of peptides presented by class I molecules, whilst the HLA-DM A and B genes are relevant to the loading of peptides in the HLA class I molecules.

The HLA class II genes are constitutively expressed on B-lymphocytes, monocytes and dendritic cells, and on activated T-lymphocytes and granulocytes (Table 14.1). HLA class II expression can also be induced on non-haematopoietic cells, for example fibroblasts and endothelial cells, as the result of activation or by the effect of certain inflammatory cytokines such as γ-interferon, TNF-α, etc.

Function

The HLA molecules play a pivotal role in the induction and regulation of the immune response. Both the phenomenon of MHC restriction and the development of tolerance learnt as T-cells go through the thymus result in the selection of a T-cell repertoire that will form the basis of an individual's capacity to respond to antigens. HLA class I molecules are primarily but not exclusively involved in the presentation of endogenous antigens to CD8+ cytotoxic T-cells, whereas the HLA class II molecules present, primarily but not exclusively, exogenous antigenic peptides to CD4+ helper T-cells. These cells, once activated, can initiate and regulate a variety of processes leading to the maturation and differentiation of cellular and humoral effector cells including the secretion of cytokines. The presentation of antigenic peptides is a highly regulated process and requires a fine interaction between the antigenic peptide, the antigen-binding groove of the HLA molecules and the T-cell receptor. Allelic variation of the HLA molecules can profoundly affect the ability to present certain peptides because of the presence or absence of critical contact residues in the peptide-binding groove.

HLA molecules on donor cells loaded with donor-derived peptides can also be recognised directly by T-cells of the host by a mechanism called allorecognition. Two pathways of allorecognition, direct and indirect, have been identified both of which lead to the strong alloimmunisation seen in patients receiving blood transfusion or a solid organ or bone marrow/stem cell transplantation.

Thus HLA molecules have become increasingly more relevant in a variety of clinical situations such as susceptibility to certain autoimmune and infectious diseases, solid organ and stem cell transplantation, and in blood cell alloimmunisation. With regard to the latter, two examples will be discussed; refractoriness for prophylactic platelet transfusion by HLA alloimmunisation (*see Figure 14.4*), and HLA class II restriction of the formation of anti-HPA-1a antibodies.

Prophylactic platelet transfusions

Prophylactic platelet transfusions are essential to prevent bleeding during intensive chemotherapy or other myeloablative therapies. Increments in the platelet count after the infusion of an adult dose of donor platelets ($>250 \times 10^9$/l) are frequently disappointing. Non-immune factors such as splenomegaly, bleeding, sepsis, fever and certain drugs (e.g. amphotericin) can compromise the beneficial effect of donor platelet infusions. In 10–20% of patients the problem of poor increments is further compounded by antibody-mediated destruction of donor platelets. Despite that, the clinical definition of refractoriness remains much disputed, clinically the picture of an increased frequency of platelet transfusions to maintain satisfactory platelet counts and effective haemostasis requires further laboratory investigations for HLA class I, and HPA alloantibodies, platelet autoantibodies or high titre anti-A or anti-B antibodies.

The ability to type donors and patients for HLA class I A and B and HPA by molecular techniques using genomic DNA (*see Molecular typing techniques, p 183*, and *The molecular basis of platelet-specific or HPA antigens, p. 192*) has resulted in a more accurate donor and patient matching, with improved platelet recovery. The algorithm currently used for the management of the alloimmunised patient with poor increments is shown in Figure 14.4.

Haemolytic disease of the newborn (HDN)

The Rh system

The Rh system is the most immunogenic red cell blood group system after the ABO system. Whilst the antigens of the latter are of carbohydrate nature, the Rh antigens are non-glycosylated proteins. Two-dimensional gel electrophoresis of trypsin digests of Rh proteins, which could be performed once human monoclonal antibodies specific for Rh alloantigens were available, provided evidence of a high level of homology between the proteins carrying the RhD, and the RhC/c and RhE/e alloantigens.

The Rh genes

Cloning of the *RhD* and *RhCE* genes (carrying the RhD, and RhC/c and RhE/e antigens, respectively) revealed a high level of sequence homology (Table 14.2), confirming the observation made by gel electrophoresis. These molecular studies suggested that the C/c and E/e antigens are localised on a single protein, the RhCE protein encoded by the *RhCE* gene and its allelic variants. The recent

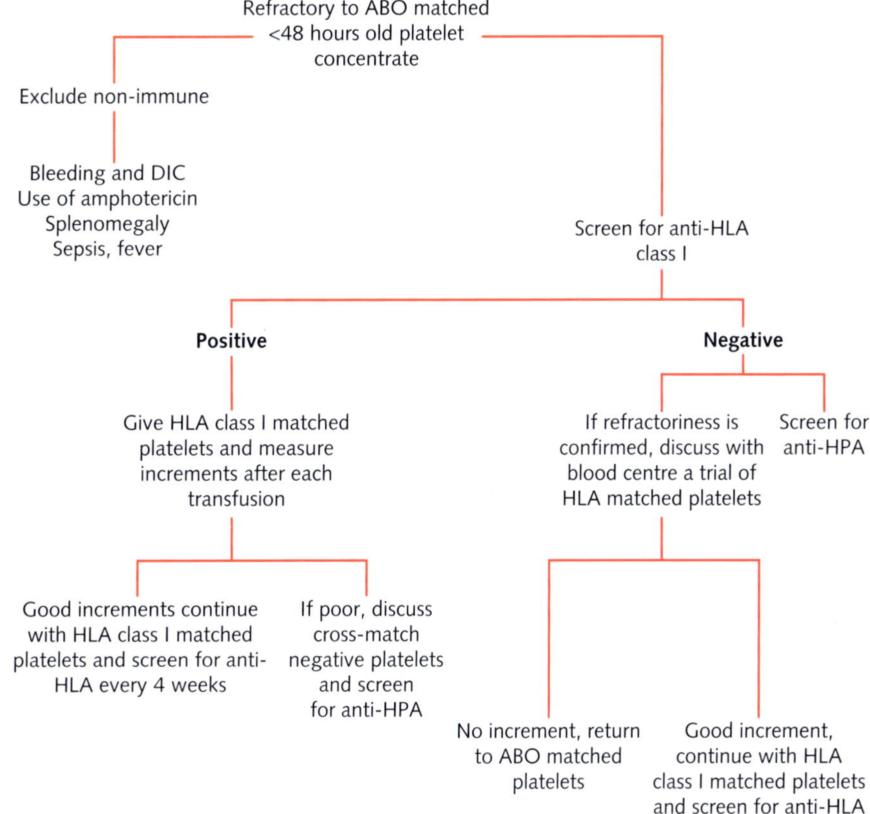

Fig. 14.4 Platelet transfusions in alloimmunised patients
An algorithm outlining the decision process for the management of alloimmunised patients refractory for random donor platelets. After confirmation of refractoriness for random donor platelets, patients are screened for HLA class I alloantibodies and, if positive, HLA class I matched platelets are transfused. In 20–30% of patients increments with HLA class I matched platelets are poor and screening for HPA antibodies should follow. Also, the possible presence of potent anti-A or anti-B should be excluded since platelets do carry ABO blood group antigens. In case there are no detectable HLA class I antibodies, a 'trial' of HLA matched platelets and screening for HPA antibodies should be considered (right arm of algorithm).

Table 14.2 Amino acid sequence of the RhD and RhCE proteins.

CE	MSSKYPRSVRRCLPLWALTLEAALILLFYFFTHYDASLEDQKGLVASYQVGQDLTVMAALGLGFLTSNFRRHSWSS
D	---I-------S--------
	VAFNLFMLALGVQWAILLDGFLSQFPPGKVVITLFSIRLATMSAMSVLISAGVLGKVNLAQLVVMVLVEVTALGT
	--------------------------S-----------------L-----VD----------------------N
	LRMVISNIFNTDYHMNLRHFYVFAAYFGLTVAWCLPKPLPKGTEDNDQRATIPSLSAMLGALFLWMFWPSVNSPLL
	----------------MM-I---------S----------E----K--T----------------I----F--A--
	RSPIQRKNAMFNTYYALAVSVVAISGSSLAHPQRKISMTYVHSAVLAGGVAVGTSCHLIPSPWLAMVTLGVAGLI
	----E----V------V-----------------G---K------------------------------------
	SIGGAKCLPVCCNRVLGIHHISVMHSIFSLLGLLGEITYIVLLVLHTVWNGNGMIGFQVLLSIGELSLAIVIALTS
	-V----Y--G--------P-S-I-GYN----------I-------D--GA--------------------------
	GLLTGLLLNLKIWKAPHVAKYFDDQVFWKFPHLAVGF
	-----------------E-------------------

Amino acids are given in single letter code. Identicity has been underlined.

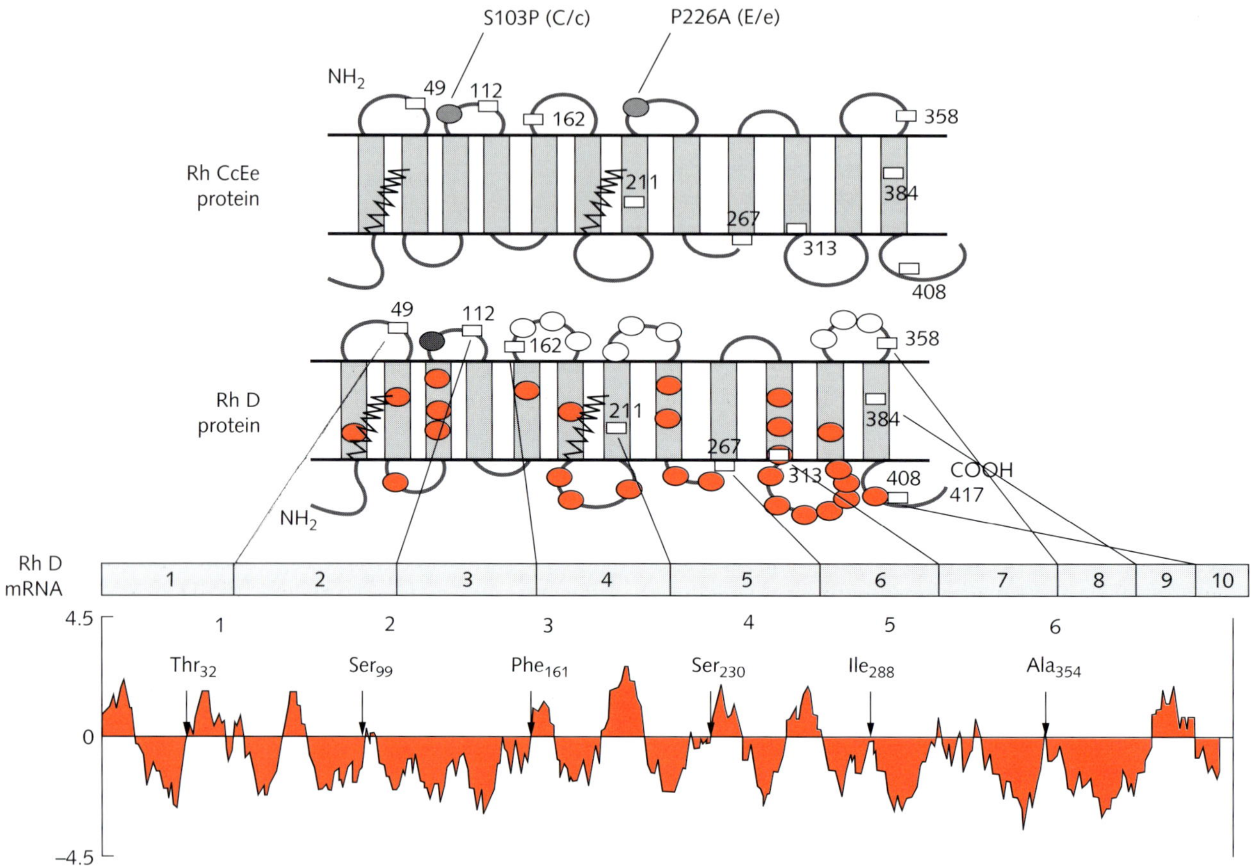

Fig. 14.5 RhD and RhCE proteins
Schematic representation of the topography of the RhCE (upper figure) and RhD (lower figure) proteins. Both 30 kD non-glycosylated proteins traverse the red cell membrane 12 times. The difference between RhD and CE is defined by 36 of the 417 amino acids (black circles are RhD-specific residues, red circles indicate C/c and E/e polymorphisms). The square boxes (1–10) indicate position of exon–exon boundaries in the *RhD* mRNA, and a hydropathy plot of the RhD protein is shown at the bottom.

expression of the *RhD* and *RhCE* genes in K562 cell lines by retroviral transfection provided the ultimate proof that the RhD, and RhC/c and E/e alloantigens are localised on two distinct proteins encoded by these two genes and their respective allelic variants.

The 75 kb spanning RhD gene with 10 exons encodes a 30 kDa non-glycosylated protein of 417 amino acids of unknown function which traverses the red cell membrane 12 times (Figure 14.5). The gene is deleted in RhD-negative individuals (15% of the Caucasian population). The RhC/c and E/e alloantigens are carried on the highly homologous 30 kDa RhC/cE/e protein, which differs by only 36 of the 417 amino acids from RhD (Table 14.2). The difference between RhC and Rhc is associated with six nucleotide substitutions of which four result in a replacement. One of these, residue 103, is exofacial and seems to be the most critical one of the C/c polymorphism. The difference between RhE and Rhe is defined by a single proline–alanine-226 replacement in the fourth extracellular loop of the RhCE protein (Figure 14.5).

Immunogenicity of RhD and prevention of immunisation

The absence of the RhD protein in RhD negatives is the most plausible explanation of its relatively high immunogenicity, as the immune system has not been tolerised by a lookalike RhD protein encoded by an allele of the *RhD* gene. Until the late 1960s the formation of anti-D in RhD-negative pregnant women had a high incidence and was associated with significant neonatal morbidity and mortality because of hydrops fetalis and kernicterus. The discovery that the formation of anti-D could be prevented by the administration of passive immunoglobulin G (IgG) anti-D combined with a much reduced family size has led to a steep decline in

HDN-associated mortality. It is estimated that, per annum in the UK, approximately 150–200 cases of severe RhD immunisation require intrauterine treatment. The officially reported annual mortality for RhD HDN is nine cases, but estimates from screening laboratories suggest that this figure is closer to 50.

The knowledge of the structure of the *RhD* gene makes it now possible to give better support to RhD immunised women as the fetal *RhD* genotype can be determined in the first trimester from amniocyte DNA or from maternal serum. The former is now routinely used in cases of severe RhD immunisation with a RhD (D/d) heterozygous partner, whilst the latter technique which is non-invasive will need further validation before routine application in genetic counselling. The immunogenicity of RhE in RhE-negative individuals is low and the change of severe HDN because of anti-E is infinitely small when compared with anti-D. Its poor immunogenicity is best explained by the relatively small difference between self and non-self. The greater sequence difference between RhC and Rhc is reflected in a greater risk of potent alloantibody formation during pregnancy, albeit severe HDN by anti-C and anti-c antibodies is relatively uncommon.

The Kell system

The K antigen of the Kell system is, after RhD, the second most immunogenic protein blood group alloantigen system on the red cell membrane. The Kell alloantigens K and k are carried on a 93 kDa, type II transmembrane protein of 732 amino acids. The *KEL* gene spans about 21.5 kb with 19 exons and has sequence homology with genes of the protein family of zinc-binding endopeptidases, like the CALLA (CD10) antigen or human common acute lymphoblastic leukaemic antigen. The difference between K and k is based on a single base change in exon 6 causing a methionine–threonine-193 replacement. It is of interest to note that, despite this minor difference between the two forms, K is one of the most immunogenic blood group substances. This is possibly explained, although not proven, by the absence of an N-glycosylation site in the k protein at residue 191.

Immunogenicity of K and mechanism of fetal anaemia

Transfusion frequently triggers the formation of anti-K. As anti-K antibodies can cause severe HDN, it is recommended to transfuse K-negative blood to all girls and women of childbearing age. In K alloimmunisation, fetal anaemia seems to be mainly caused by antibody-mediated inhibition of erythroid maturation. The question why anti-K downregulates erythropoiesis has not been answered, but it points at a possible regulatory role of the K carrying endopeptidase in erythroid differentiation and maturation. Owing to the aplastic nature of the anaemia, the degree of fetal anaemia cannot be assessed by the measurement of bilirubin levels in the amniotic fluid, but should be based on the obstetric history, maternal anti-K level, together with paternal K status. In case of a high-risk scenario with a K-positive partner, the fetal K type should be determined by PCR on amniocyte DNA. If the fetus is K positive, fetal anaemia should be assessed and treated by peri-umbilical blood sampling (PUBS).

Red cell alloantigens other than Rh and K

Similarly to the Rh and K systems, the molecular structure of the majority of other blood group alloantigens has been resolved over the last two decades. Detailed discussion of these systems is beyond the scope of this chapter, but PCR-based typing can now be performed for most clinically relevant blood group systems (e.g. Duffy, Jk, M/N and S/s). This knowledge is of use when blood group alloantibodies are associated with severe HDN. These users include patients with thalassaemia, in whom blood transfusion has been given before a complete red cell phenotype was established.

The high level of sequence homology between the *RhD* and *RhCE* genes, and the occurrence of crossing-over events which are often associated with reduced expression of the Rh antigens, requires ample expertise in the use of PCR for prenatal diagnosis. Therefore, such tests should be performed in laboratories with a scientific interest in blood group genetics.

Haemolytic disease of the newborn (HDN)

Frequency

Of all pregnant women 1–1.5% screen positive for red cell alloantibodies. In roughly half, the antibodies are of possible clinical significance, and antibody potency needs monitoring during pregnancy to determine the risk of significant haemolysis requiring therapy. Severe disease with intrauterine intravascular transfusion therapy occurs in approximately 1 in 5000 pregnancies and is mainly due to anti-D or anti-K.

Pathology

Maternal alloantibodies can be formed against a blood group alloantigen present on the fetal red cells but absent from the maternal ones. RhD, K, Rhc, RhC are the main culprits with respect to HDN. Red cell alloantibodies of the IgG class can cross the placenta, bind to the fetal red cells and shorten their survival. In K immunisation, hyperbilirubinaemia is a less reliable parameter to predict severity of fetal anaemia, and these pregnancies can be complicated by early fetal loss.

Treatment of HDN

An increased concentration of unconjugated bilirubin in the neonate poses the risk of kernicterus. Treatment of severe haemolytic anaemia and hyperbilirubinaemia in the post-delivery setting is by exchange transfusion with compatible donor red cells. When a pregnancy was preceded by one with a history of severe HDN, intrauterine intravascular transfusion of compatible donor red cells by PUBS is the treatment of choice with good outcome in 90% of cases. Genetic counselling of couples with a heterozygous partner has been greatly helped by the discovery of the *Rh* and *K* genes (*see The Rh genes, p. 188*, and *The Kell system, p. 191*).

Prevention of HDN

Before the introduction of anti-D prophylaxis, the majority of HDN cases were caused by RhD immunisation. The routine RhD testing of all pregnant women, combined with anti-D prophylaxis for RhD negatives carrying a RhD-positive infant, has been extremely successful in lowering HDN-associated morbidity and mortality. Screening for clinically significant red cell alloantibodies in pregnant women is the standard of care in most European countries and cases of possible severe disease should be identified early in pregnancy allowing the prevention of morbidity or mortality.

Neonatal alloimmune thrombocytopenia

Platelet-specific or HPA alloantigen systems

Besides the alloantigens shared with other blood cells (e.g. HLA class I A and B alloantigens), platelets also express alloantigens which are carried on proteins uniquely expressed on platelets but not on other blood cells (Table 14.1). Alloimmunisation against platelet-specific antigens or HPA is associated with three clinical syndromes:

1 Neonatal/fetal alloimmune thrombocytopenia (NAITP).
2 Post-transfusion purpura (PTP).
3 Refractoriness for platelet transfusions (PR).

NAITP was first described by van Loghem in 1959 and was initially thought to be a rare disorder. Prospective screening studies in pregnant (Caucasian) women have shown that 1 in 1100 neonates have severe thrombocytopenia ($<50 \times 10^9$/l) due to maternal anti-HPA-1a, confirming the notion that the most frequent cause of severe thrombocytopenia in the term newborn is maternal alloantibodies against a fetal HPA alloantigen.

This serious clinical condition is caused by the destruction of fetal/neonatal platelets by maternal HPA alloantibodies of the IgG class. Cerebral bleeds in the perinatal period are the most concerning complication, which either occur *in utero* or during delivery. In cases of severe thrombocytopenia ($<20 \times 10^9$/l), there remains a small but definite risk of this serious complication in the first days of life, warranting treatment. For proper clinical management, the cause of severe thrombocytopenia in an otherwise healthy term neonate should be determined with urgency and correction of a count $<20 \times 10^9$/l by platelet transfusion is of utmost importance. This should precede the outcome of platelet antibody investigation, as this can be time-consuming.

The molecular basis of platelet-specific or HPA antigens

So far, 19 platelet-specific alloantigen systems have been described. All are bi-allelic and have been mapped to certain membrane proteins. Eleven of the 19 alloantigen systems are on the integrin heterodimer $\alpha_{IIb}\beta_3$ or GPIIb/IIIa (Table 14.3 and Figure 14.6); of the remaining eight, three are on GPIb/IX/V, two on the integrin $\alpha_2\beta_1$ or GPIa/IIa and one each on GPIV, GPV and CD109. With the advent of PCR, the molecular basis of all but five of the systems has been resolved in the last decade. With the exception of one system, the difference between the two alleles is a single nucleotide substitution in the gene encoding the relevant glycoprotein (Table 14.3). Amplification of genomic DNA by PCR-SSP (*see PCR-SSP, p. 185*, and *Figure 14.7*) can be used to type donors and patients, even when the latter are thrombocytopenic.

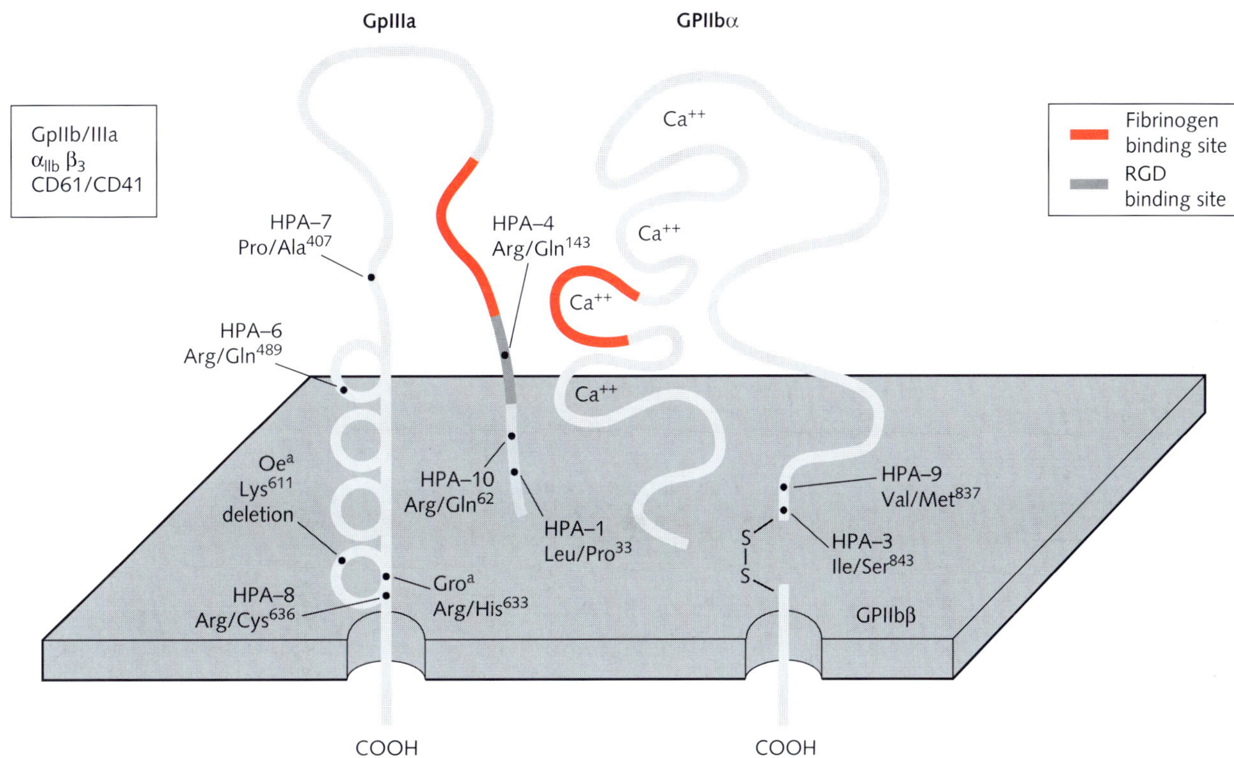

Fig. 14.6 Schematic presentation of GPIIb/IIIa
A schematic presentation of platelet GPIIb/IIIa or the $\alpha_{IIb}\beta_3$ integrin. GPIIIa is recognised by murine monoclonal antibodies of the CD61 cluster and the heterodimer by antibodies of the CD41 cluster. The amino acid substitutions arising from the allelic variation of the GPIIb and GPIIIa genes are depicted by black dots and the name of the HPA system is noted. Amino acids are given in three-letter acronyms. The fibrinogen-binding site is in 'red' and the Arg/Gly/Asp (RGD)-binding site is in 'dark grey'. The RGD peptide is the minimal fibrinogen-derived peptide which binds GPIIb/IIIa.

Immunogenicity and immune response restriction

As the difference between self and non-self is defined by a single amino acid substitution, the immunogenicity of the HPA alloantigens is relatively poor, when compared with that of some of the other blood cell alloantigens (e.g. RhD and HLA class I). The two most clinically relevant HPA antigens are HPA-1a and HPA-5b on the β_3 and α_2 integrins, platelets GPIIIa and GPIa, respectively. Alloantibodies against other HPA alloantigens are observed infrequently in pregnancy but do occur, albeit at a low frequency, in haemato-oncological and other patients on long-term prophylactic platelet transfusion.

The HPA-1a and 1b alloantigens are based on a cytosine for guanidine mutation in the GPIIIa gene resulting in leucine–proline-33 mutation. Why the immunogenicity of HPA-1a (leucine-33) is magnitudes higher than that of its anti-thetical antigen HPA-1b (proline-33) was initially not well understood. In the early 1980s, it was discovered that the formation of anti-HPA-1a in pregnancy was positively associated with the HLA haplotype A1, B8, DR3. Further study revealed that nearly all antibody formers were positive for the 0101 allele of the DRB3 gene (DRB3*0101 or DR52a, *see HLA class II genes*, p. 187, and *Figure 14.8*). A prospective study in 25,000 pregnant women showed that this class II marker has an odds ratio of 140, which makes it one of the most reliable HLA associations reported to date, with an equally negative predictive power as HLA B27 in ankylosing spondylitis. A differential in the efficiency of presentation of the GPIIIa-leucine-33 (HPA-1a)-derived oligopeptide between DRB3*0101-positive and negative antigen-presenting cells to CD4-positive T-cells is the most likely explanation of this restriction in alloimmunisation. The frequency of the HLA DRB3*0101 allele in Caucasians is 33% and this marker has therefore a high negative predictive value but a low positive one for anti-HPA-1a formation.

Allele frequencies

In Caucasians, the allele frequency for the majority

Table 14.3 Platelet-specific alloantigen systems.

System	Antigen	Alternative names	Glycoprotein	Nucleotide change	Amino acid change
HPA-1	1a	Zw^a, Pl^{A1}	GPIIIa	T^{196}	$Leucine^{33}$
	1b	Zw^b, Pl^{A2}		C^{196}	$Proline^{33}$
HPA-2	2a	Ko^b	GPIbα	C^{524}	$Threonine^{145}$
	2b	Ko^a, Sib^a		T^{524}	$Methionine^{145}$
HPA-3	3a	Bak^a, Lek^a	GPIIb	T^{2622}	$Isoleucine^{843}$
	3b	Bak^b		G^{2622}	$Serine^{843}$
HPA-4	4a	Yuk^b, Pen^a	GPIIIa	G^{526}	$Arginine^{143}$
	4b	Yuk^a, Pen^b		A^{526}	$Glutamine^{143}$
HPA-5	5a	Br^b, Zav^b	GPIa	G^{1648}	Glutamic $acid^{505}$
	5b	Br^a, Zav^a, Hc^a		A^{1648}	$Lysine^{505}$
HPA-6w			GPIIIa	G^{1564}	$Arginine^{489}$
	6bw	Ca^a, Tu^a		A^{1564}	$Glutamine^{489}$
HPA-7w			GPIIIa	C^{1267}	$Proline^{407}$
	7bw	Mo		G^{1267}	$Alanine^{407}$
HPA-8w			GPIIIa	T^{2004}	$Arginine^{636}$
	8bw	Sr^a		C^{2004}	$Cysteine^{636}$
HPA-9w			GPIIb	G^{2603}	$Valine^{837}$
	9bw	Max^a		A^{2603}	$Methionine^{837}$
HPA-10w			GPIIIa	G^{281}	$Arginine^{62}$
	10bw	La^a		A^{281}	$Glutamine^{62}$
			GPIIIa	G^{1946}	$Arginine^{633}$
		Gro^a		A^{1946}	$Histidine^{633}$
		Iy^a	GPIbβ	G^{141}	$Glycine^{15}$
				A^{141}	Glutamic $acid^{15}$
		Oe^a	GPIIIa		
		Va^a	GPIIb/IIIa		
		Gov^a	CD109		
		Gov^b			
		Pl^T	GPV		
		Vis	GPIV		
		Pe^a	GPIbα		
		Sit^a	GPIa		

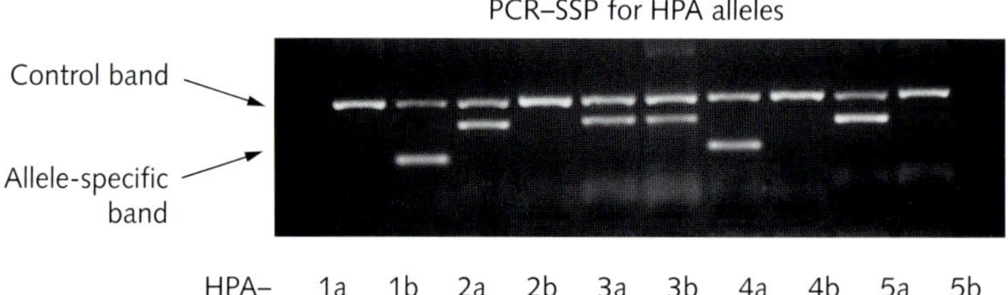

Fig. 14.7 PCR-SSP for HPA alleles
Results of the agarose gel electrophoresis of PCR products obtained by amplification of segments of the GPIIIa, GPIbα, GPIIb and GPIa genes using allele-specific primers for the 'a' and 'b' alleles of the HPA-1, -2, -3, -4 and -5 systems. The results on this donor are HPA-1b1b, 2a2a, 3a3b, 4a4a and 5a5a. Products of the allele-specific amplification are the lower bands. In all reactions a set of control primers has been included to produce an amplicon (upper band) derived from the growth hormone gene.

of HPA systems is skewed towards the 'a' allele. The allele frequencies vary between populations, for example GPIIIa-proline-33 (HPA-1b) is extremely rare or absent in the Far East, whilst the opposite is the case for the GPIIIa-glutamine-143 form (HPA-4b).

Incidence of NAITP

Alloantibodies against the HPA-1a (Pl^{A1}, Zw^a) alloantigen occur in 1 in 365 pregnancies and cause severe thrombocytopenia with a neonatal platelet count $<50 \times 10^9$/l in 1 in 1100 term neonates.

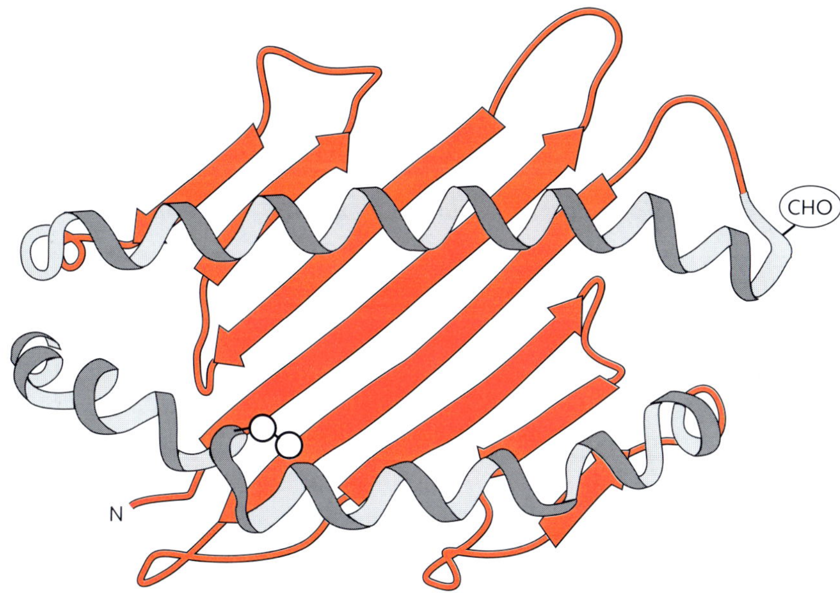

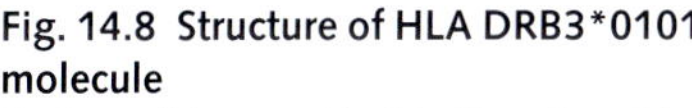
Fig. 14.8 Structure of HLA DRB3*0101 molecule
A view of the peptide-binding site of the HLA class II DRB3*0101 molecule as seen by the T-cell receptor of a T-lymphocyte. Two α helices (see Figure 14.1b) are resting on a base of anti-parallel running β pleated sheets. The antigen-derived peptide is not shown, but in our example of immune response restriction an oligopeptide derived from fetal GPIIIa-Leu33 will be juxtaposed between the two helices. The presence of this peptide defines the difference between self and non-self and triggers the proliferation of GPIIIa-Leu33 (HPA-1a) alloantigen-specific helper T-cells.

Pathology

Maternal IgG alloantibodies against a fetal HPA alloantigen can cross the placenta, bind to the fetal platelets thus reducing platelet survival. HPA-1a and HPA-5b are the two clinically most relevant alloantigens.

Characteristics

Presents in the otherwise healthy newborn as petechiae or ecchymoses or is found coincidentally by a whole blood count. Severe cases can present with neurological symptoms because of cerebral bleeds or with hydrops fetalis or cerebral cysts. Diagnosis is based on the detection of HPA alloantibodies in the maternal serum combined with a parental HPA incompatibility as determined by PCR-SSP.

Inheritance

All systems described to date are bi-allelic with co-dominant expression of both alleles. Homozygous women can produce alloantibodies against a paternally inherited platelet alloantigen present on the fetal platelets but absent from the maternal ones. In cases where the partner is homozygous for the relevant alloantigen, there is a 100% chance that his future offspring will be at risk, whilst in the case of heterozygosity, 50% will be affected.

Treatment

A neonatal platelet count $<20 \times 10^9$/l should be corrected immediately, preferably with HPA-1a and 5b-negative donor platelets, as these will be compatible with the maternal HPA alloantibody in over 95% of cases. In cases of absence of HPA compatible ones, initial transfusion of random ABO/RhD compatible platelets should be considered, followed by the transfusion of compatible ones if the platelet count dips again. In a typical case the platelet count should recover to normal within a week, although a more protracted recovery can occur.

In a subsequent pregnancy a decision needs to be taken on whether treatment of the fetus, the mother or both is indicated, or whether conservative management is acceptable. In cases of the latter, the pregnancy should be closely monitored, and the mother advised to avoid any non-steroidal anti-inflammatory drugs as well as aspirin. The delivery needs careful planning between obstetric and paediatric teams in close consultation with the consultant haematologist. Treatment during pregnancy should be reserved for the cases in which the estimated risk of severe fetal/neonatal thrombocytopenia is considerable and treatment should be in collaboration with a fetal medicine unit. The available treatments during pregnancy are (i) intrauterine intravascular transfusion of compatible platelets by PUBS at weekly intervals or just before delivery, (ii) intravenous IgG (ivIgG) or corticosteroids, or a combination of both, to the mother. As no randomised trials have been performed on either therapy, firm evidence of efficacy is lacking. However, weekly platelet transfusions by PUBS, although invasive and technically demanding, has shown good outcome in families with previously severely affected children. Repeated infusion of ivIgG to the mother remains highly controversial as the initial report of its possible effectiveness made use of a historical control group. The costs are high and there remains a small but definite risk of transmission of infectious agents by a protein concentrate obtained from large plasma pools. The precise mechanism of action, if any, of corticosteroids administered to the mother on the severity of fetal disease is poorly understood.

Counselling

Counselling of couples with an index case about the risks of severe fetal/neonatal thrombocytopenia in a next pregnancy needs to be based on the severity of disease in the index case and the outcome of immunological investigations. The following should be taken into account:

- Thrombocytopenia in subsequent cases is as, or generally more, severe.
- Antibody specificity and titre have some correlation with severity, for example HPA-5b antibodies generally cause mild thrombocytopenia, which rarely results in a cerebral bleed. The latter is generally associated with HPA-1a antibodies.
- A high titre HPA antibody is more likely to be associated with severe thrombocytopenia, but cerebral bleeds also occur with low titres.

Neonatal alloimmune neutropenia

Maternal alloimmunisation against neutrophil-specific alloantigens on fetal/neonatal neutrophils is rare, although there are no precise prevalence figures. Clinical presentation is one of mainly bacterial infection with a selective neutropenia on a whole blood cell count. The number of well-characterised neutrophil-specific alloantigen systems is limited.

The NA system

The most immunogenic, bi-allelic NA alloantigen system is localised on the neutrophil FcRγIIIb (CD16), one of the two low-affinity receptors (R) for the constant domain (Fc) of human IgG (γ). The difference between the two alleles is based on four amino acids with an arginine/serine, asparagine/serine, aspartate/asparagine and valine/isoleucine at positions 36, 65, 82 and 106. This polymorphism results in a molecular weight shift between the two isoforms because of the loss of a glycosylation site in the NA1 protein (50–65 kDa, FcγRIIIb-NA1 and 65–80 kDa, FcγRIIIb-NA2). Two other FcγRIIIb associated alloantigens have been reported. The LAN antigen, which was associated with neonatal alloimmune neutropenia in an Aboriginal family, and SH which is based on an alanine–asparagine-78 mutation of a FcγRIIIb isoform encoded by an additional FcRγIIIB gene which is present in 10% of Caucasians. The latter is associated with an increased expression of the FcγRIIIb.

The FcγRIIIb 'null' phenotype is rare and is based on a double deletion of the FcγRIIIb gene, and is in some associated with a deletion of the FcγRIIc gene. The deficiency for the most abundant Fc receptor on neutrophils does not seem to be associated with an obvious clinical phenotype. This is in contrast with a mutation in the *FcγRIIIa* gene, which encodes a leucine–histidine-48 substitution in the first extracellular domain of the NA cell FcγRIIIa which, although only described in one infant, was associated with recurrent and serious respiratory tract viral infection from birth. The FcγRIIIb 'null' phenotype can cause immune neutropenia in the newborn due to maternal anti-FcγRIIIb isoantibodies.

PCR techniques can be used to determine the NA, SH and FcγRIIIb 'null' genotypes, and transfectants expressing the FcγRIIIb NA allotypes are useful probes for alloantibody detection.

NB alloantigens

Of the two NB alloantigens, NB1 and NB2, the former is localised on a 58–64 kDa secondary granule protein and is expressed as a glycosyl–phosphatidyl–inositol anchored surface membrane glycoprotein on neutrophils. The percentage of neutrophils expressing the NB antigens varies between individuals, and anti-NB alloantibodies can give a typical bi-modal fluorescence profile when granulocytes from a donor with partial NB expression are used. The gene encoding the NB protein has not been cloned and NB alloantigen typing is based on the use of human immune antisera and immunofluorescence.

Alloantigens on CD11a and CD11b

The genes encoding the αL and αM subunits of the β2 integrin or CD11a and CD11b are polymorphic. The alloantiserum Ond^a defines an arginine–threonine-766 mutation in αL (CD11a) and the Mart^a alloantiserum an arginine–histidine-61 mutation in αM (CD11b). Alloantibody formation against these two polymorphisms has been observed in transfusion recipients, but no neonatal neutropenia due to anti-CD11a or CD11b has been reported. This is best explained by the wide tissue distribution of these proteins.

In addition to neonatal neutropenia, neutrophil-specific antibodies are implicated in non-haemolytic febrile transfusion reactions, transfusion-related acute lung injury and autoimmune neutropenia. Severe but reversible neutropenia in the newborn might require treatment with antibiotics to control bacterial infection. So far, there is minimal to no evidence that the mutations in the FcγRIIIb protein have any functional consequences exemplified by the recently described FcγRIIIb 'null' phenotype which is not linked with an obvious pathological phenotype. In sharp contrast, the single amino acid mutation in the NK cell FcγRIIIa gene, which might be rare, might be associated with a more grave clinical condition.

Conclusions

The molecular basis of the majority of blood cell alloantigens, including those of the HLA system, has been discovered over the last two decades. The use of molecular techniques allows their reliable definition at high resolution, replacing previous less reliable techniques which were based on the use of polyclonal antibody reagents. This new body of knowledge has already made a significant contribution to current clinical management. On the one hand, first trimester fetal typing for blood cell-specific alloantigens can now be used in cases of severe maternal alloimmunisation to prevent fetal and neonatal morbidity, and improved selection of HLA and HPA matched donor platelets aids the management of haemato-oncological patients. On the other hand, it is envisaged that in the near future bone marrow and solid organ transplants across apparent mismatches can progress because of the identification of so-called 'permissive mismatches', and better HLA matching will allow accommodation of the graft at lower levels of immune suppression. Finally, a more complete understanding of the molecular rules defining a subject's immune response status should lead to the identification of 'high responders' in order to target these for a more specific manipulation of their immune system with the aim of establishing alloantigen-specific non-responsiveness.

Further reading

Bennett PR, Le Van Kim C, Colin Y *et al.* (1993) Prenatal determination of fetal RhD type by DNA amplification. *New England Journal of Medicine*, **329**, 607–610.

Deo YM, Graziano RF, Repp R, van de Winkel JG. (1997) Clinical significance of IgG Fc receptors and Fc gamma R-directed immunotherapies. *Immunology Today*, **18**, 127–135.

Gruen JR, Weissman SM. (1997) Evolving views of the major histocompatibility complex. *Blood*, **90**, 4252–4265.

Howell WM, Navarrete C. (1996) The HLA system: an update and relevance to patient–donor matching strategies in clinical transplantation. *Vox Sanguinis*, **71**, 6–12.

Huizinga TW, Roos D, von dem Borne AE. (1990) Neutrophil Fc-gamma receptors: a two-way bridge in the immune system. *Blood*, **75**, 1211–1214.

Kuijpers RW, von dem Borne AE, Kiefel V *et al.* (1992) Leucine33–proline33 substitution in human platelet glycoprotein IIIa determines HLA-DRw52a (Dw24) association of the immune response against HPA-1a (Zwa/PIA1) and HPA-1b (Zwb/PIA2). *Human Immunology*, **34**, 253–256.

Le van Kim C, Mouro I, Cherif Zahar B *et al.* (1992) Molecular cloning and primary structure of the human blood group RhD polypeptide. *Proceedings of the National Academy of Sciences (USA)*, **89**, 10925–10929.

Madrigal JA, Arguello R, Scott I, Avakian H. (1997) Molecular histocompatibility typing in unrelated donor bone marrow transplantation. *Blood Reviews*, **11**, 105–117.

Maslanka K, Yassai M, Gorski J. (1996) Molecular identification of T cells that respond in a primary bulk culture to a peptide derived from a platelet glycoprotein implicated in neonatal alloimmune thrombocytopenia. *Journal of Clinical Investigation*, **98**, 1802–1808.

Mouro I, Colin Y, Cherif Zahar B, Cartron JP, Le Van Kim C. (1993) Molecular genetic basis of the human Rhesus blood group system. *Nature Genetics*, **5**, 62–65.

Newman PJ, Valentin N. (1995) Human platelet alloantigens: recent findings, new perspectives. *Thrombosis and Haemostasis*, **74**, 234–239.

Smythe JS, Avent ND, Judson PA *et al.* (1996) Expression of RHD and RHCE gene products using retroviral transduction of K562 cells establishes the molecular basis of Rh blood group antigens. *Blood*, **87**, 2968–2973.

van Loghem JJ, Dorfmeyer H, van de Hart M, Schreuder F. (1959) Serological and genetical studies on the platelet antigen (zw). *Vox Sanguinis*, **4**, 161–169.

Vaughan JI, Manning M, Warwick RM *et al.* (1998) Inhibition of erythroid progenitor cells by anti-Kell antibodies in fetal alloimmune anemia. *New England Journal of Medicine*, **338**, 798–803.

von dem Borne AE, de Haas M, Roos D, Homburg CH, van der Schoot CE. (1995) Neutrophil antigens, from bench to bedside. *Immunological Investigation*, **24**, 245–272.

von dem Borne AE, Ouwehand WH. (1989) Immunology of platelet disorders. *Baillieres Clinical Haematology*, **2**, 749–781.

Warkentin TE, Smith JW. (1997) The alloimmune thrombocytopenic syndromes. *Transfusion Medicine Reviews*, **11**, 296–307.

Williamson LM, Hackett G, Rennie J. (1998) The natural history of fetomaternal alloimmunization to the platelet-specific antigen HPA-1a (PlA1, Zwa) as determined by antenatal screening. *Blood*, **92**, 2280–2287.

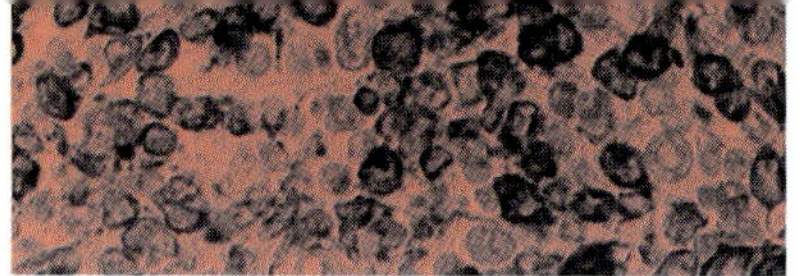

Chapter 15 Haematopoietic growth factors

Graham Molineux & Rosemary Mazanet

Introduction

It has been known since ancient times that the blood system responds to specific stimuli in order to preserve homeostasis. To provide for ongoing replenishment of short-lived cellular blood elements, as well as prompt and specific differentiation of target cells in response to stress states such as blood loss or infection, is the process of *haematopoiesis*. Haematopoiesis is regulated on several levels; the cells themselves have differing maturation potentialities (Figure 15.1), the extracellular matrix within which haematopoiesis occurs is known to have more than a merely permissive role, and there exists also a series of glycoprotein hormones termed the haematopoietic growth factors (HGFs). The mechanisms used to effect regulation of haematopoiesis involve complex cellular interactions as well as responses to circulating HGF and may result in apoptosis, mitosis and differentiation of specific subsets of haematopoietic progenitor cells.

The development of semisolid culture systems over three decades ago allowed normal haematopoietic progenitor cells to proliferate *in vitro* and form recognisable colonies when conditioned media (containing various sera or extracts) were used. Because the specific protein factors that induce colony growth were initially identified in the sera through these colony formation assays, they were named *colony-stimulating factors*, or CSFs. Considerable progress followed quickly to determine the cell types contained within the haematopoietic colonies and in characterising the different CSFs in both murine and human systems. The *in vitro* assays continue to be refined and have identified the lineage hierarchy of normal haematopoietic progenitor cells, and the CSFs involved at each level.

In addition to the CSFs, many interleukins (ILs, originally immune cell to immune cell signalling molecules) have been identified which are active in the haematopoietic cascade. Some ILs can be, or originally were, considered to be single-lineage HGFs, such as IL-2 (T-cell growth factor), IL-5 (eosinophil differentiation factor), IL-7 (B-lymphocyte progenitor cell growth factor) and IL-12 (natural killer-cell stimulatory factor), although in general they are now believed to be quite pleiotropic.

Many of these cytokines are produced by marrow stromal cells and are undoubtedly involved in haematopoietic stem cell development at specific sites within the marrow. Indeed, several examples of interactions with specific extracellular matrix materials have emphasised that CSFs often are localised very specifically and may effect their actions via locally determined mechanisms. We now know that the CSFs induce proliferation of haematopoietic progenitor cells, activate mature blood cells, enhance mature effector cell function and initiate the production of other HGFs.

Molecular cloning

The use of improved biotechnology tools led to the isolation, cloning and expression of these factors to produce large quantities for pharmacological use, but the challenges early investigators faced were substantial. We will illustrate a few examples below.

Murine IL-3, the first HGF to be cloned, was also known as multi-CSF from its demonstrated activity as a T-cell stimulatory factor, mast cell-growth factor, eosinophil CSF, erythroid megakaryocyte-stimulating factor, and granulocyte and macrophage stimulating activities in murine systems. When murine cDNA clones were used to probe for the human gene, they were unable

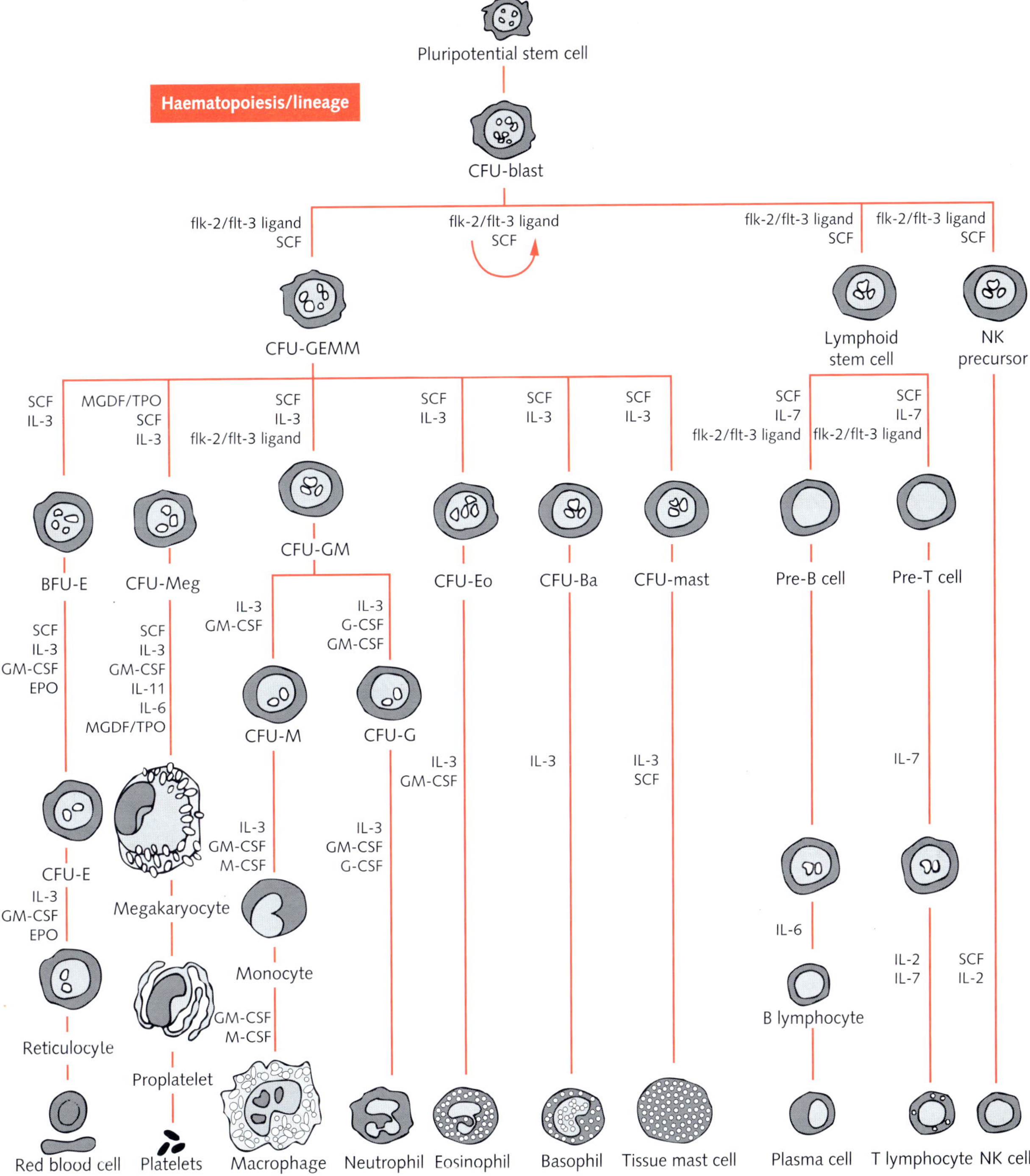

Fig. 15.1 Scheme of haematopoiesis including some of the growth factors that influence the production of blood cells
Key: CFU-GEMM, multilineage colony-forming cell; BFU-E, erythroid burst-forming cell; CFU-GM, granulocyte-macrophage colony-forming cell; CFU-M, macrophage colony-forming cell; CFU-Eo, eosinophil colony-forming cell; CFU-Ba, basophil colony-forming cell; IL, interleukin; SCF, stem cell factor; G-CSF, granulocyte colony-stimulating factor; GM-CSF, granulocyte-macrophage colony-stimulating factor; M-CSF, macrophage colony-stimulating factor; TPO, thrombopoietin; MGDF, megakaryocyte growth and development factor; EPO, erythropoietin.

to hybridise human DNA leading to the conclusion that there was only minor homology between the two molecules. It was later learned that there is only 29% homology between murine and human IL-3 proteins, with no cross-reactivity, prohibiting their use in assays for each other.

The cloning of erythropoietin (EPO), the first HGF to become commercially available, provides interesting insight into the challenges involved in the field of biotechnology research. Following its purification from the urine of aplastic anaemia patients, there was a limited amount known about the primary structure of human erythropoietin (EPO) and no known source of erythropoietic mRNA. No cell lines had been described that produced significant amounts of EPO that could be useful as a source of mRNA.

The human *EPO* gene was cloned in two laboratories using similar techniques. It was necessary to use several methods to isolate a single copy gene from a genomic library with multiple DNA probes. Once the technology was developed and the appropriate DNA probe sequences were identified, however, it was possible to clone the human, monkey and mouse genes for EPO. The choice of cell line (Chinese hamster ovary, CHO) to produce a glycosylated product necessary for *in vivo* activity of EPO complicated the final stages of drug development.

Another successful commercialised use of biotechnology is G-CSF (granulocyte colony-stimulating factor), where the presence of the factor in the serum of endotoxin-treated mice was first recognised as having haematopoietic regulatory activity and was able to induce differentiation of a mouse leukaemic cell line. The human G-CSF molecule was purified from the bladder carcinoma cell line 5637 or from a squamous cell carcinoma cell line and the gene cloned. Luckily for the early investigators, G-CSF has biological activity across species (i.e. human G-CSF is biologically active in mice), probably because of close homology in functional domains (73% overall homology at the protein level between human and murine molecules) (Figure 15.2).

In contrast, GM-CSF (granulocyte-macrophage colony-stimulating factor), another myeloid lineage factor which is also commercially available, was purified from a human monocyte cell line U937 and a mouse T-lymphoma cell line ATCC-CRL-8080. Unlike G-CSF, there is no close homology between human GM-CSF and murine GM-CSF, although the molecular structure of GM-CSF is relatively highly conserved, with 56% homology at the protein level between human and murine forms, but the haematopoietic activity does not cross these species barriers (Figure 15.3). The lack of an appropriate animal model for testing may have resulted in some drug development delays.

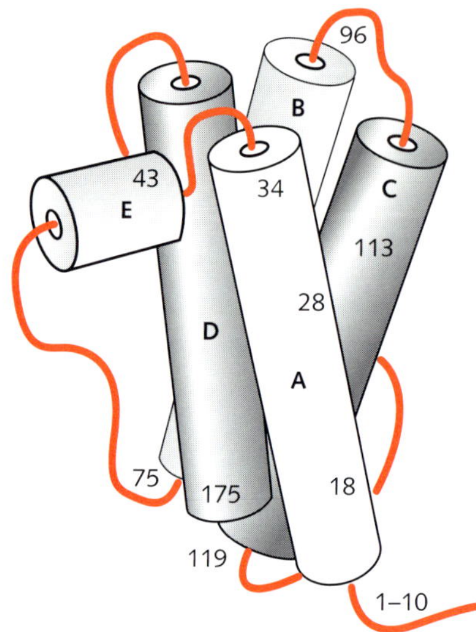

Fig. 15.2 G-CSF as an example of the structure of a cytokine
Note the four antiparallel helices. Amino acid numbers are shown in the diagram.

Thrombopoietin was long thought to exist, but demonstration of the lineage-restricted regulator of platelet production was not completed until relatively recently. The redundancy apparent in the regulators of this lineage may manifest itself in other lineages as well when a fuller understanding is gained. However, on a practical level, the overlap of many cytokines in the regulation of thrombopoiesis led to the development of numerous putative 'platelet factors' such as IL-3, GM-CSF, IL-6 and IL-11 before the lineage-restricted regulator was found. Thus blind alleys also existed to mislead the intrepid early researcher.

The results from molecular cloning have not only allowed for the production of large quantities of purified factors for further experiments, but have often provided clues on how cytokine networks interact or on how disease states may be further studied. It is interesting to note that chromosome 5q contains a family of genes involved in haematopoietic regulation. The genes for GM-CSF, IL-3, M-CSF and the M-CSF receptor (c-fms), IL-4, IL-5 and the receptor for PDGF all map to the long arm of chromosome 5 prompting speculation that additional genes involved in haematopoiesis will be discovered in this region. It is noteworthy that deletions involving chromosome 5q have been described in various haematopoietic disease states. The gene encoding G-CSF is on chromosome 17, near the t(15;17)

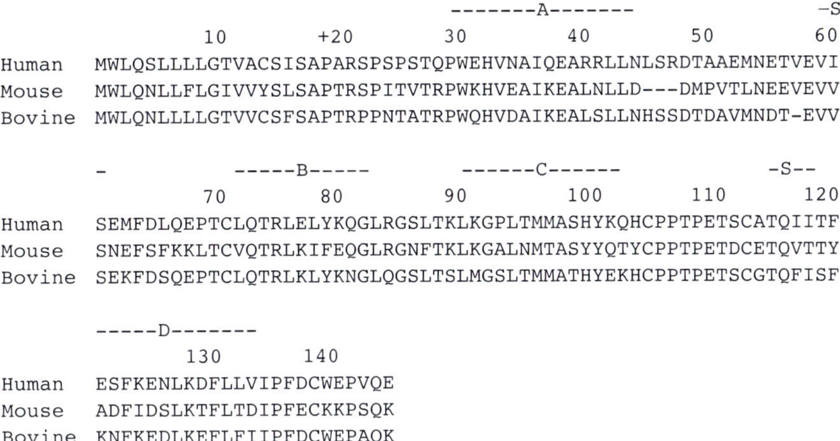

Fig. 15.3 Divergence in amino acid sequence of GM-CSF from mouse and human

translocation breakpoint characteristic of acute promyelocytic leukaemia.

Haematopoiesis *in vivo*

Expression

In the majority of mature cell types investigated, transcription of the *GM-CSF*, *G-CSF* and *M-CSF* genes is constitutive even in the absence of specific stimuli, although the transcripts are rapidly degraded in the cytoplasm and do not become useful protein unless the stabilisation of mRNAs leads to induction. There is little evidence for constitutive production of some CSFs except that fibroblast and endothelial cell lines spontaneously produce M-CSF *in vitro* (whether this occurs *in vivo* is as yet unclear), implying regulation via production in response to unknown factors. Contrasting with the myeloid growth factors is the newly described thrombopoietin, which would appear to be produced constitutively and regulated primarily via consumption rather than production. Even less is known about the mechanisms required to shut off CSF production, although there is evidence for downregulation of transcription after induction. The biological effects of cytokines are mediated through binding to a low number of high-affinity receptors on target cells. These cell surface receptors also appear to be widely expressed by abnormal haematopoietic cells and by non-haematopoietic cells. The potential significance of this ligand binding will be discussed later.

Receptor binding

Receptors consist of extracellular binding domain(s) and an intracellular domain that serves to activate cytoplasmic kinases leading to cell differentiation and proliferation. Defects in the internal domain of this receptor can alter cell behaviour to favour proliferation without differentiation, a remarkable discovery and one that has led to the suggestion of a specific lesion which predisposes severe congenital neutropenia patients to the development of acute myeloid leukaemia. G-CSF exerts its function via the activation of a membrane receptor that belongs to the superfamily of haematopoietin receptors, also referred to as class I cytokine receptors. Characteristic structural features of members of this family are the presence of four highly conserved cysteine residues and a motif of tryptophan-serine-*x*-tryptophan-serine within an approximately 200 amino acid region in the extracellular domain. This region is referred to as the cytokine receptor homology (CRH) region and is crucial for ligand binding (Figure 15.4).

There appear to be common pathways but also some unique mechanisms for signalling by these individual factors, which helps to explain the synergistic activities observed in *in vivo* and *in vitro* studies.

Some factors have been identified only as a ligand that binds to a receptor identified with a clinical consequence, as in the case of the Mpl ligands, a family of closely related HGFs that bind to the thrombopoietin receptor, c-Mpl. The name Mpl comes from the initial finding that a truncated form of this receptor, v-Mpl, was part of the transforming gene in a murine myeloproliferative leukaemia retrovirus (MPLV). The proto-oncogene (m-MPL) was later isolated and found to be present on platelets, megakaryocytes and a few earlier haematopoietic precursor cells. Subsequently, the ligand binding to it (c-Mpl) ligand) was purified from thrombocytopenic plasma, and identified as the physiologic regulator of platelet production, historically called *thrombopoietin*.

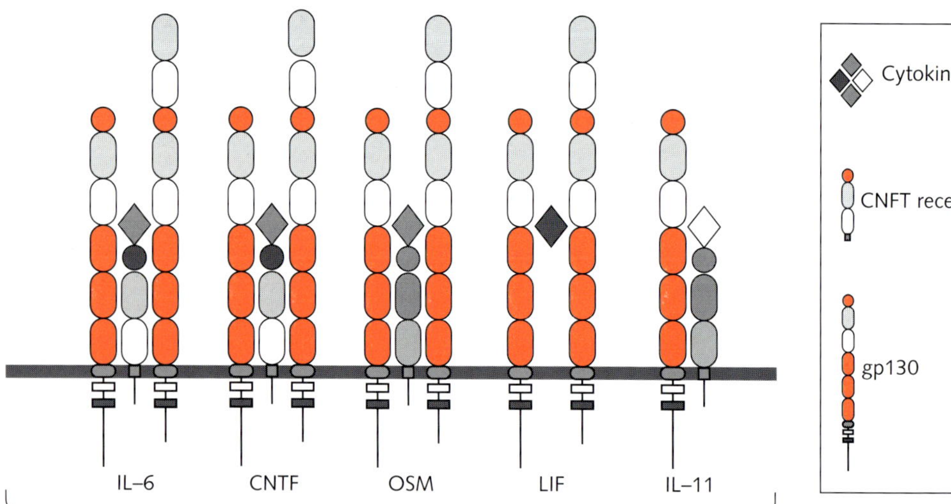

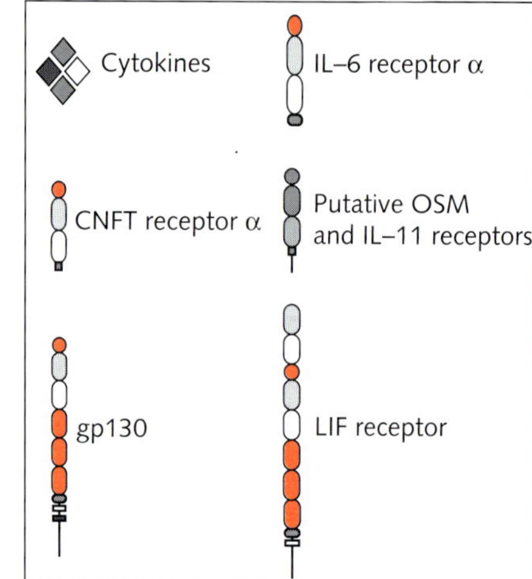

Fig. 15.4 Receptors for various cytokines showing the structural similarities between family members

Endogenous production

The most straig htforward situation for understanding clinical disease as a result of deficient HGF production is the anaemia of renal disease and the lack of EPO production by the diseased kidney. It was known that nephrectomised rats would not produce EPO in response to hypoxic stimuli, but that ureter-ligated rats would still respond normally. Subsequent studies showed that anaemic patients with chronic kidney disease also had low EPO levels, leading to the realisation that an EPO deficiency state existed, and that replacement therapy may be beneficial.

In another situation where endogenous levels correlate well with the clinical scenario, thrombopoietin (TPO or c-mpl ligand) regulates most of the normal production of platelets. Thrombopoietin is the only endogenous ligand for c-MPL and is the key regulator of platelet production. As outlined above, this lineage-restricted cytokine is probably regulated via consumption rather than induction of production.

In the case of myelopoiesis, the situation is not quite as clear. Endogenous GM-CSF is rarely found in the circulation in any clinical situation, as it is believed to be primarily a locally acting factor. In contrast, the levels of circulating endogenous G-CSF increase in a variety of pathological conditions, such as Gram-negative and fungal infections, and exposure to endotoxins. The highest G-CSF levels are found in neutropenic patients and are correlated with fever. In patients with cyclic neutropenia there are marked fluctuations in serum levels, and in patients with autoimmune neutropenia, peripheral ANC changes in parallel with the serum level of endogenous G-CSF, with a delay of 4–5 hours.

Although both G-CSF and GM-CSF are potent stimulators of myelopoiesis, the existing data suggest that G-CSF is the primary factor for the upregulation of neutrophils in infection and in various pathological conditions where the ANC level is decreased. One possible explanation for this localisation is that both G-CSF and GM-CSF are elevated during infection but that G-CSF circulates in the blood and stimulates neutropoiesis, while GM-CSF remains localised at the site of infection to help retain and activate arriving cells. The concept of regulation by consumption has been exploited in the evolution of so-called 'designer cytokines' like PEG-rHuMGDF (an artificial c-mpl ligand comprising a truncated thrombopoietin-like polypeptide and a covalently attached poly(ethylene glycol) to increase the hydrodynamic size above the threshold for renal clearance) and similarly derived G-CSFs. These materials are effectively self-regulating in as much as the target cells they induce can in turn remove the drug itself via receptor-mediated clearance.

Clues from knockout animals

Technological advances in the production of transgenic and gene deletion or 'knockout' animals have further elucidated the constitutive and reactive roles for these factors *in vivo*.

The physiologic role of IL-2, IL-4 and IL-7, IL-10 by gene knockout experiments illustrates the essential role for some growth factors in maintaining immune competent cells: somewhat surprisingly, mice deficient in IL-7 may have much more severe immune impairment than animals deficient in IL-2 or IL-4.

The mice deficient in the growth factor GM-CSF have relatively normal haematopoiesis but those deficient in G-CSF are severely neutropenic, with impaired neutrophil function. This suggests that G-CSF is required for maintaining the normal quantitative balance of neutrophil production during 'steady state' granulopoiesis *in vivo*, and indicates that GM-CSF has a role in 'emergency' granulopoiesis during infection. Data reported from double knockout (*G-CSF –/–, GM-CSF –/–*) confirmed this hypothesis (Figure 15.5).

It is interesting to note that, in mice in which the *TPO* gene has been eliminated by homologous recombination (*Tpo –/–*), the number of platelets and megakaryocytes is less than 20% of that in normal mice (*Tpo +/+*) (*reviewed in* Murone *et al.*, 1998). This paper describes a classic knockout experiment where heterozygotes had platelet counts 60% of normal. This gene dosage effect is the strongest evidence yet that the TPO gene is not regulated by the platelet count. These thrombopoietin-deficient mice grew and bred normally and had normal haemostasis.

Because megakaryocytes were present and produced platelets, it appears that thrombopoietin is not necessary for megakaryocyte differentiation or platelet shedding. Rather, it serves as an amplification system for the production of platelets.

The constitutive expression of thrombopoietin is confirmed by measured thrombopoietin mRNA levels in liver and kidneys of thrombocytopenic animals. These measurements show that there is no change in transcription rate despite a greater than 20-fold rise in the concentration of thrombopoietin in the circulation. This principle was confirmed in mice in which the thrombopoietin receptor had been eliminated by homologous recombination (*m-Mpl –/–*). Despite having a platelet count 15–20% of normal and markedly elevated thrombopoietin levels, there was no change in the thrombopoietin mRNA levels in liver and spleen in these animals. The constitutively produced thrombopoietin is bound by the avid thrombopoietin receptors on platelets and rapidly cleared from the circulation. Proof for this comes from the recent demonstration that platelets from normal, but not c-Mpl-deficient, mice bound radioactively labelled thrombopoietin which was rapidly internalised and degraded. When normal murine platelets were infused into c-Mpl knockout mice, elevated thrombopoietin levels dropped to normal values within 2 hours.

This type of gene targeting experimentation will undoubtedly provide many further advances in our understanding of haematopoietic regulation in the years ahead.

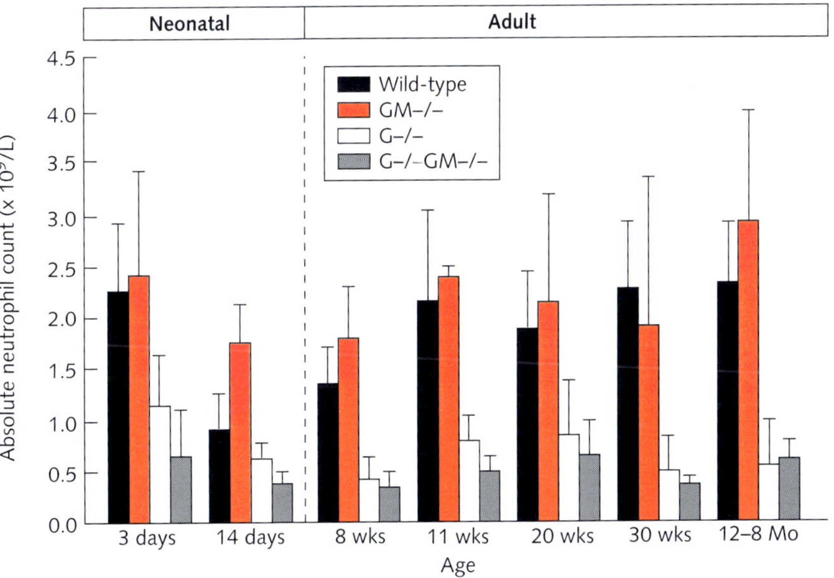

Fig. 15.5 Baseline neutrophil numbers in mice lacking G-CSF, GM-CSF or both factors
This indicates the reduction in basal neutrophil numbers in the G-CSF knockouts, but the relatively normal neutrophil numbers in GM-CSF knockout mice. The ability to respond to infection by elevating neutrophil numbers is different between the G-CSF and GM-CSF knockouts.

Drug development

The CSFs are appealing as therapeutic agents because they are used to recapitulate, on a pharmacological basis, what they are known to effect on a physiological scale. The limiting feature of HGFs is that other less-defined processes may also be triggered.

There is often great species specificity in terms of *in vitro* and *in vivo* effects. For this reason, preclinical development of HGFs may rely increasingly on the use of non-human primates and SCID (severe chronic immune deficiency) mice. As mentioned earlier, one of the major barriers in HGF research is the species specificity of these proteins, as well as the antigenicity that they, or the production products associated with their expression vector, may elicit.

The design of preclinical studies, especially for cytokines with pleiotropic actions, must carefully parallel the design of the proposed initial clinical trial, as results obtained with a recombinant human HGF administered to other species may not be transferable to the clinic.

An additional challenge as a result of HGF administration as pharmacologic agents is the possibility of eliciting both the clinical effects of the direct action of the factor, and the indirect actions due to activation of other cytokines or networks. As we have stated, over the last few years, a large number of *HGF* genes have been cloned and their products produced in bacteria or yeast. Although all of these molecules merit discussion, we will focus our attention on the CSFs in clinical use.

Erythropoietin

The recombinant form of EPO was one of the first marketed recombinant HGFs. Native EPO is a glycoprotein hormone that regulates the production of red blood cells by acting on committed erythroid progenitor cells. There are two forms of EPO marketed in Europe: epoietin alpha and epoietin beta that have different carbohydrate content and diluent constituents. EPO's greatest benefit is its ability to correct the anaemia of chronic renal failure and the treatment of chemotherapy-induced anaemia. Second generation derivatives of EPO are now under development and it remains to be seen what further advances will be made with what is the most mature of all growth factor therapeutics.

Granulocyte colony-stimulating factor

G-CSF is the major growth factor involved in the production of neutrophilic granulocytes. Severe congenital neutropenia and acute myeloblastic leukaemia are both characterised by a maturation arrest in the myeloid lineage. Although marrow cells from patients with severe congenital neutropenia frequently show a reduced responsiveness to G-CSF, neutrophilic colony formation *in vitro*, as well as neutrophil production *in vivo*, can usually be induced with G-CSF. Patients with severe congenital neutropenia have an increased risk of developing acute myeloblastic leukaemia, which suggests that the same functionally related defects may be involved in the pathogenesis of the disease.

G-CSF has been extensively studied *in vitro* and in clinical trials. There are many benefits to cancer patients attributed to the use of this factor, including: reduction in febrile neutropenia, documented infections, intravenous antibiotic use, and reduction in hospitalisations due to infections. Other benefits are reduction in mucositis which hampers eating, reduction in antibiotic-induced diarrhoea, the ability to administer full-dose chemotherapy on time, completion of chemotherapy sooner, and the ability to intensify chemotherapy. (Neupogen® package insert, Amgen, Thousand Oaks, California.)

Neupogen® (rmetHuG-CSF) is approved for the support of myelosuppression in severe congenital neutropenia, and as a result of chemotherapy in acute myeloid leukaemia, non-myeloid malignancies and bone marrow transplantation. In addition, it is approved for the mobilisation of peripheral blood progenitor cells (PBPC). More than 1.5 million patients have received this product and it is approved in 46 countries. Antigenicity has been reported with rHuGM-CSF. Whether this is due to the glycosylation or to its effect on antigen-presenting cells is unclear.

c-mpl ligand or thrombopoietin

The Mpl ligands are a family of closely related HGFs that bind to the thrombopoietin receptor, c-Mpl. In addition to the endogenous Mpl ligand, thrombopoietin, two recombinant Mpl ligands, recombinant thrombopoietin and pegylated megakaryocyte growth and development factor (PEG-MGDF), are under investigation.

When recombinant thrombopoietin or PEG-MGDF is administered to normal animals or humans, there is a dose-dependent increase in the platelet count, but no effect on leucocytes or erythrocytes. When administered following chemotherapy in animal models of humans, Mpl ligands reduce the duration, and sometimes the degree, of thrombocytopenia. The Mpl ligands may also be effective in reducing the thrombocytopenia in patients with HIV infection, liver disease, myelodysplasia, or for plateletpheresis.

The c-Mpl ligand has moved rapidly through its preclinical studies and initial trials in human subjects.

It appears to be a very powerful agent for the treatment of thrombocytopenia. The preclinical animal models clearly demonstrate that Mpl ligands have modest multilineage effects as well as their major thrombopoietic effect, with this response being, in part, at the level of the marrow. Numerous *in vitro* studies have demonstrated that recombinant thrombopoietin can enhance proliferation of erythroid and myeloid progenitors.

Detailed examination of both TPO-l-mice and c-Mpl-l-mice also demonstrated the cross-lineage effects of TPO. This may be the best demonstration of the multilineage effect of thrombopoietin, as the bone marrow precursors for megakaryocytes were decreased in all of the mice, but precursors for all other lineages were decreased for the mice as well, despite no effect on the leucocyte and erythrocyte counts. Administration of recombinant thrombopoietin to the thrombopoietin-deficient, but not to the c-Mpl-deficient, mice corrected the precursor cell defect.

Interleukin-11 (IL-11)

IL-11 is a good example of a growth factor with pleiotropic actions which has been developed for clinical use in thrombocytopenia (Figure 15.6).

Human and mouse IL-11 share 88% amino acid identity and are cross species reactive. Similar in sequence and gene structure to IL-6, G-CSF, oncostatin-M (OSM), leukaemia inhibitory factor (LIF) and growth hormone, IL-11 signals through gp130, which was originally identified as a component of the IL-6 receptor.

Administration of IL-11 to normal mice causes an increase in circulating platelet levels likely mediated via its demonstrated effects on megakaryocyte maturation alone or in combination with other growth factors such as IL-3 and stem cell factor (SCF). This ability has led to a development programme culminating in Food and Drug Administration (FDA) approval for IL-11 in thrombocytopenia. Despite the appearance of relative lineage fidelity implied by its effects upon predominantly a single circulating cell type, the discovery of IL-11 was facilitated by its actions upon a different cell type—plasmacytoma cells. Among the other properties of IL-11 are abilities to weakly or indirectly influence B-cell development, augmentation of antibody responses, induction of hepatic acute phase proteins, promotion of erythroid colony growth *in vitro*, protection of intestinal mucosa from cytotoxic damage *in vivo*, influences upon bone metabolism and inhibition of adipogenesis. Among this myriad of effects, boosting platelet numbers led most quickly to registration; whether other properties of this material will eventually lead to other indications is as yet unclear. None the less, IL-11 represents a good example of a growth factor which was isolated and purified based on one activity, yet finally found a therapeutic niche in a different setting. How the growth factor is used clinically may also be expected to change in the face of development of what is widely held to be the true physiological regulator of platelet production—thrombopoietin. Perhaps the other distinctive properties of IL-11 will support continuation of its use, or possibly its lifetime as a front-line platelet factor will be limited by the emergence of thrombopoietin-like regulators.

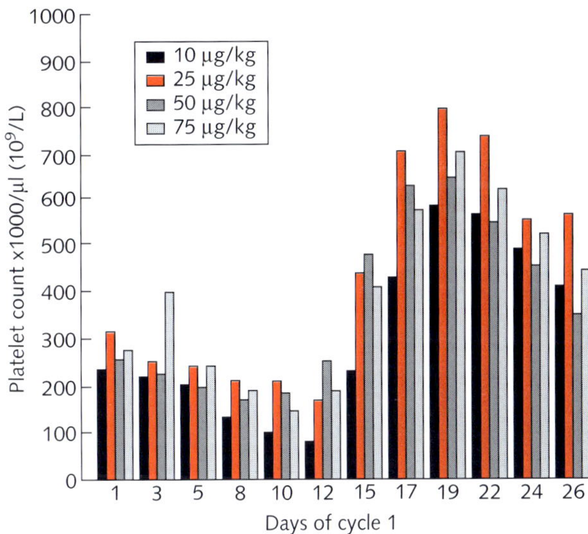

Fig. 15.6
The ability of interleukin-11 to raise platelet counts after cancer chemotherapy has led to its approval for this use.
IL-11 is a pleiotropic cytokine and has many other systemic effects in addition to improving platelet numbers.

Stem cell factor

SCF enhances the proliferation of early haematopoietic cells, particularly in combination with a variety of agents, particularly Mpl ligands such as thrombopoietin and MGDF. It works in concert with other HGFs to potentiate the effects of these cytokines, with the resultant haematopoietic phenotype determined by the precise combination.

Mobilisation of stem cells

Although SCF in combination with other growth factors can promote proliferation and development of primitive multipotent and putative stem cells *in vitro*, it was somewhat surprising to find that SCF *in vivo* (even by itself) could induce significant emigration of these and other progenitor cells from the bone marrow to the blood

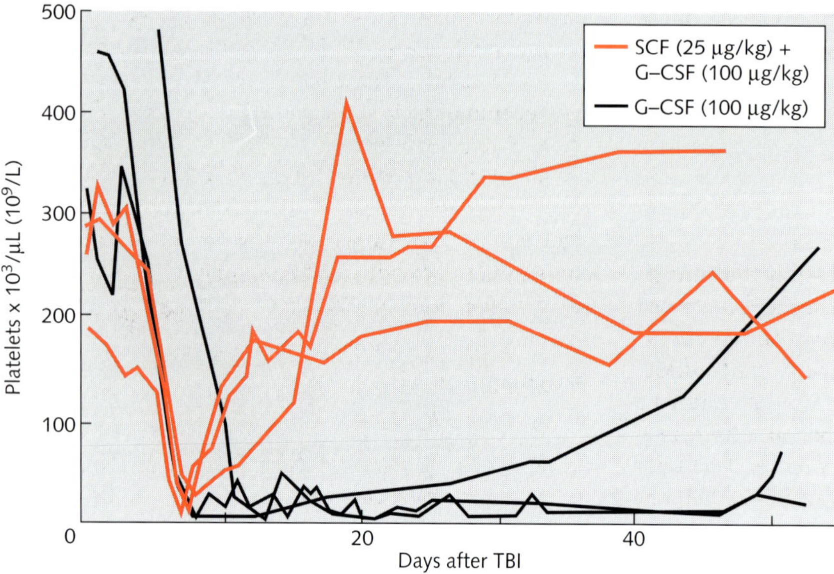

Fig. 15.7
The ability of SCF to enhance the *in vivo* response to G-CSF has been documented in several preclinical models. Here, the ability of G-CSF to mobilise haematopoietic progenitor cells into the blood is exaggerated by the inclusion of G-CSF in baboons.

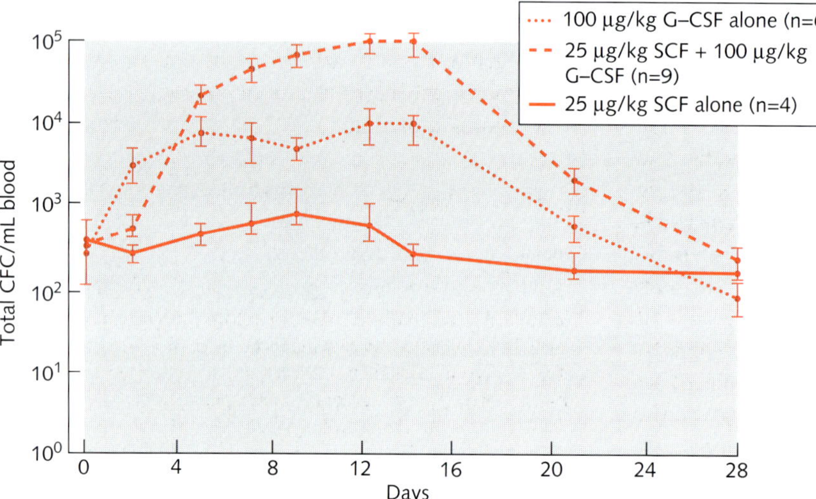

Fig. 15.8
The progenitor cells mobilised by G-CSF can successfully engraft a transplanted baboon. The cells mobilised by G-CSF + SCF promote more rapid recovery, probably as a result of the increased numbers seen in Figure 15.7, but there is also indirect evidence that the cells are of higher quality.

(Figure 15.7). Moreover, data also suggest that the total 'body load' of primitive progenitor cells increases in both mice and humans treated with SCF.

However, perhaps much more significant from the therapeutic viewpoint was the finding that the interaction between SCF and G-CSF, that was observed for progenitor cell development *in vitro*, also occurred *in vivo* in terms of mobilisation of haematopoietic progenitor cells into the blood. In man, low doses of SCF (≥10 mg/kg/day) in combination with G-CSF mobilise approximately threefold more CD34+ cells than G-CSF alone, confirming data obtained in primates (Figure 15.8). Furthermore, the quality of these cells in respect to their capacity to engraft lethally irradiated animals appears to show an improvement over that seen with G-CSF alone. In other words, the combination of SCF and G-CSF preferentially mobilises the most primitive haematopoietic cells. This has been confirmed in humans at least with respect to multipotential and megakaryocyte precursors.

The therapeutic potential of these findings is obvious, particularly since equivalent cells, induced by more conventional agents such as chemotherapy and/or G- or GM-CSF, have proven useful in transplant settings, both as a means of haematopoietic support for myelosuppressed patients and as a source of cells capable of re-establishing haematopoiesis in myeloablated animals and patients. In fact, the speed of recovery of, for example platelets, after transplantation either with PBPC alone, or in support of marrow transplantation, has indicated that PBPC offer superior performance to equivalent marrow populations particularly in the short term.

Clinical adoption

HGFs can reduce the morbidity and possibly the mortality from some types of cancer treatment and from other HGF-deficiency states. Reductions in hospitalisation and supportive care (transfusion requirements and antibiotics) have been documented in several trials and can reduce total care costs. However, the cost is substantial, and these drugs are one of the many new expensive pharmacy purchases, prompting payers to ask whether the cost is warranted by the benefit.

Economic and clinical analyses of CSFs have mostly been complimentary. The use of CSFs is justified on economic grounds in those cases in which the most clinical benefit has been observed, i.e. for primary prophylaxis of febrile neutropenia when the rate is high, for peripheral stem cell mobilisation, and for haematopoietic reconstitution after stem cell transplantation.

The high acquisition costs of HGFs have attracted substantial attention from purchasers, providers and health economists. Initial economic studies evaluating the use of growth factors demonstrated that their use is cost saving when the risk of febrile neutropenia is >40%. In these cases the savings in hospitalisation and treatment costs are larger than drug acquisition costs. At lower risk levels use of HGF has been shown to partially offset the drug acquisition costs, the level of the offset depending on the level of risk for febrile neutropenia, the daily charge for hospitalisation and the duration of febrile neutropenia.

The American Society for Clinical Oncology (ASCO) published clinical practice guidelines for the use of growth factors in 1994 which recommended the use of HGF when the risk of febrile neutropenia was >40% coinciding with the results of the economic analysis. Revised guidelines from ASCO issued in 1996 did not change the recommendation for HGF use.

Lyman revised his initial cost estimates in 1996. The new analysis added to the direct costs of the treatment of febrile neutropenia the indirect and intangible costs. When indirect costs are included HGF costs are offset when the risk of febrile neutropenia is at about 30%, and when intangible costs are added HGF costs are offset when the risk of febrile neutropenia is at ~20%. Recent economic analysis of HGF use has shifted the emphasis from cost offset to cost effectiveness studies where costs of treatment are balanced against clinical outcomes. Silber *et al.* (1998) modelled the use of growth factors in early breast cancer patients where standard dose chemotherapy is associated with survival benefit. The use of growth factors for the 50% of patients most at risk for chemotherapy dose modification was associated with a cost per year of life saved of about $35,000—well within the range of cost effectiveness ratios considered to provide good economic value in the delivery of conventional medical care.

Conclusions

The development of recombinantly produced endogenous proteins for pharmacologic delivery remains one of the most important medical advancements of the decade. In the new millennium, the promise of screening the human genome for additional novel proteins with therapeutic potential looms large. Additional proteins or small molecule mimics may require some engineering to optimise compounds whose natural function may not be the same protein therapeutic target. Continued mining of the genome combined with molecular techniques should provide therapeutics for many important diseases in the coming millennium.

Further reading

General

Burgess A, Metcalf D. (1980) Characterization of a serum factor stimulating the differentiation of myelomonocytic leukemic cells. *International Journal of Cancer*, **319**, 415–418.

Cebon J, Layton JE, Maher D, Morstyn G. (1994) Endogenous haemopoietic growth factors in neutropenia and infection. *British Journal of Haematology*, **86**, 265–274.

LeBeau M, Lemons R, Espinosa R. (1989) Interleukin-4 and interleukin-5 map to human chromosome 5 in a region encoding growth factors and receptors and are deleted in myeloid leukemias with del(5q). *Blood*, **73**, 647–650.

The American Society of Clinical Oncology. (1996) Update of Recommendations for the Use of Hematopoietic Colony Stimulating Factors: Evidence-Based Clinical Practice Guidelines. *Journal of Clinical Oncology*, **14**, 1957–1960.

Erythropoietin

Besarah A, Flaharty KK, Erslev AJ *et al.* (1992) Clincial pharmacology and economics of recombinant human erythropoietin in end-stage renal disease: the case for subcutaneous administration. *Journal of the American Society of Nephrology*, **2**, 1405–1416.

Egrie JC, Browne JK. (1991) The molecular biology of erythropoietin. In: Erslev AJ, Adamson JW, Eschbach JW, Winearls CG, eds. *Erythropoietin Molecular, Cellular and Clinical Biology*. Baltimore: Johns Hopkins University Press, pp. 21–40.

Eschbach JW, Abdulhadi MH, Browne JK *et al.* (1989) Recombi-

nant human erythropoietin in anemic patients with end-stage renal disease; results of phase III multicenter clinical trial. *Annals of Internal Medicine*, **111**; 992–1000.
Eschbach JW, Kelly MR, Haley NR, Abels RI, Adamson JW. (1989) Treatment of the anemia of progressive renal failure with recombinant human erythropoietin. *New England Journal of Medicine*, **321**, 158–163.
Evans RW, Rader B, Mannienen DL, the Cooperative Multicenter IPO Clinical Trial Group. (1990) The quality of life of hemodialysis patients treated with recombinant human erythropoietin. *Journal of the American Medical Association*, **263**, 825–830.
Jacobs K, Shoemaker C, Rudersdorf R *et al.* (1985) Isolation and characterization of genomic and CDNA clones of human erythropoietin. *Nature*, **313**, 806–810.
Lin F, Suggs S, Lin C *et al.* (1985) Cloning and expressions of the human erythropoietin gene. *Proceedings of the National Academy of Sciences (USA)*, **82**, 7580–7584.

G/GM-CSF

Burgess AW, Begley CG, Johnson GR *et al.* (1987) Purification and properties of bacterially synthesized human granulocyte-macrophage colony-stimulating factor. *Blood*, **69**, 43–51.
Cantrell MA, Anderson D, Cerretti DP *et al.* (1985) Cloning, sequence, and expression of a human granulocyte/macrophage colony-stimulating factor. *Proceedings of the National Academy of Sciences (USA)*, **82**, 6250–6254.
Ernst T, Ritchie A, Demetri G, Griffin J. (1989) Regulation of granulocyte and monocyte colony stimulating factor mRNA levels in human blood monocytes is mediated primarily at a post-transcriptional level. *Journal of Biological Chemistry*, **264**, 5700–5703.
LeBeau MM, Westbrook CA, Diaz MO *et al.* (1986) Evidence for the involvement of GM-CSF and FMS in the deletion (5q) in myeloid disorders. *Science*, **231**, 984–987.
Nagata S, Tauchiya M, Asano S *et al.* (1986) Molecular cloning and expression of cDNA for human granulocyte colony-stimulating factor. *Nature*, **319**, 415–418.
Rapoport AP, Abboud CN, DiPersio JF. (1992) Granulocyte-macrophage colony-stimulating factor (GM-CSF) and granulocyte colony-stimulating factor (G-CSF): receptor biology, signal transduction, and neutrophil activation. *Blood Reviews*, **1**, 43–57.
Zhan Y, Lieschke GJ, Grail D, Dunn AR, Cheers C. (1998) Essential roles for granulocyte-macrophage colony-stimulating factor (GM-CSF) and G-CSF in the sustained hematopoietic response of Listeria monocytogenes-infected mice. *Blood*, **91**, 863–869.

Stem cell factor

Bodine D, Seidel N, Zsebo K, Orlic D. (1993) *In vivo* administration of stem cell factor to mice increases the absolute number of pluripotent hematopoietic stem cells. *Blood*, **82**, 445–455.
Molineux G, Migdalska A, Smitkowski M, Zsebo K, Dexter TM. (1991) The effect on hematopoiesis of recombinant stem cell factor (ligand for c-kit) administered *in vivo* to mice either alone or in combination with granulocyte colony-stimulating factor. *Blood*, **78**, 961–966.
Okada S, Nakauchi H, Nagayoshi K *et al.* (1992) *In vivo* and *in vitro* stem cell function of c-kit- and Sca-1-positive murine hematopoietic cells. *Blood*, **80**, 3044–3050.
Tong J, Gordon M, Srour E *et al.* (1993) *In vivo* administration of recombinant methionyl human stem cell factor expands the number of human marrow hematopoietic stem cells. *Blood*, **82**, 784–791.

Thrombopoietin

Bartley TD, Bogenberger J, Hunt P *et al.* (1994) Identification and cloning of a megakaryocyte growth and development factor that is a ligand for the cytokine receptor mpl. *Cell*, **77**, 1117–1124.
de Sauvage FJ, Hass PE, Spencer SD *et al.* (1994) Stimulation of megakaryocytopoiesis and thrombopoiesis by the c-Mpl ligand. *Nature*, **369**, 533.
Kaushansky K, Lok S, Holly RD *et al.* (1994) Promotion of megakaryocyte progenitor expansion and differentiation by the c-Mpl ligand thrombopoietin. *Nature*, **369**, 568.
Lok S, Kaushansky K, Holly RD *et al.* (1994) Cloning of murine thrombopoietin cDNA and stimulation of platelet production *in vivo*. *Nature*, **369**, 565.
Murone M, Carpenter DA, De Sauvage FJ. (1998) Hematopoietic deficiencies in c-mpl and TPO knockout mice. *Stem Cells*, **1**, 1–6.
Silber JH, Fridman M, Shpilsky A *et al.* (1998) Modeling the cost-effectiveness of granulocyte colony-stimulating factor use in early-stage breast cancer. *Journal of Clinical Oncology*, **16**, 2435–2444.
Wendling F, Maraskovsky E, Debill N *et al.* (1994) c-Mpl ligand is a humoral regulator of megakaryopoiesis. *Nature*, **369**, 571.

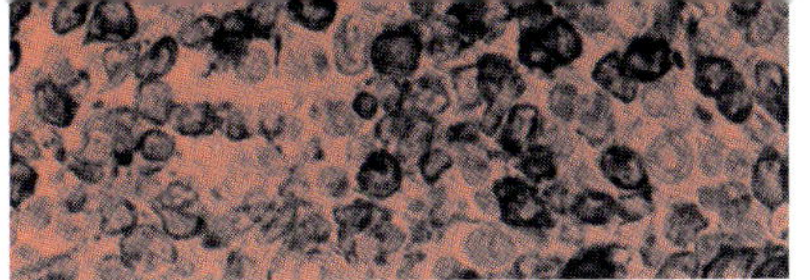

Chapter 16 Molecular therapeutics in haematology

A Keith Stewart

Introduction

Clinical investigation of gene transfer in humans began with the seminal trials of Rosenberg *et al.* (1990) and Anderson (1992) involving gene transfer of genetically altered lymphocytes into patients and was closely followed by studies of gene transfer using human bone marrow. Studies of the blood system have therefore been pivotal in the early development of human gene therapy. Gene marking or gene therapy protocols are now under intensive investigation worldwide with over 2000 patients treated in more than 250 trials by the end of 1997. Since haematology has contributed so much to the genesis of human gene therapy, it is the purpose of this chapter to reiterate both the inherent promise and the remaining obstacles posed by the application of gene transfer using haematopoietic cells.

Gene transfer strategies

An ever increasing array of techniques has been described to facilitate gene transfer into blood cells. These techniques can be broadly grouped as *physical methods* or *viral vectors*.

Physical means of gene delivery

Physical methods of gene transfer are generally of low efficiency and provide only transient gene expression in the absence of selection. The advantages of these systems are that genes are transferred without viral sequences which may affect the biology of the target cell, large or multiple genes can be transferred and gene transfer is independent of the proliferative status and cell surface receptor profile of the target cell. Those methods of physical gene transfer which have been used in the clinical setting include *electroporation* (electric fields which create channels in cell membranes allowing passage of DNA into the cell), *particle bombardment* (microscopic gold beads labelled with DNA which are forced through the cell membrane by CO_2-driven pressure) or *liposomal encapsulation* of DNA. Liposomal gene delivery has gained most acceptance in the clinical arena, driven by the relatively high gene transfer efficiencies obtained with newer liposomal formulations and by safety considerations as an alternative to viral vector gene delivery. Other non-viral gene delivery systems which include use of plasmid DNA alone, so-called 'naked' DNA, synthetic polymers and bacterial gene delivery systems are among the many other methods which have been developed and are entering clinical trials. The use of plasmid DNA alone is surprisingly efficient at gene transfer, particularly in specific tissues such as muscle. Thus DNA-based gene delivery is gaining in popularity in malignancy, infectious disease and in applications directed towards the vascular bed. In cancer, DNA-based vaccines are in clinical trials where the antigen is encoded by the plasmid with or without an immunostimulatory gene.

Physical methods such as electroporation, direct DNA transfer and liposome-mediated transfer have been used with varying levels of success in transferring genes into haematopoietic cells. However, genes rarely integrate with physical methods of transfer and the vectors are lost in multiplying cells, and thus are generally of little value to long-term stable gene transfer applications. Nevertheless, when transient gene replacement is sufficient, such as in cancer immunotherapy applications, physical methods of gene transfer seem likely to find a niche.

Viral vectors for gene transfer

Viral gene transfer methods take advantage of the normal virus life cycle in which genetic material is transferred into a host cell. For viral gene transfer vectors, the viral genome is modified by deleting most viral genes and inserting therapeutic or marker genes in their place. The viral gene products necessary for the production of recombinant viral particles are then provided *in trans* by packaging cell lines which have been transfected with plasmids carrying the viral genes missing from the vector. Recombinant viral vectors are transfected into the packaging cells, and replication incompetent recombinant viral particles are produced. Replication incompetent viruses are safe for clinical applications because they transduce target cells only once, and are unable to cause a secondary infection because of the absence of viral genes required for replication (Figure 16.1).

The most commonly used viral backbones are based on the murine retroviruses and human adenoviruses;

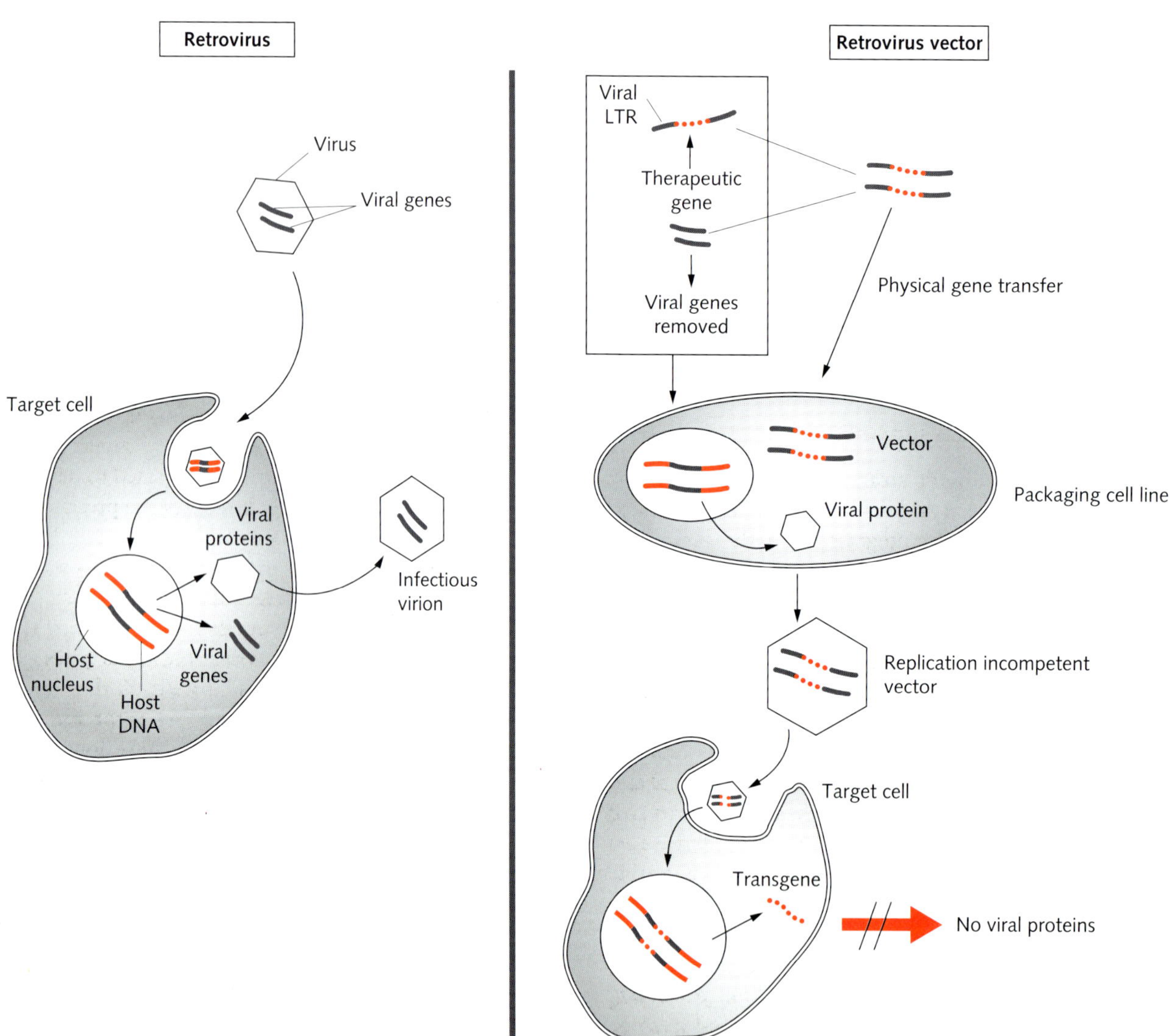

Fig. 16.1 Retroviruses bind cell surface receptors before internalisation
After random integration into the host genome viral proteins are produced which encapsulate viral RNA. In a retroviral vector the *gag*, *pol* and envelope encoding genes have been removed allowing space for cloning of the gene of interest. To make an infectious virus the vector is introduced into a packaging cell line expressing *gag*, *pol* and *env* genes. The packaged vector can then bind to, and be internalised by, a target cell where integration into the host genome occurs and the vector transgene is produced. Since the target cell lacks the genes necessary to make a new virion the vector is not infectious.

Table 16.1 Viral vectors.

	Retrovirus	Adenovirus	Helper-dependent adenovirus	Adeno-associated adenovirus (AAV)	Herpes	Lentivirus	Pox viruses
Advantages	Efficient gene transfer Integrates	Very efficient gene transfer High transgene expression	Large cloning capacity Not immunogenic	Integrates Cell cycle independent Safe	Very efficient gene transfer Cell cycle independent	Integrates	Efficient gene transfer
Disadvantages	Cell cycle dependent Promoter silencing Safety issues	Immunogenic Transient expression	Technically cumbersome Helper virus contamination Transient expression	Limited cloning capacity Helper virus contamination	Helper virus contamination Transient Cytotoxic	Safety issues	Transient expression Immunogenic
Potential applications	Stem cell gene therapy, e.g. haemophilia, Gaucher's, immunodeficiency	Cancer immunotherapy Cystic fibrosis	Gene replacement therapy	Cancer immuno-therapy Gene replacement therapy via muscle	Cancer immuno-therapy	Gene replacement therapy targeting non-dividing cells	Cancer immunotherapy

however, herpes, pox, vaccinia, adeno-associated viral (AAV) and lentiviral vectors are also being developed and evaluated. The relative merits and disadvantages of each vector system are outlined in Table 16.1.

Retroviral gene transfer systems

Retroviruses are double-stranded RNA viruses. The RNA genome is reverse transcribed into double-stranded DNA, which randomly integrates into the target cell genome of cycling cells. Retroviral vectors derived from the Moloney murine leukaemia virus (MMLV) and other murine oncoviruses are most commonly used for gene transfer into haematopoietic cells.

In gene transfer vectors the wild type retroviral genome is modified by deleting most *gag*, and all *pol* and *env* sequences. Viral sequences which are retained in the retroviral vector include the packaging signal and long terminal repeats (LTRs) which are necessary for viral integration. These modifications render the vectors replication incompetent while making 6–8 kb available for the insertion of desired genes.

Retroviral packaging cell lines have been engineered to minimise the chance of accidental replication competent retrovirus (RCR) production. The packaging plasmids are based on the wild type retroviral genome but have extensive deletions of retroviral sequences, such as the packaging signal and 3′ LTR, and deliberately split the genes encoding essential viral packaging proteins into two plasmids. These modifications have minimised recombination-prone homologous sequences between the gene transfer vector and the packaging plasmids, thereby significantly reducing the chance of recombination leading to RCR. Another measure of safety is present in retroviral gene transfer systems as recombinant retroviruses packaged in murine packaging cell lines are rapidly inactivated by human serum.

In addition to the safety features of retroviral gene transfer systems described above, all viral supernatants and patient samples which have been exposed to retroviral supernatant are extensively tested for the presence of RCR prior to infusion into patients.

In addition to the relative safety of retroviral vectors, other advantages include integration of vector into the host cell genome allowing long-term expression of the LTR-driven transgene in the host cell and its progeny. Disadvantages include the requirement of the target cells to be in cycle, the specificity of receptor binding and silencing of transgene expression. Since long-term expression of transgenes is a requirement for most haematopoietic stem cell-based gene therapies, many viral vectors use viral promoters, such as the endogenous MMLV/LTR which can direct high levels of expression. Nevertheless, such promoters are frequently silenced. There are several mechanisms of such downregulation including cytokine-mediated promoter suppression, DNA methylation, genetic environment of integration sites or position within the retroviral vector. Thus, even if efficient gene transfer is achieved, transgene expression, and thus therapeutic impact, may be low. Newer retroviral vectors have demonstrated significantly higher and longer expression than conventional retroviral vectors. For example MSCV, MND and MFG vectors have been designed with multiple modifications to the

MMLV backbone which more efficiently enable genes to be expressed in murine, primate and human haematopoietic cells.

Retrovirally encoded transgenes can also be expressed in a cell-specific manner using cellular promoters which allow for regulated expression. For example, expression in leucocytes can be enhanced by CD11b, CD18 or major histocompatibility complex (MHC) I promoters, while expression in erythroid cells can be greatly enhanced by the β-globin promoter and locus control region. Furthermore, viral transgene expression may be regulated by inducible promoter systems such as the *tet* operon system which uses exogenous tetracycline to transactivate the gene of interest. Such regulated and cell-specific systems may prove of utility in therapeutic applications by providing a control mechanism for the expression of potentially toxic gene products.

Other viral gene transfer systems

Recombinant adenoviral gene transfer systems are commonly used for some applications. Adenoviruses infect cells efficiently *in vitro* and *in vivo*, express high levels of transgene, can infect both cycling and stationary cells and exhibit wide tissue tropism. Adenoviral vectors have been used to efficiently transfer genes into a variety of human cancers and into haematopoietic progenitor and malignant cells. Nevertheless, circulating B- and T-lymphocytes have generally proven resistant to adenoviral-mediated gene transfer. The receptor for adenoviruses has recently been identified and will now be of utility in determining the mechanism of adenoviral binding and cell entry. Adenoviral vectors do not integrate into the genome and are lost from cycling target cells within weeks of transduction. First generation adenoviral vectors may incite potent immune responses due to viral genes encoded on the vectors resulting in the elimination of transduced cells and thus preventing successful re-administration of adenoviral vectors. Adenoviruses are therefore ideal vectors if an immune response and/or short-term high transgene expression is desired; however, they are not suitable for therapies which require long-term transgene expression or integration of the transgene. In an attempt to overcome these limitations new generations of adenoviral vectors have either retained immunosuppressive sequences in E3, eliminated all viral sequences except the necessary inverted terminal repeats (ITRs) or are based on a helper-dependent system with low levels of contaminating helper virus. Lytic adenovirus vectors which replicate only in permissive cells have been developed and hold promise for the treatment of solid tumours, for example one such vector system only replicates in cells defective in the tumour suppressor gene p53.

The human parvovirus, AAV, is also being evaluated as a vehicle for gene transfer. AAVs are non-pathogenic to humans and establish a latent infection in the absence of adenovirus. Wild type AAV integrates with high efficiency into human chromosome 19q13.3-qter, which appears to be a benign genomic site. Only the AAV ITRs are required for recombinant AAV vectors, which allows ~4 kb for inserts. However, both the efficiency and specificity of integration are lost without the wild type genes. A number of studies are focused on determining the sequences responsible for the specific integration site, and preliminary results suggest that the rep protein is necessary for integration. AAVs have titres of $\sim 10^6$/ml, and can be concentrated up to 10^9/ml. Recombinant AAV particles can integrate into both stationary and cycling cells, although they do not do so very efficiently.

Integration of a recombinant AAV vector carrying the human β-globin gene into murine haematopoietic stem cells (HSCs) was demonstrated by the presence and expression of the human β globin in primary and secondary murine bone marrow transplant recipients for up to 9 months. Human CD34+ cells have also been stably transduced with recombinant AAV vectors, with up to 80% of colony-forming units (CFU) carrying the transgene.

Herpes simplex-based viral vectors or amplicons are also now being developed for human use. Like adenovectors, herpes virus-based vectors exhibit a high efficiency of gene transfer into a wide variety of cell types but are not integrated. These vectors are distinguished by their wide tissue tropism and large cloning capacity. Such vectors have been demonstrated to be highly efficient at transfecting HSCs with 80–100% gene transfer efficiency.

As discussed above, MMLV-based retroviral vectors only integrate into cells undergoing mitosis, which precludes their use for delivery to target cells that are non-dividing, such as the majority of HSCs. This has led to the development of replication incompetent viral vector systems based on lentiviruses and foamy viruses which can integrate into stationary cells. Foamy viruses have a large genome, do not cause any known disease and can be used for *in vivo* gene transfer because foamy viruses are not inactivated by human serum. Lentiviral vectors also show promise as gene transfer vehicles. Current vectors contain less than 25% of the HIV-1 genome, are therefore relatively safe, stably integrate into stationary cells and maintain long-term expression of transgene. There is currently considerable optimism that lentiviral and/or foamy viral vectors will overcome the

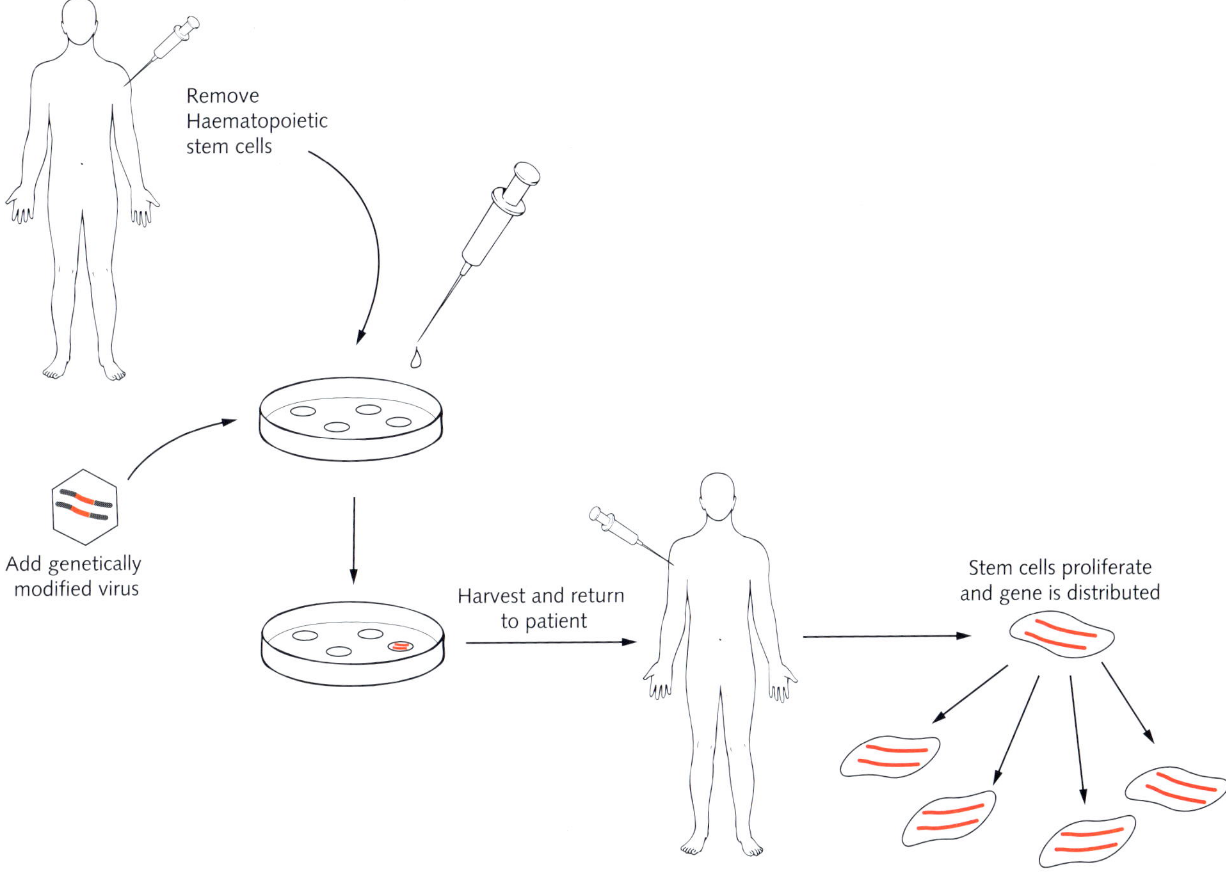

Fig. 16.2
Haematopoietic stem cells can easily be harvested from patients and retrovirally transduced. The transduced cells are returned to the patient where all blood cells maturing from the gene-modified stem cell retain and express a copy of the transgene. In theory, this gene transfer method could help distribute the gene product throughout the body at clinically relevant levels.

shortcomings of MMLV-based retroviruses by delivering genes to a wide spectrum of cell types, including quiescent HSCs. Preliminary studies show that these vectors mediate gene transfer into murine, baboon and human haematopoietic cells at comparable levels to MMLV.

Stem cell gene delivery in haematology

Pluripotent HSCs cells are attractive targets for gene therapy in humans because of their capacity for self renewal and the wide systemic distribution of their progeny (Figure 16.2). Sustained expression of transgenes at clinically relevant levels in the progeny of HSCs would result in novel and potentially curative treatments for a wide range of blood diseases including haemophilia A and B, haemoglobinopathies, hereditary immune deficiencies or storage diseases of childhood. Even the partial correction of such blood diseases would have substantial impact on the transfusion needs of the affected populations. Nevertheless, despite the inherent promise of HSC gene transfer, successful long-term engraftment of genetically marked HSCs in humans has proved an elusive goal.

Gene marking of haematopoietic stem cells

Gene marking of HSCs facilitates study of the long-term distribution and survival of transplanted cells (*in vivo*). In most applications, the cells to be tagged are incubated *ex vivo* with a replication-defective retrovirus bearing a reporter gene. The reporter gene used exclusively in clinical studies to date is the bacterial neomycin phosphotransferase (*neo*) gene which, when expressed, confers resistance to the neomycin analogue G418. Other marker genes are now available and include murine heat stable antigen, human CD24 antigen, the truncated nerve growth factor receptor, modified CD4 or green fluorescent protein (Plate 16.1, facing page 128). The stable and unique integration pattern of proviral DNA in the genome of marked cells can provide a permanent marker for individual haematopoietic or malignant cells and their clonal descendants. Clinical applications in which gene marking has provided new and important information include the infusion of retrovirally marked, autologous, tumour-infiltrating lymphocytes (TIL) into patients with advanced melanoma and the infusion of retrovirally marked bone marrow or peripheral blood into patients with myeloid leukaemia, myeloma and neuroblastoma. The study of such patients offers three important lines of investigation: (i) is retroviral-mediated gene transfer safe?; (ii) do genetically altered bone marrow or blood stem cells contribute to long-term haematopoiesis?; (iii) do malignant cells or their precursors contribute to the high relapse rates observed after myeloablative therapy and autologous HSC transplantation?

A number of groups have reported the consequences of infusing gene-marked bone marrow cells into humans and the contribution of contaminating tumour cells in the graft to disease recurrence. The first important observation is that retroviral-mediated gene transfer as currently practised appears safe. No detrimental effects, either on the autograft or in patients, have been reported. Replication competent virus has not been detected. The second important observation is that HSCs contribute to long-term haematopoiesis, albeit at relatively low levels (Table 16.2).

In the first reported studies in children, 2–15% of clonogenic haematopoietic progenitor cells were marked after ABMT (*see* Brenner *et al.*, 1993). The marker gene was detectable for up to 4 years after transplant and was found in granulocytes, B-cells and T-cells, at least by PCR. In the adult gene marking studies reported to date however, retroviral transduction of marrow or peripheral blood stem cells has resulted in detection of vector integration in only 0.01–0.1% of peripheral blood cells (Figure 16.3). Although the marker gene persisted for up to 2 years, *neo*-positive cells could only be detected intermittently with a sensitive PCR reaction.

Recent work by a number of groups suggested that modification of the transduction protocols would result in a significant improvement in the engraftment of genetically modified HSCs. A second generation of gene marking trials therefore attempted to increase levels of gene transfer in adult human HSCs. For example, since preclinical experience indicated that the use of bone marrow stroma enhances gene transfer into HSCs this approach was evaluated in a clinical trial. However, the results of this trial have proved no better than those discussed above and, in general, are very similar to those of the paediatric gene transfer studies. Although there is a high level of gene-marked progenitors in the early post-transplant period with a mean of 12% gene-marked bone marrow colonies (CFU-GM), the level drops to 3% by 2 years post-transplant (Figure 16.4), and only 0.01% of the blood cells in the periphery are marked. Recent primate gene marking studies using novel cytokine combinations to induce HSC cycling, fibronectin-assisted virus–cell co-localisation and pseudotyped retroviruses are more encouraging and suggest that the successful application of human gene transfer will eventually be achieved.

Gene-marked relapse

In total, data on 34 patients enrolled on gene marking studies during bone marrow transplant for AML, neuroblastoma, CML, breast cancer or myeloma have been presented (Table 16.3). Of the 14 relapsed patients, gene-marked tumour cells have been detected in nine,

Table 16.2 Summary of reported results from gene marking trials.

Centre	Cells	Protocol	*In vitro* CFU-GM gene transfer	*In vivo* results
St Jude Children's Hospital	BM	1 exposure 6 hours	5–20%	2–15% bone marrow CFU at 1 year
NIH	MPB CD34+ BMCD34+	3 exposures 3 days +cytokines	21%	0.01–0.001% blood cells +ve at >18 months
University of Toronto	BM	2 exposures 21 days stroma	37%	3% CFU +ve at 2 years 0.01% blood +ve at 2 years

MPB, mobilised peripheral blood; BM, bone marrow.

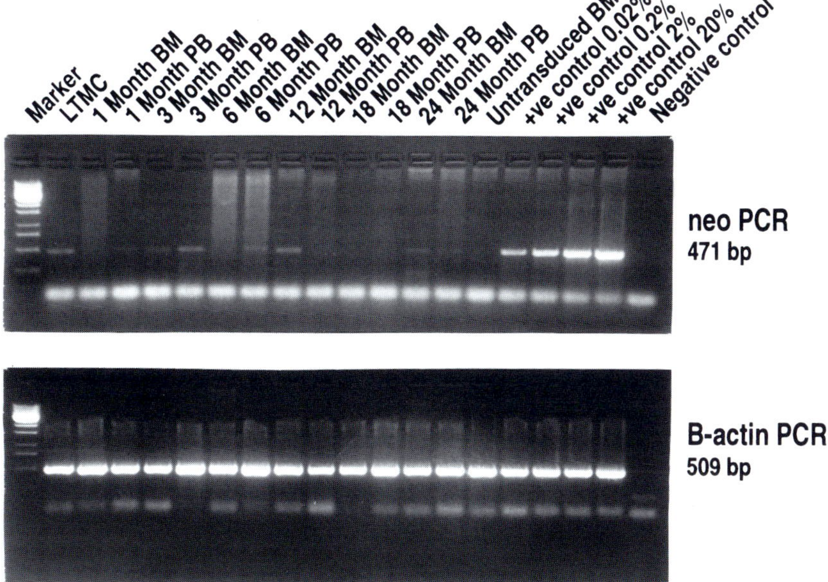

Fig. 16.3
Gene marking of peripheral blood (PB) and bone marrow (BM) is shown over a 2-year period for a patient who received gene-marked bone marrow cells grown on stroma during retroviral infection. Although the *neo* resistance marker gene is readily detectable for 2 years, the levels of gene transfer are low.

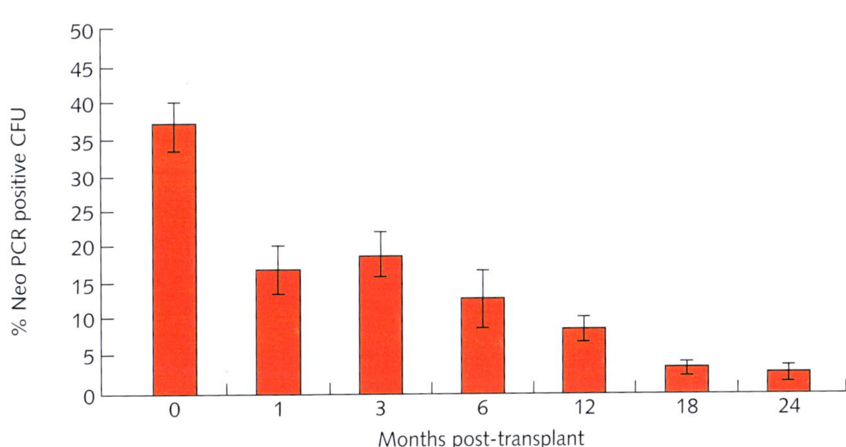

Fig. 16.4
The number of colonies arising from bone marrow which contain the neo marker gene falls with time after gene transfer. Shown here are the average number of PCR-positive colonies from 15 patients on a gene marking trial. By 2 years post-transplant less than 5% of colonies are gene marked. Note that the number of positive CFU far exceeds the percentage of cells in the blood (Figure 16.3) that are gene marked raising the possibility that gene-marked bone marrow progenitors do not differentiate normally in the patient, or are immunologically cleared.

Table 16.3 Gene marking studies.

	Patients	Relapse	Marked
AML	12	4	2
Neuroblastoma	9	5	4
CML	2	2	2
Myeloma	6	0	0
Breast cancer	5	3	0

and if patients with breast cancer are excluded a remarkable nine of 11 patients with leukaemia or neuroblastoma had gene-marked relapse. In one AML patient the simultaneous detection of a cytogenetic marker along with the *neo* gene confirmed that gene-marked cells contributed to relapse. A second critical observation was made when Rill *et al.* (1994) reported that a multiplicity of neuroblastoma cells in the graft contributed to relapse. The high frequency of gene-marked relapse, despite the very low frequency of transfused malignant cells, strongly suggests that a large percentage of tumour cells in the graft contribute to relapse or, alternatively, that tumour cells susceptible to retroviral gene marking are uniquely capable of engraftment and clonal expansion.

In adults, Diesseroth *et al.* (1994) at MD Anderson have examined tumour relapse in the HSC malignancy, CML. Again, by demonstrating that clonogenic cells at relapse contain both the *neo* marker gene and the tumour-specific *BCR-ABL* oncogene rearrangement, this group demonstrated that infused gene-marked tumour cells can contribute to relapse.

The final published report of gene marking haematopoietic cells in cancer patients is from Dunbar *et al.* (1989) at the NIH. In 11 patients with breast cancer or myeloma, CD34+ bone marrow or peripheral blood haematopoietic progenitor cells were isolated and marked. None of the six myeloma patients have demonstrated gene-marked relapse nor have CD38 bright (plasma cells) in the marrow of two patients contained the marker gene as determined by PCR at 1 year post-transplant. Similarly, in three breast cancer patients who have relapsed no evidence for the *neo* gene has been found in tumour biopsies.

Future directions

The exciting observations made in the early gene marking studies described above raise as many questions as they answer. Most importantly, the long-term engraftment of genetically altered haematopoietic cells must still be optimised and the functional expression of therapeutic genes at clinically relevant levels demonstrated. Nevertheless, these studies set the stage for the investigation of a multiplicity of manoeuvres designed to increase gene transfer efficiency and long-term gene transfer using HSCs. Some strategies being pursued are described in Table 16.4 and include increasing the cell to virus contact by incorporating HSC selection, retroviral envelope targeting or co-localisation of vector and cell on stromal elements into gene transfer protocols. New vector systems improving on both retroviral and lentiviral backbones and incorporating envelope pseudotyping may increase gene transfer efficiency, while novel growth factor combinations may more efficiently, induce stem cell cycling thus allowing retroviral integration. Further investigation of traditional and novel purging mechanisms in the prevention of gene-marked relapse is underway and clinical trials of gene replacement with therapeutic intent have begun.

Chemoprotection

Preclinical and early clinical studies discussed above demonstrate that HSCs can be safely genetically altered using retroviral vectors, and such cells can, following autologous transfusion, engraft and be maintained in the donor bone marrow for at least 2 years. Together, these results suggest that normal bone marrow cells could be removed, transduced with a retroviral vector containing a drug resistance gene and returned to untreated patients with no toxicity. Theoretically, such cells would expand clonally after chemotherapy treatment and confer a relative resistance to toxic chemotherapy allowing further chemotherapy dose escalation and potentially cure of some patients. Furthermore, such drug resistance genes

Table 16.4 Strategies for optimisation of gene transfer into HSCs.

Strategy	Method
Inducing cells to cycle	*Ex vivo* cytokine stimulation Collection of cells during recovery phase after myeloablation or mobilisation Culture on stromal layers
Increased cell–virus contact	Centrifugation of cells and virus during transduction Viral supernatant flow through systems Coat dishes with fibronectin Higher viral titres and multiple exposures
Increase viral receptor on target cells	Increase levels of amphotropic receptor by phosphate depletion Transfer amphotropic receptor into cell by adeno or adeno-associated virus Target cells that have high levels of receptors
Pseudotyped recombinant retroviruses	GALV receptor for entry into target cells VSV-G envelope for entry into target cell
Modified viral vectors to target non-cycling cells	Lentivirus and foamy virus vectors
Positive selection of transduced cells	Add positive selectable marker to vector

may serve as selectable markers allowing concentration of gene-marked cells and selection for a second therapeutic gene product.

Gene products may confer chemoprotection

Numerous potential mechanisms of cellular resistance to chemotherapy agents have been described. Candidate gene products for chemoprotection (and their substrates) include P-glycoprotein (anthracyclines, taxol, etoposide, vinca alkaloids), MRP (anthracyclines, etoposide, vinca alkaloids), cytidine deaminase (cytosine arabinoside), ribonucleotide reductase (hydroxyurea), topoisomerase II (etoposide), aldehyde dehydrogenase (cyclophosphamide), O^6-alkylguanine-DNA-alkyltransferase (nitrosoureas), glutathione-s-transferase (melphalan), dihydrofolate reductase (methotrexate), thymidylate synthase (floxuridine) and tubulin (vinca alkaloids).

The cDNA for the human *MDR-1* gene has been cloned and expressed in both mouse and human cells in culture. The *MDR-1* gene, when transferred into mouse and human bone marrow cells in culture using retroviral constructs, leads to drug resistance of transduced cells *in vitro*. Transplanted cells engraft and confer drug resistance to bone marrow *in vivo* and allow selection for *MDR-1* transduced cells by chemotherapy (Figure 16.5).

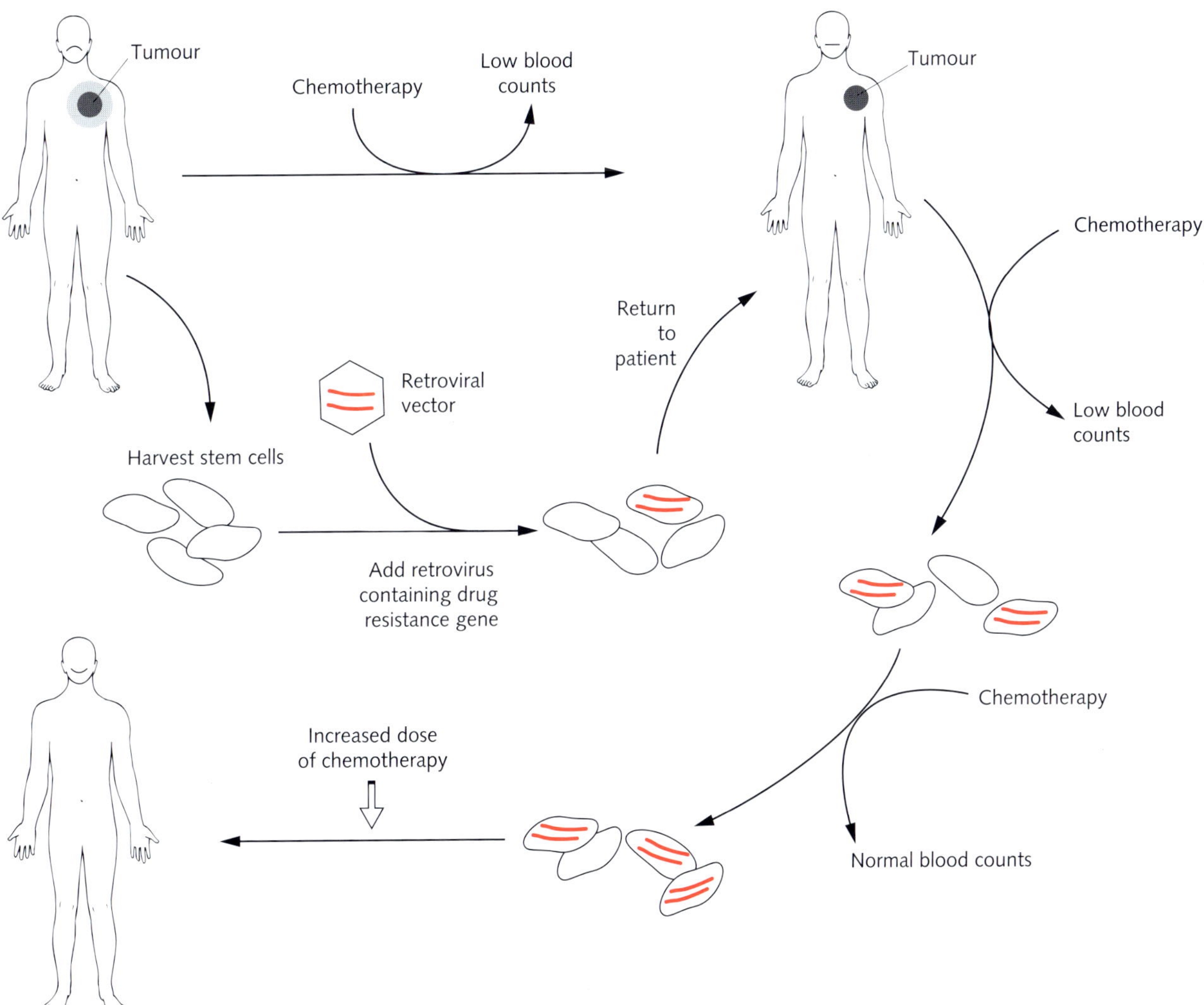

Fig. 16.5 Stem cells removed from the patient can be genetically engineered to express a drug resistance gene
Theoretically, after return to the patient, the cells are selected by chemotherapy (i.e. normal stem cells survive chemotherapy less well than the drug resistance gene expressing cells). At a certain point the number of drug resistant bone marrow cells rises to a degree which protects bone marrow from the effects of chemotherapy and thus higher doses of chemotherapy can be given without all of the usual side effects. Note, however, that systemic side effects not related to bone marrow will persist. This method could also be used to select for a second gene product expressed in concert with the *MDR-1* gene.

Human bone marrow cells have also successfully been transduced by exposure to *MDR-1* retroviral gene transduction. Using a short-term culture of whole bone marrow with supernatants obtained from a high titre MDR-1 producer line, 10–50% of the bone marrow-derived progenitor cells express the transferred *MDR-1* gene. With the best *MDR-1* retroviruses developed so far, drug concentrations up to 10 times the 50% lethal dose can be used.

Clinical trials of chemoprotection

Clinical trials of *MDR-1* gene transfer into haematopoietic cells for chemoprotection in cancer therapy are underway. The intent is to confer drug resistance to bone marrow and thus allow escalation of chemotherapy drugs without increasing myelosuppression. The approach used for gene transfer is generally similar to that used for human gene marking trials. Preliminary results indicate that infusion of *MDR-1* gene modified cells is safe and no deleterious effects of infusing gene modified cells have been observed. Neutrophil and platelet recovery times are normal following infusion of gene modified cells. Nevertheless, clinical experience in gene marking studies (*discussed above*) suggests that these trials are unlikely to demonstrate therapeutic effect as the gene delivery approaches being used have been shown in marking trials to be of limited utility in achieving clinically relevant gene transfer.

Gene replacement therapy

The first human clinical gene transfer trials for single gene disorders focused on adenosine deaminase (ADA) deficiency and are summarised in Table 16.5. Recombinant retroviruses containing the normal human *ADA* cDNA were transferred into either peripheral blood T-lymphocytes, bone marrow or cord blood cells from ADA-deficient patients. T-lymphoid cells expressing the normal *ADA* gene are expected to have a selective growth and survival advantage over ADA-deficient cells, even though patients are maintained on PEG-ADA enzyme therapy.

ADA patients who have received multiple infusions of autologous *ADA* transduced blood cells have increased levels of enzyme in their serum, and up to 20% of their peripheral blood T-cells carry provirus. In two of three trials in which patients received autologous marrow or cord blood cells transduced with *ADA*, containing retroviruses, between 12–40% of CFU were transduced, and marked cells were found for greater than 1-year post-infusion. In the one study in which provirally marked cells were not maintained for greater than 6 months, there was lower *in vitro* gene transfer efficiency of 5–12% CFU prior to transplant (*see* Hoogerbrugge *et al.*, 1996).

In the cord blood study there was evidence for a selective growth advantage of T-cells as there were higher levels of marked T-cells than myeloid cells even while the patients were maintained on progressively lower doses of PEG-ADA enzyme therapy. Enzyme therapy was withdrawn from one patient and the number of T-cells carrying the provirus increased to 30%; however, the total number of B-lymphocytes and natural killer (NK) cells dropped and the patient had reduced immune function. The patient subsequently resumed PEG-ADA treatment.

Gaucher disease, which results from a deficiency in glucocerebrosidase, has also been proposed as amenable to treatment by gene transfer into HSCs. Results from two gene transfer studies have been reported. Mobilised blood or marrow CD34+ cells from Gaucher patients were transduced with a glucocerebrosidase-containing retroviral vector and infused into non-myeloablated autologous recipients. In both studies, transduced cells were detected at low levels in blood and/or marrow

Table 16.5 Gene therapy trials for ADA deficiency.

Centre	Cells	Protocol	*In vitro* gene transfer	*In vivo* results
NIH	PB supernatant	9–12 hrs		Increased immune repertoire Number of T-cells normalised after 2 years
Italy	PB BM	Co-culture 72 hrs or supernatant	2.5–50% cells 30–40% CFU	Multilineage repopulation with marked cells Increased immune repertoire for 2 years
The Netherlands	CD34+ BM	Co-culture + IL-3	5–12% CFU	Transduced cells detected 3–6 months after transplant
Childrens' Hospital	CB CD34+	Supernatant + IL-3, + IL-6, + SCF	12.5–21.5% CFU	Multilineage repopulation with transduced cells
Japan	PB	Supernatant + IL-2	3–7% cells	Improvement in immune function10–20% of blood cells carrying provirus >1 yr

leucocytes. One patient who received cells transduced with an MFG retroviral vector had an increase in levels of enzyme corresponding to 50% of normal, maintained for 12 months post-infusion. No therapeutic benefit or increased enzyme was detected in other patients.

Collectively, the results from the gene transfer studies for genetic disease described above illustrate several points which will likely impact on the success of gene transfer for other single gene disorders: (i) the presence in patients of cells carrying the provirus for greater than 1 year has demonstrated the safety and feasibility of gene therapy; (ii) the transfer of genes which provide a growth and survival advantage can provide long-term maintenance of transduced cells; (iii) a selective advantage of transduced cells cannot compensate for poor *in vitro* gene transfer efficiency; (iv) successful gene therapy of deficiency disorders could be severely limited by immune responses in immunocompetent patients; and (v) gene delivery and expression levels will need to be increased in order to provide therapeutic benefit to most inherited diseases. Clinical gene therapy trials for other inherited single gene disorders such as Fanconi's anaemia type 'C', mucopolysaccharidosis type I, X-linked SCID, and chronic granulomatous disease are ongoing. The results from these and other studies may provide new evidence on the therapeutic potential of HSC gene transfer for single gene disorders.

Gene therapy of haematologic malignancy

A number of potential approaches to the gene therapy of haematologic malignancies can be considered (Table 16.6) and are discussed here.

Genetic immunotherapy

Many tumour cells express peptide antigens on their cell surface in association with major histocompatibility class I molecules (MHC class I), and these antigens may allow immune effector cells to distinguish tumour from normal tissue (Figure 16.6). Some of these 'tumour-associated antigens' (TAAs) have been isolated and shown to be recognised by human cytotoxic T-lymphocyte (CTL) cell lines. Nevertheless, tumour cells known to express potentially antigenic peptides manage to evade host immunosurveillance and proliferate *in vivo*. Thus, tumour cells may lack the necessary signals required to induce expression, by immune effector cells, of cytokines necessary for activation and *in vivo* expansion of CTLs. The end result is anergy, a failure of the T-cells to respond to the tumour antigen. In addition to optimal presentation of antigen to the T-cell receptor, efficient activation of naive T-cells requires a second costimulatory signal. It is now appreciated that molecules of the B7 family (B7-1/CD80, B7-2/CD86) on antigen presenting cells engaging CD28/CTLA-4 receptors on T-cells play a key role in this process, inducing autocrine IL-2 production and T-cell proliferation. Murine models have demonstrated that T-cell-mediated rejection of tumours can be induced by transduction of tumour cells with such costimulatory molecules. In the absence of costimulatory signals, it is possible to bypass this requirement by ectopic expression of cytokines, the downstream products of costimulation, and thus overcome or prevent anergy of the immune effector cells. Thus, proof of principle that cytokine gene-transduced tumour cells can prevent tumour engraftment has been obtained. Such models have also shown that transduction of the genes for various cytokines, such as IL-2, IL-4, IL-6, IL-7, IL-12, IFN-γ, GM-CSF and TNF-α into murine tumours not only led to primary rejection of the modified cells but often elicited protective immunity against subsequent tumour challenge with unmodified tumour cells. Furthermore, in such models, synergy has been demonstrated between molecules with varying mechanisms of action, for example IL-2, IL-12 and B7-1 (Figure 16.7).

Proof of concept for immunotherapy as a valid approach to the treatment of haematologic malignancy has now been provided by clinical studies which demonstrated that infusion of allogeneic T-cells can eradicate

Table 16.6 Approaches to gene therapy.

Strategy	Genes employed	Problems and merits
Gene replacement	*p53, p16, Rb*	Gene delivery to every cell required Specific to defective cancer cell
Gene inhibition	*BCR-ABL, C-MYC, cyclin D1, BCL-2*	Gene delivery to every cell required
Suicide genes	Thymidine kinase, cytosine deaminase	Immunogenicity and bystander effect contribute
Drug resistance genes	*MDR-1, DHFR*	Stem cell gene delivery required
Immunotherapy	*IL-2, IL-12, B7-1, CD40L, GM-CSF*	Systemic response, autoimmunity a theoretical problem Requires that tumour express foreign antigen

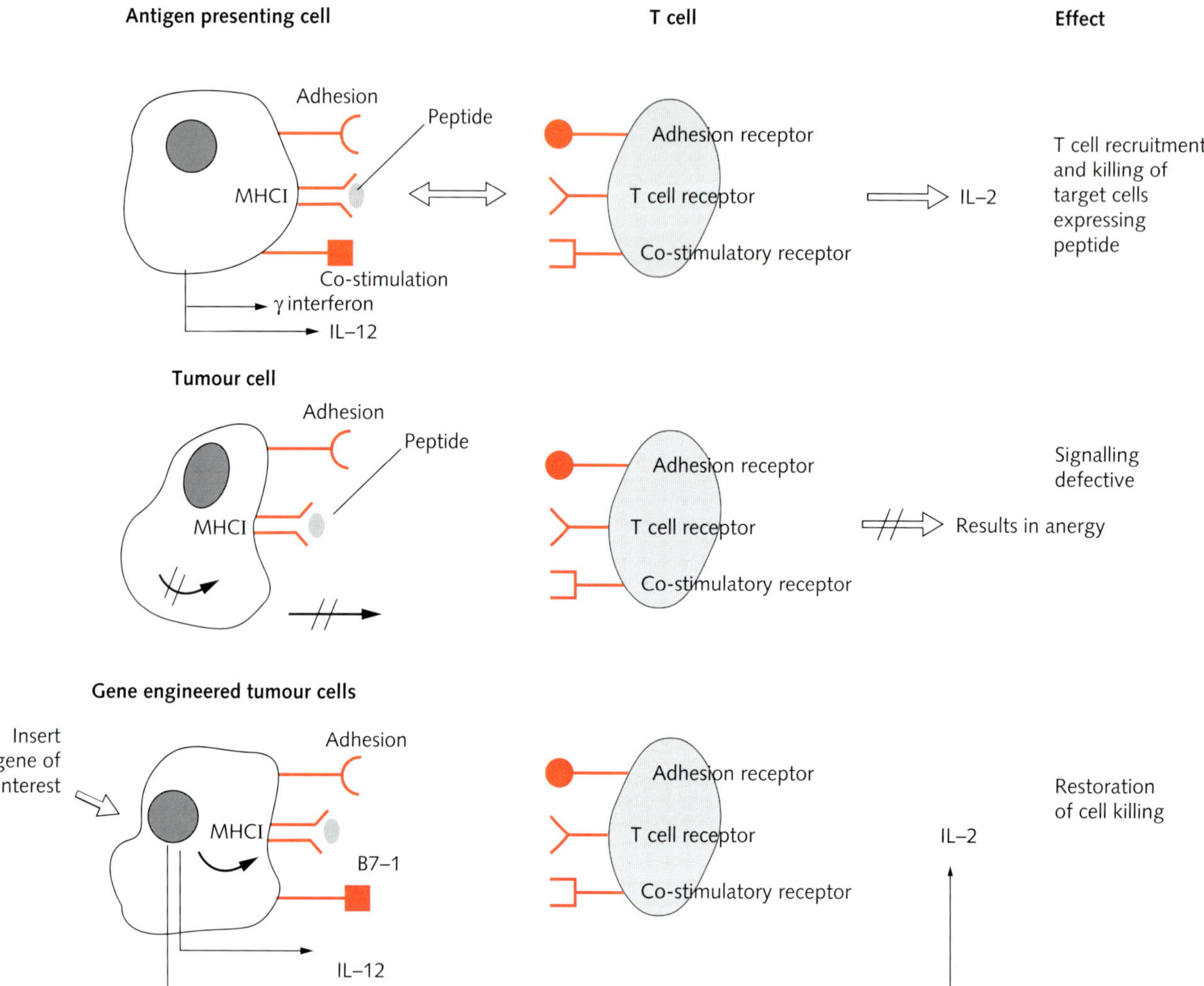

Fig. 16.6
Efficient signalling of T-cells occurs following adhesion, provision of the major histocompatibility complex (MHC class I)/T-cell receptor signal and after a costimulatory signal is received. Under normal circumstances professional antigen presenting cells (APCs) present processed peptides in the groove of the MHC I complex to T-cells. Tumour cells are often deficient in one or all of the components required to function as antigen presenting cells either because they lack an appropriate tumour antigen, cannot process the antigen or are deficient in adhesion molecules, MHC class I or costimulatory molecules required to generate a T-cell response. These missing components can be provided or enhanced using gene transfer techniques. By overcoming the deficiencies of the tumour cell the gene engineered cells can serve as autologous cancer vaccines presenting foreign antigen to the host T-cells.

minimal disease in patients relapsing after allogeneic transplant. Unfortunately, these encouraging allogeneic responses require a haploidentical T-cell donor, which is not available to the vast majority of patients. Another more widely applicable approach now entering clinical trials is the use of autologous tumour cells which have been genetically engineered to express one or more of the immune stimulatory cytokines mentioned above. Trials in myeloma, low grade lymphoma, leukaemia and chronic lymphocytic leukaemia which use this strategy are being pursued.

Cellular immunotherapy

As outlined above, the object of cancer immunotherapies is to efficiently present TAAs to the immune system. The most immunologically powerful (so-called *professional*) antigen presenting cells are bone marrow-derived dendritic cells (DCs). DCs express MHC class I and II, B7-1, B7-2, CD40, ICAM-1 and LFA-3, are capable of presenting processed antigen for days and are potent stimulators of immunity when administered as a vaccine to animals. DCs modulate immune responses in part by secretion of

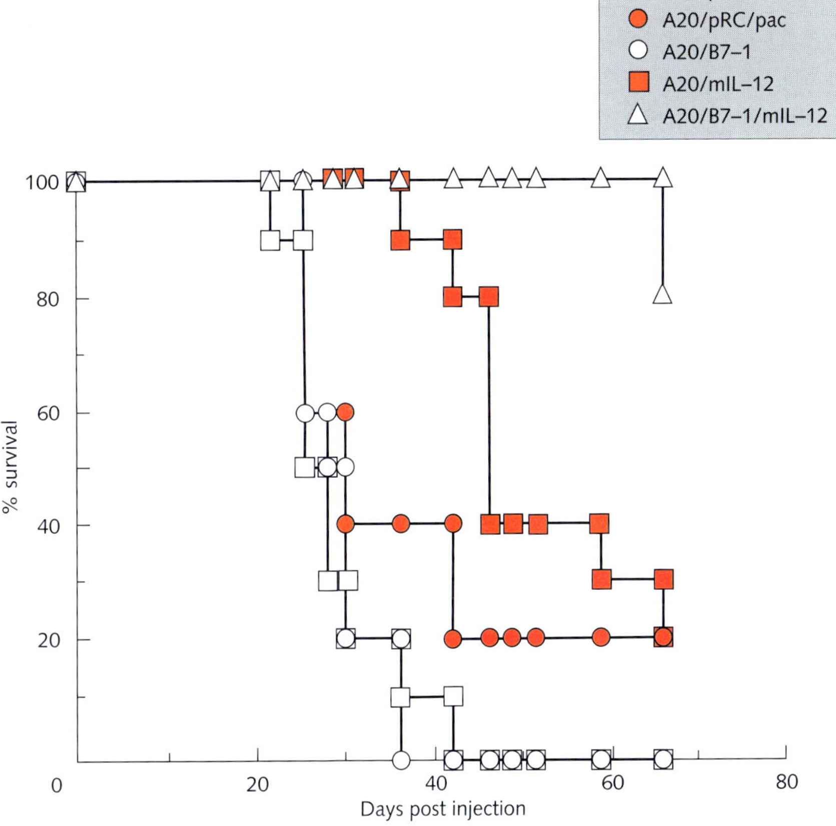

Fig. 16.7
The A20 lymphoma cell line was genetically engineered to express either B7-1, IL-12, or a combination of both. Shown in this figure, reproduced from Pizzoferrato *et al.* (1997) with permission, survival of mice inoculated with a mixture of 10^5 parental and 10^5 variant cell at the same site on day 0 is shown. Although there is a marginal increase in survival for the IL-12 cell line, clearly the majority of protected mice were vaccinated with the A20 cell line co-expressing B7-1 and IL-12.

IL-12 (hence, the notion of converting tumour cells into antigen presenting cells by introduction of IL-12 and B7-1 genes). DCs can be readily expanded from bone marrow progenitors *in vitro* using cytokine-supplemented medium (useful cytokines include Flt3L, TNF-α, GM-CSF, IL-4) and can also be propagated using GM-CSF-expressing tumour cells as a continuous source of cytokine (presumably explaining the *in vivo* anti-tumour properties of GM-CSF). Such cells may also be genetically engineered to express TAAs and thus hold great promise for the immunotherapy of haematologic malignancy.

Suicide gene therapy

The so-called suicide genes are pro-drugs which, when expressed by target cells, confer susceptibility to drug-induced cell death. The gene most commonly employed to date in clinical trials is the herpes virus–thymidine kinase gene which, when expressed, confers sensitivity to the drug ganciclovir. Use of thymidine kinase is further assisted by diffusion of the gene product into neighbouring cells and thus a *bystander effect* occurs which is mediated via the gap junctions connecting cells (Figure 16.8). The obvious limitations of this treatment approach are that not all cells targeted will be successfully gene modified and thus, even with the bystander effect, only a fraction of malignant cells will be destroyed. Nevertheless, applications of this type are in clinical trials in solid tumours and have proved to be of potential clinical relevance in the prevention of graft-versus-host disease (GVHD). In the latter approach gene-modified lymphocytes are infused into patients relapsing after an allogeneic bone marrow transplant. If signs of GVHD are noted ganciclovir is started and the lymphocytes aborted. Other approaches being explored as part of the therapeutic arsenal of cancer gene therapy include combining thymidine kinase with cytokines, use of novel cell suicide genes or use of cell death genes which are non-immunogenic.

Genetic inhibition: antisense and ribozymes

A number of oncogenes, for example *RAS*, *C-MYC*,

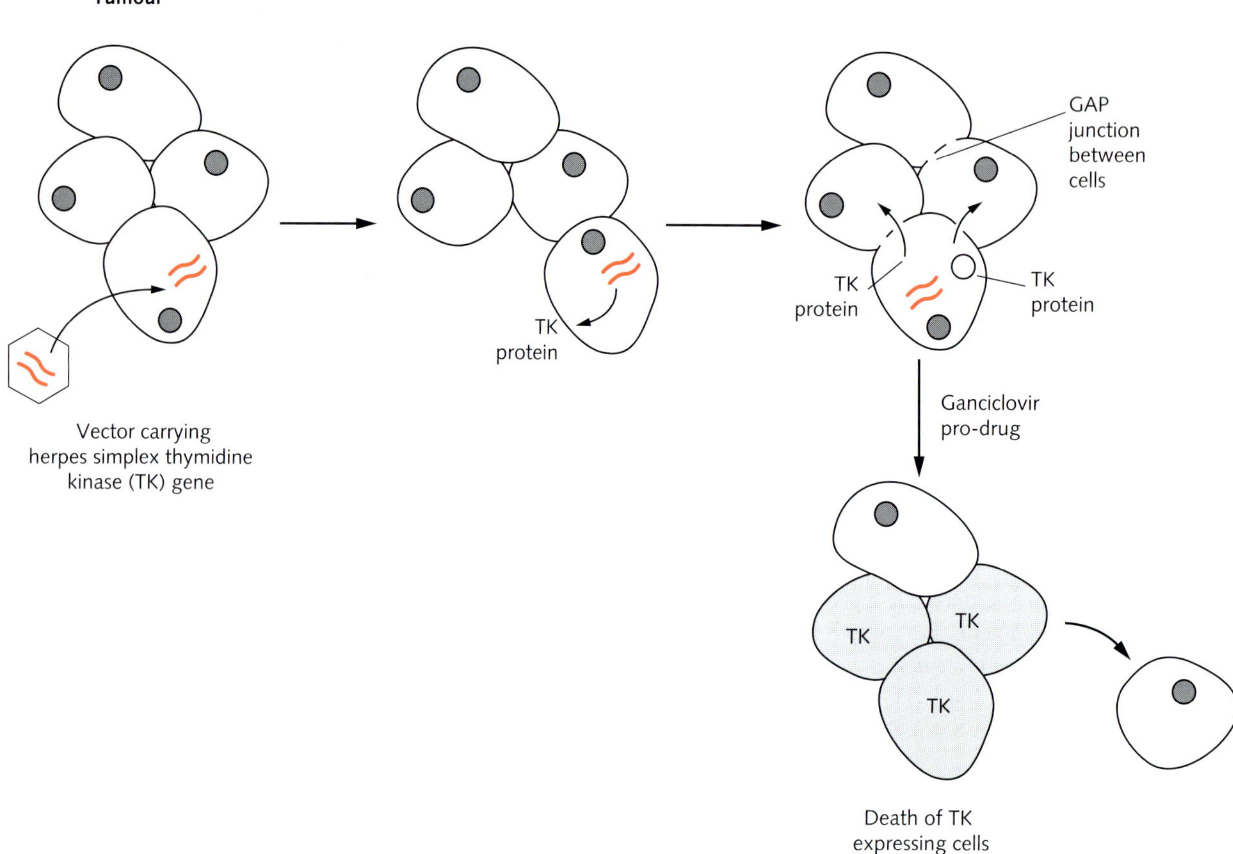

Fig. 16.8
The protein product of the thymidine kinase 'suicide' gene appears capable of diffusing into neighbouring cells via gap junctions which join the cells together. This non-specific diffusion allows for a greater cell kill than might be predicted using known gene transfer efficiency. As cells are dying and releasing tumour antigen into the local milieu of the tumour it is possible that such suicide gene therapies will synergise with immune-based treatment strategies.

cyclin D1 and *BCR-ABL*, are overexpressed in haematologic malignancy and in many cases are pivotal in the progression of malignant disease. One gene therapy approach to such malignancies is therefore the use of antisense cDNAs to bind to, and prevent transcription of, the sense target cDNA. Alternatively, RNAs with enzymatic activity—*ribozymes*—which possess highly specific RNA cleaving potential have been used. The failure of current gene transfer technology to introduce genetic material into all target cells will, however, likely limit such therapeutic strategies *in vivo* for the time being. *In vitro* strategies are now being pursued using such molecules for the 'purging' of blood or bone marrow HSC transplant products for return to patients after myeloablation.

Gene replacement therapy

A number of tumour suppressor genes, for example p53, retinoblastoma and p16, are commonly deleted in haematologic malignancies. Many of these tumour suppressor genes have been inserted in viral vectors for the purpose of gene replacement therapy. However, most haematologic malignancies are disseminated at presentation and current gene transfer technology is inadequate for widespread gene replacement *in vivo* in the majority of haematology patients. Use of gene replacement vectors *in vitro* is, however, being explored for the purpose of purging bone marrow or stem cell autografts free of tumour prior to autologous transplantation. In the future, gene transfer technology may allow the use of such genes in a more therapeutically relevant manner.

Vascular-mediated anti-tumour therapy

Since gene delivery to every cancer cell is currently limiting the application of successful gene therapy, attention has recently turned to the use of the supporting vascular epithelium as a target to inhibit tumour proliferation and dissemination. One very promising strategy is the sustained delivery of angiostatic genes with viral vectors. In this strategy, inhibitors of blood vessel growth are expressed within the tumour for sustained time periods leading to tumour regression and inhibition of metastasis. Preclinical evaluation of such strategies is only now underway.

Conclusions

Concepts and approaches to molecular therapy of diseases of the blood system which are currently popular have been described in this chapter but many other therapeutic strategies are also being developed. Indeed, the advent of human gene therapy trials combined with rapid advances in gene transfer technology and the increasingly rapid identification of novel genes by the Human Genome Project are setting the stage for a new era in human medicine. The field of human molecular medicine will surely continue to expand and make inroads in a therapeutically relevant way. It seems likely that study of the blood system, both in the laboratory and in patients, will continue to play a pivotal role in the further development of this field.

Further reading

Introduction

Anderson WF. (1992) Human gene therapy. *Science*, **256**, 808–813.

Brenner MK, Rill DR, Holladay MS *et al.* (1993) Gene marking to determine whether autologous marrow infusion restores long term haemopoiesis in cancer patients. *Lancet*, **342**, 1134–1137.

Brenner MK, Rill DR, Moen RC *et al.* (1993) Gene-marking to trace origin of relapse after autologous bone-marrow transplantation. *Lancet*, **341**, 85–86.

Miller AD. (1992) Human gene therapy comes of age. *Nature*, **357**, 455–460.

Rosenberg SA, Aebersold P, Cornetta K *et al.* (1990) Gene transfer into humans—immunotherapy of patients with advanced melanoma, using tumor-infiltrating lymphocytes modified by retroviral gene transduction. *New England Journal of Medicine*, **323**, 570–578.

Gene transfer strategies

Bergelson JM, Cunningham JA, Droguett G *et al.* (1997) Isolation of a common receptor for Coxsackie B viruses and adenoviruses 2 and 5. *Science*, **275**, 1320–1323.

Bischoff JR, Kirn DH, Williams A *et al.* (1996) An adenovirus mutant that replicates selectively in p53-deficient human tumor cells. *Science*, **274**, 373–376.

Cantwell MJ, Sharma S, Friedmann T, Kipps TJ. (1996) Adenovirus vector infection of chronic lymphocytic leukemia B cells. *Blood*, **88**, 4676–4683.

Chen HH, Mack LM, Kelly R *et al.* (1997) Persistence in muscle of an adenoviral vector that lacks all viral genes. *Proceedings of the National Academy of Sciences (USA)*, **94**, 1645–1650.

Crystal RG. (1995) Transfer of genes to humans: early lessons and obstacles to success. *Science*, **270**, 404–410.

Danos O, Mulligan RC. (1988) Safe and efficient generation of recombinant retroviruses with amphotropic and ecotropic host ranges. *Proceedings of the National Academy of Sciences (USA)*, **85**, 6460–6464.

Dilloo D, Rill D, Entwistle C *et al.* (1997) A novel herpes vector for the high-efficiency transduction of normal and malignant human hematopoietic cells. *Blood*, **89**, 119–127.

Gunzburg WH, Salmons B. (1996) Development of retroviral vectors as safe, targeted gene delivery systems. *Journal of Molecular Medicine*, **74**, 171–182.

Hallek M, Wendtner CM. (1996) Recombinant adeno-associated virus (rAAV) vectors for somatic gene therapy: recent advances and potential clinical applications. *Cytokines and Molecular Therapy*, **2**, 69–79.

Hawley RG, Lieu FHL, Fong AZC, Hawley TS. (1994) Versatile retroviral vectors for potential use in gene therapy. *Gene Therapy*, **1**, 136–138.

Kotin RM, Siniscalco M, Samulski RJ *et al.* (1990) Site-specific integration by adeno-associated virus. *Proceedings of the National Academy of Sciences (USA)*, **87**, 2211–2215.

Lever AM. (1996) HIV and other lentivirus-based vectors. *Gene Therapy*, **3**, 470–471.

Marconi P, Krisky D, Oligino T *et al.* (1996) Replication-defective herpes simplex virus vectors for gene transfer *in vivo*. *Proceedings of the National Academy of Sciences (USA)*, **93**, 11319–11320.

Miller AD, Buttimore C. (1986) Redesign of retrovirus packaging cell lines to avoid recombination leading to helper virus production. *Molecular and Cellular Biology*, **6**, 2895–2902.

Miller DG, Adam MA, Miller AD. (1990) Gene transfer by retrovirus vectors occurs only in cells that are actively replicating at the time of infection. *Molecular and Cellular Biology*, **10**, 4239–4242.

Mulligan RC. (1993) The basic science of gene therapy. *Science*, **260**, 926–932.

Naldini L, Blomer U, Gallay P *et al.* (1996) *In vivo* gene delivery and stable transduction of nondividing cells by a lentiviral vector. *Science*, **272**, 263–267.

Neering SJ, Hardy SF, Minamoto D, Spratt SK, Jordan CT. (1996) Transduction of primitive human hematopoietic cells with recombinant adenovirus vectors. *Blood*, **88**, 1147–1155.

Rollins SA, Birks CW, Setter E, Squinto SP, Rother RP. (1996) Retroviral vector producer cell killing in human serum is mediated by natural antibody and complement: strategies for evading the humoral immune response. *Human Gene Therapy*, **7**, 619–626.

Temin HM. (1993) Retrovirus variation and reverse transcription: abnormal strand transfers result in retrovirus genetic variation. *Proceedings of the National Academy of Sciences (USA)*, **90**, 6900–6903.

Yang Y, Nunes FA, Berencsi K *et al.* (1994) Cellular immunity to viral antigens limits E1-deleted adenoviruses for gene therapy. *Proceedings of the National Academy of Sciences (USA)*, **91**, 4407–4411.

Stem cell gene delivery

Brenner MK. (1996) Gene transfer to hematopoietic cells. *New England Journal of Medicine*, **335**, 337–339.

Cheng L, Du C, Murray D *et al.* (1997) A GFP reporter system to assess gene transfer and expression in human hematopoietic progenitor cells. *Gene Therapy*, **4**, 1013–1022.

Deisseroth AB, Zu Z, Claxton D *et al.* (1994) Genetic marking shows that Ph+ cells present in autologous transplants of chronic myelogenous leukemia (CML) contribute to relapse after autologous bone marrow transplant in CML. *Blood*, **83**, 3068–3076.

Dunbar CE, Cotter-Fox M, O'Shaughnessy JA et al. (1995) Retrovirally marked CD34-enriched peripheral blood and bone marrow cells contribute to long term engraftment after autologous transplantation. *Blood*, **85**, 3048–3057.

Rill DR, Santana VM, Roberts WM *et al.* (1994) Direct demonstration that autologous bone marrow transplantation for solid tumors can return a multiplicity of tumorigenic cells. *Blood*, **84**, 380–383.

Stewart AK, Sutherland DR, Nanji S *et al.* (1999) Engraftment of gene-marked hematopoietic progenitors in myeloma patients after transplant of autologons long-term marrow cultures. *Human Gene Therapy*, **10**(12), 1953–1964.

Chemoprotection

Guild BC, Mulligan RC, Gros P, Housman DE. (1988) Retroviral transfer of a murine cDNA for multidrug resistance confers pleiotropic drug resistance to cells without prior drug selection. *Proceedings of the National Academy of Sciences (USA)*, **85**, 1595–1599.

Hesdorffer C, Ayello J, Ward M *et al.* (1998) Phase I trial of retroviral-mediated transfer of the human MDR1 gene as marrow chemoprotection in patients undergoing high-dose chemotherapy and autologous stem-cell transplantation. *Journal of Clinical Oncology*, **16**, 165–172.

Sorrentino BP, Brandt SJ, Bodine D *et al.* (1992) Selection of drug-resistant bone marrow cells *in vivo* after retroviral transfer of human MDR1. *Science*, **257**, 99–103.

Ward M, Richardson C, Pioli P *et al.* (1994) Transfer and expression of the human multiple drug resistance gene in human CD34+ cells. *Blood*, **84**, 1408–1414.

Gene replacement therapy

Blaese RM, Culver KW, Miller AD *et al.* (1995) T lymphocyte-directed gene therapy for ADA-SCID: initial trial results after 4 years. *Science*, **270**, 475–480.

Hoogerbrugge PM, van Beusechem VW, Fischer A *et al.* (1996) Bone marrow gene transfer in three patients with adenosine deaminase deficiency. *Gene Therapy*, **3**, 179–183.

Kohn DB, Weinberg KI, Nolta JA *et al.* (1995) Engraftment of gene-modified umbilical cord blood cells in neonates with adenosine deaminase deficiency. *Nature Medicine*, **1**, 1017–1023.

Kohn DB, Weinberg KI, Nolta JL. (1997) PEG-ADA reduction in recipients of ADA gene transduced autologous umbilical cord blood CD34+ cells. *Blood*, **90**, 404a.

Onodera M, Ariga T, Kawamura N *et al.* (1998) Successful peripheral T-lymphocyte-directed gene transfer for a patient with severe combined immune deficiency caused by adenosine deaminase deficiency. *Blood*, **91**, 30–36.

Gene therapy of haematologic malignancies

Bonini C, Ferrari G, Verzeletti S *et al.* (1997) HSV-TK gene transfer into donor lymphocytes for control of allogeneic graft-versus-leukemia. *Science*, **276**, 1719–1724.

Guinan EC, Gribben JG, Boussiotis VA, Freeman GJ, Nadler LM. (1994) Pivotal role of the B7:CD28 pathway in transplantation tolerance and tumor immunity. *Blood*, **84**, 3261–3282.

Nanda NK, Sercarz EE. (1995) Induction of anti-self-immunity to cure cancer. *Cell*, **82**, 13–17.

Pardoll D. (1992) Immunotherapy with cytokine gene-transduced tumor cells: the next wave in gene therapy for cancer. *Current Opinion in Oncology*, **4**, 1124–1129.

Pardoll DM. (1993) Cancer vaccines. *Immunology Today*, **14**, 310–316.

Pizzoferrato E, Chu NR, Hawley TS *et al.* (1997) Enhanced immunogenicity of B cell lymphoma genetically engineered to express B7-1 and interleukin-12. *Human Gene Therapy*, **8**, 2217–2228.

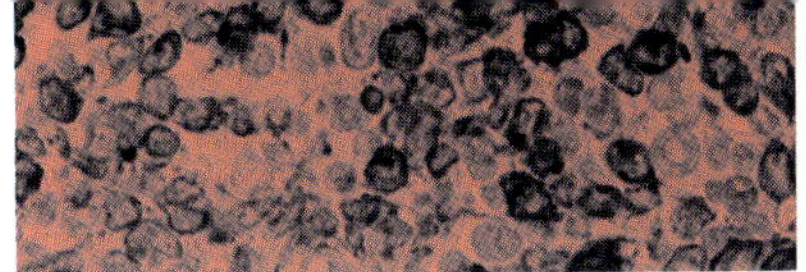

Appendix 1 Glossary

Adenine (A) Nitrogenous (purine) base, one member of the base pair A–T (adenine–thymine).

Allele Alternative forms of a gene occupying the same locus on homologous chromosomes; segregate at meiosis.

Allogeneic BMT *Allogeneic bone marrow transplantation.* Marrow from an HLA-matched donor (related or unrelated) is administered to the patient following 'conditioning' (usually chemotherapy with radiotherapy). *Cf.* autologous BMT.

Alu sequences DNA sequences recognised by the restriction enzyme *Alu I*; Alu sequences are represented ~300,000 times in the human genome.

Anergy Immunological unresponsiveness to specific antigenic re-challenge.

APC *Antigen presenting cell.* Cells capable of triggering naive T-cell response to antigen, leading to clonal T-cell expansion. APCs include dendritic cells, activated B-cells and macrophages.

Apoptosis Programmed cell death involving nuclear DNA fragmentation.

ARMS *Amplification refractory mutation system*—a PCR method that allows amplification of a single specific allele due to specific primers used, i.e. the primers bind only to the mutant allele.

Autologous BMT Patient's own bone marrow is collected following treatment (presumed disease-free) and reinfused in order to reconstitute the haematopoietic system.

Autoradiography Detection of radioactively labelled molecules on radiographic film. For analysis of nucleic acids, single-stranded DNA is immobilised onto a membrane before adding radiolabelled probe. Allows analysis of length and number of DNA fragments after separation by gel electrophoresis.

Autosome Non-sex chromosome.

BAC Bacterial artificial chromosome; allows propagation of large DNA molecules (up to 300 kb).

Base pair (bp) A pair of complementary nucleotide bases in a duplex DNA or RNA molecule.

bcl-2 Protein that inhibits apoptosis; overexpressed in, e.g., follicular NHL carrying t(14; 18).

Cap Structure at the 5′ end of mRNAs containing a methylated guanine residue.

CDR *Complementarity determining region.* Those components of Ig and TCR molecules that make contact with specific ligand; determine specificity. The CDR regions are the most variable portions of the Ig and TCR molecules.

Centromere Chromosome region to which spindle fibres attach during cell division.

Chromosome painting Labelling of whole chromosome using FISH. Involves mixture of different sequences from single chromosome.

Clonality Determination of clonal origin of cells.

Clone Population of cells or DNA molecules arising from a single progenitor.

Cloning The process of asexually producing a group of cells (clones), all genetically identical, from a single ancestor. In recombinant DNA technology, the use of DNA manipulation procedures to produce multiple copies of a single gene or segment of DNA is referred to as cloning DNA.

Cloning vector DNA molecule from a virus, a plasmid, or the cell of a higher organism into which another DNA fragment of appropriate size can be integrated without loss of the vector's capacity for self-replication; vectors introduce foreign DNA into host cells, where it can be reproduced in large quantities.

Codon DNA or corresponding RNA sequence of three base pairs that codes for a particular amino acid or termination signal.

Complementary DNA (cDNA) DNA copy of a messenger RNA generated by reverse transcriptase.

Consensus sequence DNA or amino acid sequence that specifies the most commonly found DNA base or amino acid at each position in a sequence of similar DNA or amino acid sequences.

Conserved sequence DNA or protein sequence that has remained essentially unchanged throughout evolution.

Contigs Groups of clones representing overlapping genomic regions.

Cosmid Plasmid DNA containing Cos sites to enable it to be packaged into phage particles. For example, cosmids can be packaged in λ phage particles for infection into *E. coli.* May harbour inserts of ~40 kb.

Cyclins Family of proteins that are positive regulators of cell cycle.

Cytosine (C) Pyrimidine base of RNA and DNA; one of cytosine—guanine (C–G) pair.

Diploid Cell or organism containing two complete sets of homologous chromosomes (*cf.* haploid).

DNA polymerase Enzyme that adds nucleotides to a growing chain of DNA in a 5′ to 3′ direction during DNA replication using a DNA strand as a template to copy from.

Domain In a protein this refers to a discrete region of the protein which has a specific function associated with it.

Electrophoresis Method for separating large molecules (nucleic acids or proteins) from a mixture of similar molecules using an electric current. Molecules travel through agarose or polyacrylamide gel at varying rates depending on their electrical charge and size.

Endonuclease Enzyme that cleaves nucleic acid at internal sites in the nucleotide sequence.

Epitope That part of an antigen that binds to the antigen-binding region of an antibody.

EST Expressed sequence tag.

Exon Segment of a gene which is present in the fully mature RNA after transcription, i.e. contains coding sequences (*cf.* introns).

FACS *Fluorescence activated cell sorting.* Technique used to separate cells from a population on the basis of their expression of specific antigens.

FISH Fluorescence *in situ* hybridisation. A technique used to visualise locations on chromosomes which hybridise to specific nucleotide probes. Biotin, digoxigenin or fluorescent dyes are incorporated into cDNA probes using nick-translation. Probes are then hybridised to metaphases or interphase nuclei thus defining gene number and location.

Flow cytometry Analysis of biological material by detection of the light-absorbing or fluorescing properties of cells or subcellular fractions (i.e. chromosomes) passing in a narrow stream through a laser beam. An absorbance or fluorescence profile of the sample is produced. Automated sorting devices, used to fractionate samples, sort successive droplets of the analysed stream into different fractions depending on the fluorescence emitted by each droplet.

Flow karyotyping Use of flow cytometry to analyse and/or separate chromosomes on the basis of their DNA content.

Frameshift Mutation that shifts the reading frame of triplet codons in a gene during translation of mRNA.

Gardos channel Red cell transport system accounting for selective loss of K^+ in response to increase in intracellular ionised Ca^{2+}.

G banding Technique used to visualise the band patterns of chromosomes on staining with Giemsa.

Gene Unit of heredity that specifies an RNA or mRNA. A gene will also contain intronic regions and regions that control transcription.

Gene expression Process by which a gene's coded information is converted into the structures present and operating in the cell. Expressed genes include those that are transcribed into mRNA and then translated into protein, and those that are transcribed into RNA but not translated into protein (e.g. transfer and ribosomal RNAs).

Gene mapping Construction of a map of different genetic loci based on their physical position with respect to each other.

Gene therapy Insertion of normal DNA directly into cells to correct a genetic defect.

Genetic code The sequence of nucleotides, coded in triplets (codons) along the mRNA, that determines the sequence of amino acids in protein synthesis. The DNA sequence of a gene can be used to predict the mRNA sequence, and the genetic code can, in turn, be used to predict the amino acid sequence.

Genomic library Collection of clones made from a set of randomly generated overlapping DNA fragments representing the entire genome of an organism.

Genotype The genetic make-up of a cell or organism responsible for its appearance.

Grb-2 *Growth factor receptor-bound protein 2.* Participates in downstream signalling after activation of a variety of cellular receptors. Binds to EDGF and PDGF.

Guanine (G) Purine base of RNA or DNA. One member of the base pair G–C (guanine and cytosine).

Haploid A single set of chromosomes (half the full set of genetic material), present in the egg and sperm cells of animals, and in the egg and pollen cells of plants (*cf.* diploid).

Haplotype Combination of closely linked genes. Usually inherited together as a 'block', arising from one chromosome.

Hemizygote Diploid cell or organism that contains only one allele of a gene due to loss of one chromosome of a homologous chromosome pair.

Heterodimer A complex of two non-identical moieties, e.g. proteins such as the T-cell receptor.

Heterozygote Diploid cell or organism that contains different alleles of a gene at one locus on homologous chromosomes.

Homeobox A short stretch of nucleotides whose base sequence is virtually identical in all the genes that contain it. It has been found in many organisms from fruit flies to human beings. In the fruit fly, a homeobox appears to determine when particular groups of genes are expressed during development.

Homodimer Complex of two identical moieties.

Homotetramer Tetramer comprising four identical subunits.

Hybridisation The ability of complementary single-stranded DNA or RNA molecules to form a duplex.

***In situ* hybridisation** Use of DNA or RNA probe to detect the presence of the complementary DNA sequence in cloned bacterial or cultured eukaryotic cells.

Interphase Period of the mitotic cell cycle between one mitosis and the next.

Intron Intervening sequence. Segments within the coding region of a gene which are not present in the fully mature RNA after transcription due to removal by splicing.

In vitro Taking place outside a living organism (literally '*in glass*'; *cf. in vivo*).

In vivo Taking place within a living organism ('*in life*').

Karyotype Photomicrograph of an individual's chromosomes arranged in a standard format showing the number, size and shape of each chromosome type.

Kilobase (kb) 1000 nucleotides.

Kinase An enzyme that phosphorylates a substrate.

Knockout The ability to remove a specific gene in a cell or organism by molecular techniques.

Leucine zipper Leucine-rich domain of a protein that allows protein—protein interaction.

Library An unordered collection of cloned DNA whose relationship to each other can be established by physical mapping.

Linkage The tendency for two genes in close proximity on a chromosome to be inherited together.

Locus The position of a gene on a chromosome.

LOH *Loss of heterozygosity.* Deletions believed to occur during tumour development. Identified as loss of an allele at a specific locus.

Lyonisation X chromosome inactivation in mammals. One X is randomly inactivated in each cell.

Maternal inheritance Preferential carriage of a gene by the maternal parent.

Megabase (Mb) 10^6 nucleotides.

Messenger RNA (mRNA) The mature transcript from a gene transcribed by RNA polymerase which specifies the order of amino acids during mRNA translation to protein.

Metaphase Stage in mitosis when the parental and newly synthesised chromosomes are maximally condensed but prior to their segregation to opposite spindle poles.

MHC *Major histocompatibility complex.* A polymorphic family of genes that are involved in mediating T-cell immune responses; present peptides to TCR.

Minimal residual disease Low level disease present following therapy; generally not detected using standard techniques such as light microscopy, but requires molecular techniques such as PCR for detection.

Missense mutation Single-base substitution causing incorporation of inappropriate amino acid into a protein.

Monosomy Condition in which one member of a chromosome pair is missing.

Multidrug resistance (MDR) Cell mechanism conferring drug resistance to a wide variety of chemotherapeutic agents.

Mutation A transmissible change in nucleotide sequence which leads to a change or loss of normal function encoded by that nucleotide sequence.

Nonsense mutation Mutation resulting in the premature termination during protein synthesis.

Northern blot Technique which transfers RNA molecules after size fractionation on gels to filter papers for hybridisation to specific probes.

Nucleotide A subunit of DNA or RNA consisting of a nitrogenous base (adenine, guanine, thymine or cytosine in DNA; adenine, guanine, uracil or cytosine in RNA), a phosphate molecule and a sugar molecule (deoxyribose in DNA and ribose in RNA).

Oncogene Mutated gene which is normally involved in the correct control of cell division such that disruption of the normal gene function leads to cell immortalisation and transformation.

Open reading frame Series of triplet codons in the coding region of a gene that lie between the signals to start and stop translation.

PBSC *Peripheral blood stem cell.* Following administration of chemotherapy ± growth factor, e.g. G-CSF, stem cells enter the peripheral circulation and are collected by leucopheresis.

PCR *Polymerase chain reaction.* Technique to amplify a target DNA sequence by multiple rounds of DNA synthesis. Involves a heat-stable DNA polymerase (e.g. Taq, isolated from hot spring bacterium, *Thermus aquaticus*) and two oligonucleotide primers (generally ~20 bases), one complementary to the (+) strand at one end of the sequence to be amplified and the other complementary to the (–) strand at the other end. Newly synthesised DNA can subsequently serve as additional templates for the same primer sequences, allowing a million-fold increase in DNA sequence after 30 cycles of primer annealing, strand elongation, and DNA melting.

PFGE *Pulsed field gel electrophoresis.* An electrophoretic technique to separate very large molecules of DNA by periodically altering the direction of the electric field through which the samples are migrating.

Phenotype The observable characteristics of a cell or organism resulting from the expression of the cell's genotype.

Plasmid A circular autonomously replicating, extrachromosomal DNA molecule. Some plasmids are capable of integrating into the host genome.

Pleckstrin homology domain First noted in platelet protein pleckstrin, 100 residues, function unknown.

Polymorphism DNA sequence variation among individuals. May be used as linkage marker.

Positional cloning Method for identifying the gene responsible for a genetic disease in the absence of a transcript or protein product; relies on the use of markers tightly linked to the target gene.

Primer Short oligonucleotide sequence that provides the starting point for polymerases to copy a nucleotide sequence and make a double strand.

Probe DNA or RNA molecules (single stranded) of specific base sequence, may be labelled radioactively (e.g. ^{32}P) or using non-radioactive means (e.g. digoxigenin) to detect complementary sequence on Southern blot, etc.

Promoter DNA sequence that targets RNA polymerase to a gene for transcription.

Proto-oncogene Refers to a normal gene involved in controlling cell division which, when mutated, becomes an oncogene.

Pseudogene A duplicated gene that has become non-functional.

Purine base Organic base containing two heterocyclic rings that occurs in nucleic acids (adenine and guanine in DNA and RNA).

Pyrimidine base Organic base containing one heterocyclic ring that occurs in nucleic acids. (Cytosine (C) and thymine (T) in DNA; cytosine (C) and uracil (U) in RNA.)

Q banding Banding technique to visualise the banding patterns of chromosomes using quinacrine stain.

Recombination The process by which progeny derive a combination of genes different from that of either parent. In higher organisms, this can occur by crossing over. Also occurs in non-germline cells, e.g. B-cell and T-cell during production of Ig and TCR genes, respectively.

Reporter gene A gene encoding a product which can be easily measured when introduced into cell, e.g. by transfection.

Restriction enzyme An endonuclease (usually bacterial) that recognises specific, short nucleotide sequences and cuts DNA at those sites.

Restriction enzyme cutting site Specific nucleotide sequence of DNA at which a particular restriction enzyme cuts the DNA. Some sites occur frequently in DNA (e.g. every several hundred base pairs), others much less frequently (rare-cutter, e.g. every 10 000 base pairs).

Retrovirus RNA virus that replicates by first converting its RNA genome to a double-stranded DNA copy using the enzyme reverse transcriptase.

Reverse transcriptase Enzyme used to make a DNA copy of RNA. Found in retroviruses allowing conversion of their RNA genome into double-stranded DNA which may then integrate into the host genome.

RFLP *Restriction fragment length polymorphism.* Heritable differences in the length of DNA fragments from a specific region of DNA generated by restriction enzymes due to DNA sequence differences.

Ribozyme An RNA molecule with properties of RNAse; cleaves single-stranded RNA.

RNA polymerase Enzyme that makes an RNA copy of a DNA template.

RNA splicing Removal of introns from transcribed RNA to generate a mature mRNA.

RT-PCR *Reverse transcriptase polymerase chain reaction.* Amplification of RNA by PCR after copying of the RNA → cDNA by reverse transcription.

Sequencing Determination of the order of nucleotides (base sequences) in a DNA or RNA molecule or the order of amino acids in a protein.

Somatic mutation Mutation arising in a somatic cell.

Southern blot Technique which transfers DNA molecules after size fractionation on gels to filter papers for hybridisation to specific probes.

Src homology 3 (SH3) domain Protein domain on oncoprotein Src; binds to proline-rich domains on other proteins.

Syngeneic Genetically identical (e.g. identical twins).

Taq polymerase Heat-stable DNA polymerase used for DNA amplification (*see* PCR). More recent heat-stable polymerases include VENT and Tth.

TATA box Also called Hogness Box; DNA sequence found in many eukaryotic promoters that binds the TATA binding protein in order to recruit RNA polymerase for transcription. Consensus sequence TATAAAA; specifies position where transcription is initiated.

T-cell receptor Membrane protein complexes that are expressed on T-lymphocytes and recognise specific antigens when associated with MHC molecules.

Telomere Specialised structures at the ends of chromosomes involved in the replication and stability of linear DNA molecules.

Thymine (T) Nitrogenous base, one member of the base pair A–T (adenine–thymine).

Tolerance Reduced ability to mount an immune response to specific antigens *in vivo*.

Transcription Process by which a DNA template (a gene) is copied to RNA by RNA polymerase.

Transcription factor Proteins, other than RNA polymerase, that are required for transcription of all genes.

Transfection The introduction of DNA into cells in culture.

Translation The mechanism by which mRNA is used as a template to synthesise protein on the ribosome.

Tumour suppressor gene A gene that negatively regulates cell division such that mutation in these genes results in uncontrolled cell division and tumour progression, e.g. Rb, p53 genes.

Tyrosine kinase Enzymatic activity catalysing the attachment of phosphate group to tyrosine residue within a protein molecule.

Uracil (U) Pyrimidine base that replaces the DNA base thymine in RNA molecules; forms base pair with adenine (A–U).

Vector DNA molecule in which DNA sequences can be cloned; agent used to deliver genes for gene transfer.

VNTR Variable number of tandem repeats. Variations in numbers of tandem repeat DNA sequences found at specific loci in different populations. May be used as genetic markers.

Western blot A technique which transfers protein molecules after size fractionation on gels to filter papers for analysis with antibodies.

X inactivation Inactivation of one of the X chromosomes in female somatic cells.

YAC Yeast artificial chromosome. Plasmid DNA which contains DNA sequences that allow plasmid maintenance in yeast cells permitting cloning of very large regions of DNA.

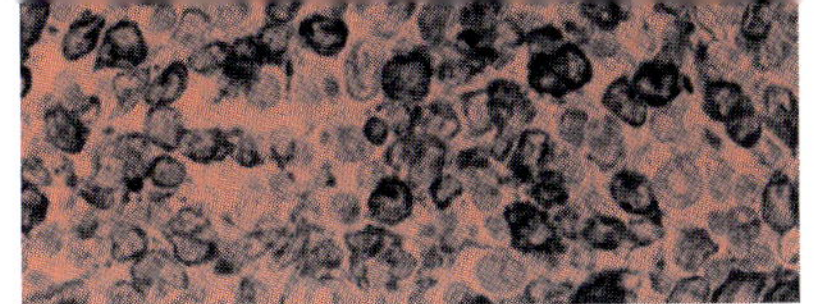

Appendix 2 Cytogenetic glossary

add Addition of chromosomal material of unknown origin to another chromosome
der Derivative of a chromosomal rearrangement
del Deletion of chromosomal material
dup Duplication of chromosomal material; extra copy of part of a chromosome
cen Centromere
Hypo/hyperdiploid Human karyotype with <46 or >46 chromosomes, respectively
i Isochromosome; chromosome whose arms are mirror images of each other
ins Insertion of chromosomal material
inv Rotation of chromosome segment by 180°
mar Marker chromosome. Signifies any structurally rearranged chromosome
p Short (petit) arm of chromosome
q Long arm of chromosome
p+/q+ Addition of DNA to short/long arms, respectively
p–/q– Deletion of DNA from short/long arms, respectively
t Translocation; chromosome segment moves from one chromosome to another. May or may not be reciprocal
ter Terminus (end); e.g. pter, qter = short arm and long arm ends, respectively
+/– Gain/loss of chromosomal material, respectively

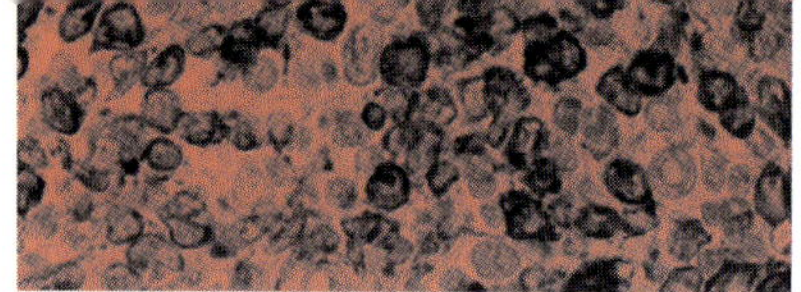

Appendix 3 Cluster designation (CD) antigens used in this book

CD	Expression	Comments
CD1a, b, c	Thymocytes, dendritic cells	Ligand for some γδ T-cells
CD3	T-cells	Complex of molecules that transduce signals from T-cell receptor
CD4	T-cells, monocytes, tissue macrophages, microglial cells, EBV-transformed B-cells	Binds HLA class II Receptor for HIV env gp120
CD5	Thymocytes and T-cells, most T-cell malignancies, B-CLL	Binds to CD72
CD8	T-cell subset	Binds MHC class I
CD10	T- and B-cell precursors, BM stromal cells, pre-B ALL	Zinc metalloproteinase, marker for pre-B-cell ALL (also termed common ALL antigen, cALLa)
CD15	Neutrophils, eosinophils, monocytes	Also called Lewis-x (Le^x)
CD19	B-cells, B-cell malignancies	Function unknown
CD20	B-cells, B-cell malignancies	Function unknown
CD21	Mature B-cells, follicular dendritic cells	Complement control protein. Receptor for complement C3d, EBV
CD23	Mature B-cells, activated macrophages, eosinophils, follicular dendritic cells, CLL	Low affinity receptor for IgE
CD28	T-cell subsets, activated B-cells	Receptor for costimulatory signal, binds CD80 (B7-1) and CD86 (B7-2)
CD34	Haematopoietic precursors, capillary endothelium	Ligand for CD62L (L-selectin)
CD38	Early B- and T-cells, activated T-cells, germinal centre B-cells, plasma cells	Function unknown
CD43	Leucocytes (except resting B-cells)	Binds CD54 (ICAM-1)
CD55	Haematopoietic and non-haematopoietic cells	Decay accelerating factor (DAF). Binds C3b
CD56	NK cells	Isoform of neural cell adhesion molecule (N-CAM)
CD59	Haematopoietic and non-haematopoietic cells	Binds complement C8 and C9
CD79a, b	B-cells	Component of B-cell antigen (analogous to CD3)
CD80	Antigen presenting cells	Costimulation. Ligand for CD28 and CTLA- 4
CD86	Antigen presenting cells	Costimulation. Ligand for CD28 and CTLA- 4

Abbreviations: see list on p. xiii

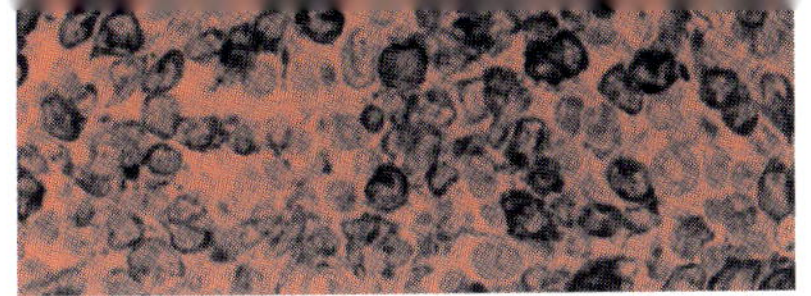

Index

Page numbers in *italics* indicate figures; those in **bold** indicate tables.